The 150

Healthiest

15-Minute Recipes

on Earth

The Surprising, Unbiased Truth about How to Make
the Most Deliciously Nutritious Meals at Home
in Just Minutes a Day

Jonny Bowden, Ph.D., C.N.S., and Jeannette Bessinger, C.H.H.C.

Text © 2011 Jonny Bowden, Ph.D., C.N.S., and Jeannette Lee Bessinger, C.H.H.C.

First published in the USA in 2011 by
Fair Winds Press, a member of
Quayside Publishing Group
100 Cummings Center
Suite 406-L
Beverly, MA 01915-6101
www.fairwindspress.com

15 14 13 12 11   1 2 3 4 5

ISBN-13: 978-1-59233-442-1
ISBN-10: 1-59233-442-3

Library of Congress Cataloging-in-Publication Data is available

Cover design Fair Winds Press
Book production: Sporto
Photography: Richard Fleishman
Food stylist: Rachel Sherwood

Printed and bound in Singapore

The information in this book is for educational purposes only. It is not intended to replace the advice of a physician or medical practitioner. Please see your health-care provider before beginning any new health program.

From Jonny:

I dedicate this book to everyone who is working to improve the health and welfare of our children with better nutrition. And to Michael Pollan, whose work has been so important in raising our consciousness about food. And to nutritionist and humanitarian Robert Crayhon, who continues to inspire so many people every single day.

From Jeannette:

I dedicate this book to my Real Food Moms partner Tracee Yablon Brenner, to my cousin Jodi Bass, to my bestie Lisa Kerr, and to all the other moms and wives like us who are doing what we can to keep getting delicious, nourishing food on the table night after night (after night, after night…!).

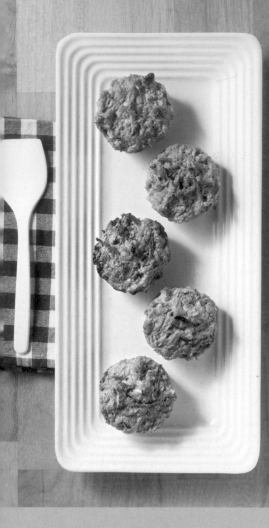

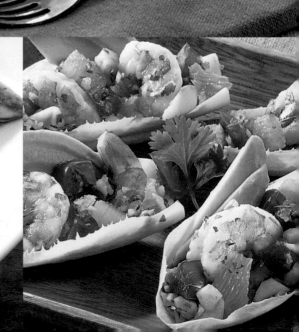

Clockwise from top left:
A Healthier Meatloaf with Chutney,
page 179; Anytime Fast Fruity Skillet
Cake, *page 162*; 15-Minute Low-Cal
Shrimp and Citrus Ceviche, *page 86*
Lean and Light Sesame Thai Chicken
and Broccoli, *page 30*

CONTENTS

THE RECIPES

1 | Fast, Fabulous, and Healthy Meals from Prep to Plate in 15 Minutes

2   25 Tasty 15-Minute Prep It and (Almost) Forget It Meals

3   The 25 Healthiest Quick Snacks

How to Create the Healthiest, Quickest, and Most Delicious Meals on Earth

If you're reading this book, there are two things I know about you:

One, you're interested in healthy food for you and your family.

Two, you're in a time crunch.

Usually, *healthy* and *fast* don't go together. "Healthy fast food" is almost an oxymoron, and most people have to choose one or the other. And when you've got a family to take care of, guess which one wins most often?

Years of private practice with nutrition clients (and even more years speaking to audiences around the country, writing books, and running a website that gets a ton of mail) have taught me that people are genuinely perplexed when it comes to food. They truly want to make smart and healthy choices, but those choices are usually very labor intensive (and often, though not always, expensive to boot).

Jeannette Bessinger has had the same experience, and she's even more "in the trenches" than I am. She works with busy families, providing nutrition education, and helping them improve both their eating habits and everyday food preparation. Many of these families are also on a budget, and all of them are time-crunched, stressed out, and overcommitted. They don't have time to investigate every food, read up on every health benefit, dissect every label, evaluate different claims, and then cook every meal from scratch. So Chef Jeannette is all-too-aware of the day-to-day challenges faced by the average person wanting to feed his or her family the best food possible in the least amount of time.

Hence, this book.

Let me say right off the bat that you're not crazy—it's sometimes very difficult to make healthy food quickly. You didn't imagine that, it's a fact of life, and we need to acknowledge that from the beginning.

But it's not impossible.

Far from it.

So we approached this cookbook as a huge challenge. How do we put together meals that are rich in nutrients (like vitamins, minerals, phytochemicals from plants, omega-3 fats, and so on), contain a good mix of protein, healthy fat, and good carbohydrates, don't break the caloric "bank," and can still be assembled from start to scratch in a reasonable amount of time?

We think we solved the problem.

Is every single recipe perfect? No. Occasionally there's a shortcut or two (like using a prepared store-bought sauce or dressing). Not every single ingredient is organic (doesn't really have to be, actually). And once in a while the recipes will spill over 15 minutes a bit, but this is, after all, real life!

So let me tell you some of the things we looked at when we created these recipes. It may help you to understand why it's actually possible to eat healthy food that can be prepared in no time. You just have to know what you're looking for.

Here's what we were looking for:

1. Nutrient Density

When I evaluate a food, I'm looking at the costs versus the benefits. Chocolate cake has a very high cost: lots of calories, lots of sugar, and almost nothing that's nutritionally good for you. Now granted, it *does* have the benefit of being delicious, but that's what evaluation is about: weighing the benefits against the cost.

When you think about it, evaluating food isn't much different than evaluating anything else you shop for. If I go into the store and see a nice shirt, I might look at the price and say, "Hmm, the shirt is okay, but I'll only wear it twice a year and it costs $300." The benefit of looking nice twice a year is not enough to compensate for the outrageous cost, especially when I can find an equally nice shirt for a fraction of the price.

To put this way of thinking into the context of food, I might think to myself, "Chocolate cake tastes really good (benefit) but really screws up my blood sugar, gives me no nutrients to speak of, and is very high in calories (cost)." Now if there were no other way to get that delicious taste, I might splurge and go for the cake. But the fact is that with some creative recipe development (the kind in which Chef Jeannette excels) I can get fabulous taste at a fraction of the cost. Not only that, but I can get nutrients that support my health, protect my waistline, and give me the building blocks for everything my body needs.

So when we nutritionists speak of "nutrient density" we're talking about the balance between nutrients and calories.

Here's an example. Spinach is a really nutrient-dense food. One cup of raw spinach has 30 mg of calcium, 24 mg of magnesium, 167 mg of potassium, 8.4 mg of vitamin C, 1,688 mcg of beta-carotene, 2,813 IUs of vitamin A, and a whopping 3,659 mcg of lutein and zeaxanthin (two superstar nutrients for eye health).

Want to know how many calories that cup of spinach has?

Seven.

See where I'm going with this? When you can eat a few cups of a food for fewer than 50 calories and get a ton of minerals, vitamins, and phytochemicals, you're eating a nutrient-dense food. There are a lot of nutrients densely packed into a small caloric package. Compare that to a tiny serving of commercially prepared chocolate cake that has about 54 IUs of vitamin A and not much more—not a single milligram of C, D, E, K, or any B vitamin (except for a tiny amount of folate). It's got a ton of sugar, 35 grams of processed carbs, and comes at a caloric cost of about 235 calories, and that's for a serving that wouldn't satisfy anyone but a squirrel.

So maybe spinach and chocolate cake represent two extremes. But the best-kept secret in the world is that when it comes to healthy food, you can actually have your cake and eat it too. Chef Jeannette has worked her kitchen magic to concoct recipes that feature nutrient-dense food at a reasonable caloric cost and that taste delicious too.

2. Glycemic Load

Okay, here's another technical-sounding concept that's easy to understand once you cut away all the scientific jargon—glycemic load. Here's what it means:

When you eat food, your blood sugar goes up. That's normal and natural and expected. But you don't want it to go too high. When blood sugar goes up, the body responds by secreting the hormone *insulin*, the job of which is to escort some of that extra sugar into the cells where it can be burned for energy. But when blood sugar rises too high (and stays up there), you need a lot of insulin to get it back down. Insulin, also known as the "fat storage" hormone, is a perfectly fine and important hormone, but when you have too much of it floating around, it can contribute to all sorts of health problems such as obesity and diabetes.

When blood sugar gets too high, it creates a separate set of problems not unrelated to the ones that come from high levels of insulin. The insulin eventually brings your blood sugar down, but sometimes it goes down too low, resulting in cravings, mood swings, and overeating. So keeping blood sugar in a nice, healthy range, which also keeps insulin in a nice, healthy range, is a major goal of healthy eating.

The glycemic index is a measure that researchers use to evaluate the effect of a given amount of food on blood sugar. (The glycemic load is an even more accurate measure of the same thing.) When foods have a high glycemic impact, they tend to create blood sugar problems. (Just for reference, foods with the highest glycemic impact include pure sugar, white bread, cornflakes, and most processed carbohydrates.) Clearly, we want to choose foods that are reasonably low glycemic, have minimal effect on our blood sugar and keep cravings, hunger, and mood swings at bay.

That's why Chef Jeannette and I always talk about foods that are "low glycemic." Translated, that means they're low in sugar or processed carbs, and won't contribute to the myriad health problems associated with too much sugar in the diet. Foods that are high in fiber (beans, for example), high in healthy fats like omega-3 (salmon), and higher in protein (grass-fed beef, chicken, and fish) all fit the bill. And almost every vegetable on the planet, and most fruits, are pretty low glycemic as well, not to mention nutrient dense!

3. Fiber

Speaking of fiber, it's one of the most important constituents of your diet, and most Americans simply don't get enough of it.

Fiber slows down digestion in the stomach and small intestine, which helps stabilize blood sugar levels. It increases our feeling of fullness, making it less likely we'll overeat. It reduces cholesterol. It may help prevent colon cancer, and it definitely helps prevent constipation and hemorrhoids. It's good for digestive disorders. High-fiber diets are associated with reduced rates of heart and kidney disease as well as lower rates of diabetes and obesity.

So Chef Jeannette and I pay attention to fiber. And we try to make sure it's in every recipe whenever possible. It's definitely one of the components of a healthy diet. Most responsible health organizations recommend that we get between 25 and 38 grams of fiber a day, but the average American only gets between 4 and 8 grams. Interestingly, most high-fiber foods are also nutrient dense and low glycemic!

Are you beginning to see a pattern here?

4. Free-Range Meats and Wild-Caught Fish

We make a pretty big deal about grass-fed meat and wild fish, and with good reason. Let's start with meat. Some studies have shown that high levels of meat consumption are associated with higher rates of cancer and heart disease, leading many people to simply avoid meat altogether. But the truth about meat eating is a bit more complicated than you might think.

Most of the meat we get in the supermarket comes from what are called factory farms. If you're an animal lover you don't want to visit a factory farm. (In fact, it's next to impossible. Factory farms are notoriously secret about their meat-processing practices and almost never allow visitors to observe—with good reason.) The cows are kept in tiny, confined spaces and fed a diet of grain. This is a problem. Cows don't digest grain very well; the stomach of a ruminant is not suited to grain, and it causes terrible acidity. Not only that, grain diets are very inflammatory, and the meat of factory-farmed beef is high in proinflammatory omega-6 fats. And if the grain-based diet weren't enough to make the cows sick (it usually is), the crowded conditions in which they live ensures that most of them won't be the healthiest specimens. As a result, factory farms routinely shoot their animals full of antibiotics, which winds up in their meat, which winds up on your table.

That's not all they're shot full of. Factory-farmed meat routinely contains hormones (such as bovine growth hormone) and steroids used to fatten the cows up and hasten the time to slaughter. These are in addition to whatever pesticides and chemicals they're exposed to in their cheap grain diet. The result is a meat "product" that is anything but healthy.

Contrast that to a grass-fed cow. Cows were meant to live on pasture. Grass is their natural diet. When they are grass fed, their meat is higher in the amazingly healthy omega-3 fats (the same fat found in cold-water fish such as salmon). Their meat also contains a cancer- and obesity-fighting fat called CLA that is conspicuously absent in the fat of factory-farmed beef. And grass-fed cows are almost always raised organically.

Studies that show ill effects from meat eating look at populations that consume large amounts of processed meats. That includes deli meats, which, in addition to all the problems stated above, also contain nitrates and high levels of sodium.

Interestingly, just as this book was going to press, a new study came out that looked at meat eating and heart disease. In this study, however, researchers didn't just lump all "meat eaters" together. They compared people who ate nonprocessed meat, such as burgers and steaks, with people who ate high amounts of processed deli meats. The results were interesting. While processed meat eaters did indeed have significantly higher risk for heart disease, the people eating nonprocessed meat did not. I suspect that if researchers actually compared those eating grass-fed meat (and wild game) to those eating processed meat, the results would be even more dramatic.

So meat has gotten a bad name, but perhaps unfairly. Real, grass-fed meat with no antibiotics, steroids, or hormones is a very different food than store-bought, factory-farmed meat. We realize it's not always possible to get grass-fed, but we feel strongly that whenever possible you should try to do so. It really makes a difference. When we do use deli meats in these recipes (only once or twice, actually), we always suggest nitrate-free and low-sodium varieties—this eliminates two of the most problematic compounds in processed meats and significantly reduces the dangers associated with eating it.

Similarly, farmed fish is fed an unnatural diet of corn and grain, which leads to problems similar to those encountered when cows are fed an all-grain diet. Wild fish such as salmon naturally dine on krill, mackerel, and crustaceans. Wild fish has lower levels of inflammatory omega-6s and higher levels of health-giving omega-3s—it's also high in antioxidants (such as astaxanthin), which are provided from their natural diet.

Although there is always concern about mercury in ocean fish, the truth is that farmed fish have an even bigger problem—PCBs. PCBs are polychlorinated biphenyls, a really nasty toxin that's been spilled into the environment since the early twentieth century and persists today, even though PCBs are now outlawed. The toxin accumulates in the fat of animals and fish, and today, according to the nonprofit Environmental Working Group, farm-raised salmon is the most PCB-contaminated protein source in the American diet.

So we recommend wild salmon whenever possible. Farmed salmon isn't going to kill you and is a compromise between eating wild salmon and not eating salmon at all, but when you can get it, wild fish is the way to go—at least where salmon is concerned!

5. Organic Versus Nonorganic

I'm always amused by the way the media spins studies on organic food. They love to trumpet headlines about studies that show no nutritional advantage to organic fruits and vegetables when, in fact, that's only part of the story. It's true that studies have been mixed about whether organic food has more nutrients than nonorganic (sometimes yes, sometimes no; it never has less). But the fact is we eat organic food *not* just because it may have a little more vitamin C or folate, but because of what it *doesn't* have—chemicals.

We believe that it makes sense to try to reduce our daily exposure to the more than 80,000 unregulated chemicals that exist in the environment (many of which come to us via the food supply). We also recognize that organic food in general is harder to find and somewhat more expensive than nonorganic. As private citizens, Chef Jeannette and I both choose our battles on the organic front. Some foods (strawberries, for example), are more contaminated and sprayed than others so when buying those particular foods, we choose (and recommend) organic. Other foods (pineapples) are pretty clean, so for those it doesn't matter as much. (For a complete and current list of the "dirtiest" and "cleanest" foods, go to www.food-news.org.)

A WORD ABOUT SHORTCUTS

First of all, let's be clear about something: *Compromise* isn't a dirty word. We're living in the real world, and, as mentioned earlier, it's not always going to be possible or practical to choose perfect, fresh, organic, local ingredients and cook them from scratch. To accomplish our bigger goal of providing you with healthy meals in 15 minutes, we made a few small compromises. We occasionally used processed products to stay under 15 minutes, but we feel that on balance, the health benefits of the recipes in which this was done still far outweigh the minor negatives associated with a small amount of processed food.

In general, when using processed or prepared foods (sauces, wraps, and the like), it's best to go for the highest-quality versions (fresh, clean ingredients, whole grain, etc.) and nix things that have too many chemicals, too much refined sugar or flour, or multiple artificial ingredients whose names you can't pronounce. We tried to be conscious of sodium content as well, and fiercely conscious of trans fats (hydrogenated oils), which we simply did not use no matter what.

What we did do was front-load the recipes with whole foods, which come from what I have referred to as the Jonny Bowden Four Food Groups—food you fish for, hunt, gather, or pluck.

As long as these foods make up the bulk of your diet, you will be way ahead of the game. Those foods account for the majority of the ingredients in the recipes that follow.

Finally we'd like to suggest that your whole diet shouldn't be composed of these quick and easy meals. If you can, try to make some time for slow food—food that may not come together in 15 minutes, but whose taste, texture, flavor, complexity, and nutritional benefits are worth the extra time needed to prepare it. We offer nutrient or flavor "bonus tips" in several of the recipes themselves for when you have an extra 5, 10, or 30 minutes.

If your diet consists of a good balance of slow food and the truly healthy fast food featured in this cookbook, you should be in very good shape indeed.

We hope reading these recipes (and the introductions) will help you make a shift in your relationship to food. Food, after all, is fuel for your body and brain, but it is more than that. It is celebration, sharing, and giving. It is meditative, mindful, and sensual. It is a source of joy and community. It is both nutritious and recreational.

It is essential.

Why not make the most of it?

Enjoy the journey.

—Jonny Bowden
Woodland Hills, CA, 2010

KEY TIPS ON HOW TO MAKE SPEEDY, TASTY WHOLE FOODS MEALS AT HOME

The average amount of time an American family spent cooking meals in the 1980s was about two hours a day. Today those two cooking hours have dwindled down to an average of 20 minutes—for all three meals! Clearly many of us have been leaning on prepared, takeout, and restaurant food to get ourselves fed. But, as Dr. Jonny so eloquently tells us, the quality of that high-calorie/low-nutrient-density food is poor and the health cost of eating so much of it has been dear, as evidenced by the epidemic of obesity we're facing (and all the other issues that have come along for the ride, such as type 2 diabetes, hypertension, and heart disease).

So if fast food isn't worth the health toll, and we no longer have two hours a day at our disposal for cooking, we need to get smarter about the raw ingredients we buy, and the way we use our time in the kitchen. Following are tips for getting healthy, tasty meals on the table fast. I've recommended a few key pieces of equipment to help cut your prep time, shopping tips, core pantry staples for the speedy whole foods kitchen, general time-saving tips for food preparation, and simple things to you can do to ensure delicious and varied flavors in your meals.

ABOUT THE 150 QUICKEST AND HEALTHIEST RECIPES

The recipes are divided into three chapters. Chapter 1 is the heart of the book, with about 100 recipes (mainly entrées with a few breakfast dishes) that will take you about 15 minutes from set up (see Organize Your Kitchen on page 22) to prepare and cook, with suggested speedy sides to complete your meal. Among the selections are about 25 recipes that require little to no actual cooking. Many of them are more like assembly meals that you can get from pantry to placemat in 15 minutes or less. Chapter 2 offers about 25 delicious entrées that require only 15 minutes or less of preparation, but need a little more time for cooking (never more than 45 minutes). Chapter 3 contains 25 tasty and innovative balanced snack ideas, most of which can be made in a flash, and many of which can serve as mini-meals in a pinch.

Dr. Jonny introduces all the recipes and highlights the special health qualities of particular ingredients or nutrients in his Nutritional Notes throughout the book. The recipes in the first two chapters suggest side dishes to complete the meal, superspeed tips that will trim even more time off the prep, ideas for enriching your dish if you have 5, 10, or 30 extra minutes of time, and variation tips for ingredient substitutions to make the dishes more versatile.

The Planned Leftover tag indicates that a recipe includes planned leftovers. Planned leftover meals allow you to prepare two meals in the same amount of time as one, so you can eat fresh that night and freeze another meal to eat at any time over the next two months. Follow our directions for flawless freezing, then thaw the dish overnight in the refrigerator before the evening you would like to eat it. The next night it's ready to simply heat and eat! Include a PL meal in your repertoire once a week and you will soon have a stock of high-quality, frozen prepared meals on hand for those evenings when you're too tired to lift a finger for food prep, but still need to feed the family. One more thing: If a non-PL dish freezes well, and most of them do, you can transform it into PL by simply doubling the amount of the original recipe and freezing one of the meals. (See the note on batching later this introduction.)

★ THE STARS

Though we love all the recipes in the book, we wanted to note those that were outstandingly healthy and delicious—the best of the best. It was a challenge deciding which ones to give a star to, and we're sure you could argue that some deservedly good ones didn't get stars. Remember, everything in this book is a star in its respective category—the ones we chose soar above the rest in terms of the nutrition they provide your body and the outstanding flavor they deliver to your taste buds. Enjoy!

THE EQUIPMENT TODAY'S SPEEDY HOME COOK NEEDS

These are the pieces of cooking equipment that I return to again and again when I need to get a dish together quickly. Investing in good kitchen tools that allow you to prepare fresh food fast will save you scads of money over time in less expensive home-cooked meals versus pricier packaged or restaurant food.

Food processor (with attachments for slicing and grating). The food processor is a simply indispensable tool for high-speed grating, slicing, and chopping. It is all you need to make sauces, dressings, raw-food bars, soups, and "instant" puddings (see chapter 3).

High-powered blender. A powerful blender can grind nuts into milk or butter, chop fruit and ice and blend it into smoothies, and even make a quick soup from raw veggies, all in a few seconds to a couple of minutes. Dr. Jonny and I love our Vita-Mix blenders.

Immersion blender. The immersion blender is a portable wand with a blender and mixer attachment. Pureeing a soup in the blender or food processor requires cooling time and usually takes multiple messy batches to get the job done. With an immersion blender you can drop it in your pot of soup (or eggs, batter, or dressing ingredients) and get the dish to the consistency you desire in seconds, with a super quick cleanup.

Mandoline. The mandoline allows you to quickly, thinly, and evenly slice or julienne firm fruits and vegetables (such as apples, carrots, beets, turnips, celery root, etc.) more safely than using a kitchen knife, and with less cleanup than a food processor.

Double mesh sieve and colander. Double mesh sieves and colanders allow for quick rinsing and draining of almost any ingredient that gets wet, including tiny grains, such as quinoa or amaranth. They are also terrific for use with delicate pastas, like rice noodles, and the best thing out there for draining and rising canned beans in no time flat. Look for stainless-steel varieties to prevent rusting.

Multiple nesting mixing bowls, measuring cups,and spoons. One of the skills of a speedy whole foods cook is preparing multiple dishes at once. To do this efficiently, have several different bowls you can use simultaneously and more than one set of measuring spoons and cups, so you don't need to wash between every use. These are inexpensive, so it won't set you back much to purchase additional sets if you already have some you like. My favorite bowls are my cheapest steel ones because they are light and shallow, easy to use and manipulate, and super fast to clean.

Tempered glassware with rubber lids. Dr. Jonny and I both advocate cooking and storing foods in glass over plastic. Glass is a better environmental choice than plastic, it's more sanitary, does not transfer flavors or colors among different dishes, and does not leach anything scary into your food when heated. Not all plastics contain BPA and other unpleasantries, but why take the risk when glass is so great in so many other ways? A tempered glass product (we like Pyrex) will not shatter in the freezer or oven, so it can travel from hot to cold without needing a container transfer, saving you time and effort. Being able to snap a lid over leftovers to refrigerate them or to batch extras for freezing is a great, time-saving convenience.

Sharp chef's and paring knives and a sharpener. Investing in one high-quality chef's knife and one high-quality paring knife (good steel, full tang, sharp edge) will save a great deal of slicing and dicing time over the years. Most slips and struggles with cutting occur because of working with a dull blade. Buy an electric sharpener or a sharpening stone, or take your knives to a sharpening service, which is usually inexpensive. By the way, that rod in a knife block doesn't actually sharpen, it's just for smoothing out any burrs on an already sharp edge.

SPEEDY SHOPPING TIPS AND PANTRY STAPLES

One of the secret keys to being able to get meals on the table quickly is keeping a well-stocked larder. If you have a good collection of staple ingredients on hand at all times, you will always be able to pull a quick meal out of your hat. Try these tips:

- **Make a list.** It's much more efficient to spend 10 minutes making a good list of what you need to restock your pantry and to make the dishes for that week, than to get to the grocery store and try to figure it out as you wander the aisles. Take a quick look in your fridge and pantry for staples. Jot down what's getting low. Then think for a minute about what dishes you know you would like to make for the next few days. Scan the recipes and write down any special ingredients you will need. For long lists, group similar items according to the area of the store where you'll find them (frozen food, produce, etc.) This will also save you time in the store by preventing the need to double back over an aisle you've already passed.

- **Get groceries to go.** Another neat time-saving strategy is to use an online grocery service. Some allow you to send them your list and then you pick up the bagged groceries yourself, while others deliver the goods straight to your door. The cost for these services varies, but most options for the larger-chain stores are quite reasonable.

- **Let the grocer do it for you.** There are plenty of whole food products out there that will save several prep steps in the kitchen. Prewashed greens, preshredded or diced veggies and cheese, precubed meat, sliced mushrooms, and prepared garlic are a few key staples.

- **Stock up on these speedy whole foods staples.** Choose high quality, "clean" items with no additives, or chemical or other artificial ingredients.

  - **Produce.** Opt for organic produce, and, whenever possible, choose fruits and vegetables that are in season. In addition to fresh produce, we also use dried fruits in this book—choose unsulphured, unsweetened, or juice-sweetened varieties, when possible.

  - **Canned and jarred foods.** When selecting canned and jarred foods, always choose high quality options with no additives or preservatives, such as sodium or any unfamiliar ingredients you can't pronounce.

  - **Condiments, oils, sweeteners, seasonings, and baking items.** Some of the lesser known ingredients used in this book include high-heat oils such as unrefined virgin coconut oil, macadamia nut oil, peanut oil, rice bran oil (neutral flavor), and ghee (clarified butter); sweeteners such as xylitol or erythritol, Sucanat, and stevia extract; seasonings such as unrefined high-quality sea salt (SI or Himalayan pink), Bragg Liquid Aminos, low-sodium tamari, umeboshi plum vinegar, miso paste, and mirin; and baking items such as whole wheat pastry flour, stone-ground corn meal, oat bran, wheat germ, and kudzu.

- **Meat and seafood.** Whenever possible, choose fresh organic, cage-free chicken breast, tenders and boneless skinless thighs; organic, nitrate-free chicken sausage; very lean grass-fed beef; and fresh or frozen, wild-caught cold-water fish.
- **Vegan meat substitutes.** We use refrigerated or frozen "chicken" breast and strips, "beef" crumbles, and "sausage" patties in these recipes.

ORGANIZE YOUR KITCHEN

To save an enormous amount of time, lay out your kitchen in an orderly fashion. Even if you have limited space, you can still save time if you store your ingredients and equipment efficiently.

Start by grouping related pantry items together in categories that make sense to you, such as baking ingredients together, herbs and spices in a single area, and so on. This is also important in the fridge as you don't want to waste time hunting around for the mustard every time you need it. To help, consider using external wall racks so you can readily see important and often-used items. In addition, keep your most-used kitchen tools (food processor, blender, immersion blender, mixer, knife block) on the counter and plugged in. Keep smaller hand tools either on wall-mounted hooks or shelves or in easy-to-reach containers.

Let the French expression *mise en place*, which means "everything in its place," guide you in laying out all the ingredients and tools you will need to make a dish before you begin. Because my kitchen is so well organized and many staples are visible, this step takes me only minutes. It is a crucial step for speed, however, and also has the double benefit of letting you know if you're missing an ingredient before the dish is half cooked!

TIME TO COOK

When you're running in from work, the kids are screaming, and the dog needs to go out, this is not the time to contemplate creating a luxurious five-course meal. Instead, think simple: one or two dishes that will cover all the macronutrients (carbohydrates, protein, and fats), provide many micronutrients (vitamins, minerals, phytonutrients, etc.), and feel satisfying to you and your family. One-pot meals, featured in this book, are perfect, both for easy prep and easy cleanup.

For entrées that don't stand alone, keep a ready stock of dishes that will provide a quick and tasty complementary side, such as mixed frozen veggies, salad fixings, fresh fruits, and quick-cooking grains. You can mix and match fruits, veggies, and grains with different seasonings to keep things interesting. Try a little dried fruit and baby greens stirred into parboiled brown rice in the last minute of cooking time. Or pour a little salad dressing or cooked marinade over simple steamed veggies for a flavor twist. A sprinkling of toasted nuts adds flavor variety, crunch, and healthy nutrients to salads, veggies, or grains.

Although many people use the microwave oven to help them get dinner on the table in minutes, Dr. Jonny and I both use it as little as possible. Microwaved food tastes flat to me, and doesn't have the same freshness of cooking with external heat. I prefer to reheat leftovers using the steamer and toaster oven, but there's just no denying that the microwave can be a meal-saver in a time crunch. There is no other way to get steaming, baked sweet potatoes on the table in ten minutes. So while we use it sparingly, there are a few recipes that call for its use.

We hope the information and recipes in this book will give you new ideas for preparing tasty, healthy meals in less time, or inspire you to return to home cooking if you have strayed from the kitchen.

To your good health!

—Jeannette Bessinger
Portsmouth, RI, 2010

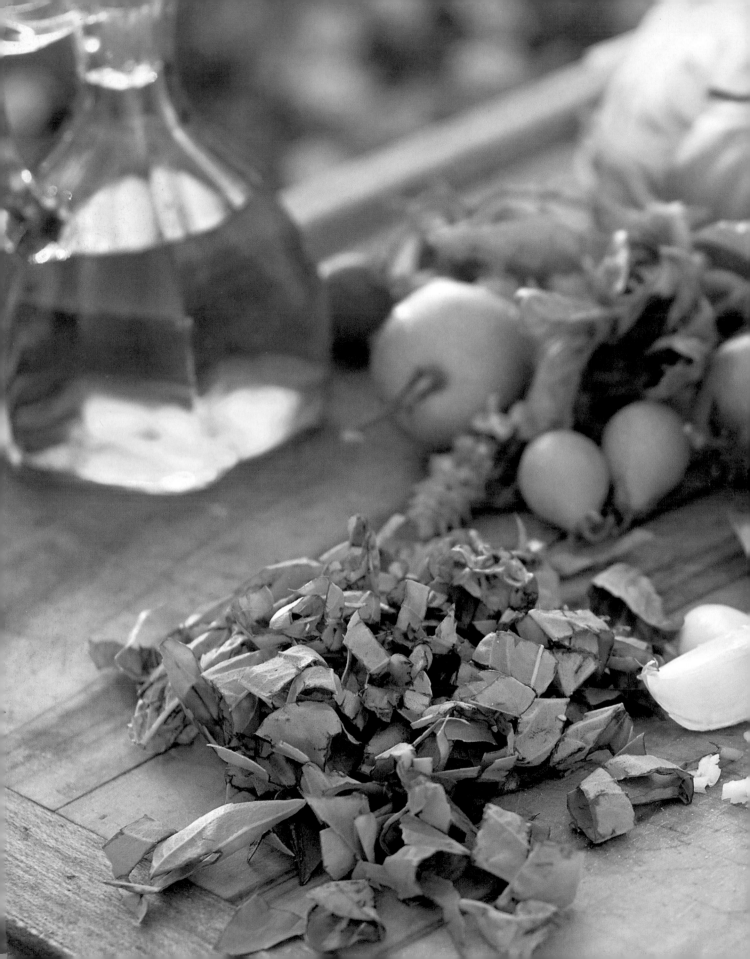

1 | Fast, Fabulous, and Healthy Meals from Prep to Plate in 15 Minutes

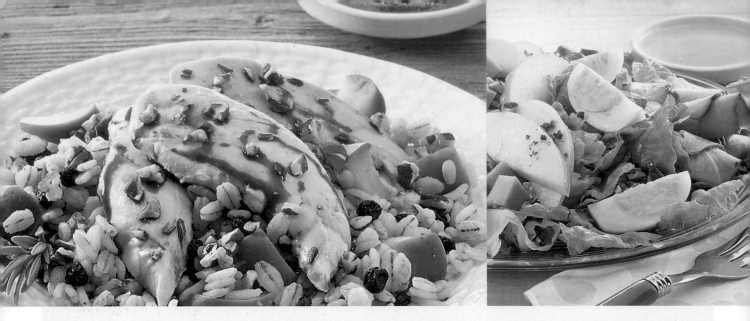

Poultry

Chicken and turkey are terrific sources of protein. A typical portion has only a couple of hundred calories and delivers more than 30 grams of protein, plus a reasonable amount of important B vitamins and almost half the daily value of selenium. But there's a world of difference between free-range and factory-farmed poultry. Choose the former whenever possible—it's much better for you!

Speedy and Spicy Curried Apricot Chicken Salad

Ingredients

- ⅓ cup (77 g) plain low-fat yogurt
- ¼ cup (60 g) high-quality mayonnaise (we like vegan varieties such as Nayonaise or Vegenaise)
- 1 to 2 tablespoons (20 to 40 g) raw honey, to taste
- 1 tablespoon (6.3 g) curry powder
- 3 cups (420 g) cooked chicken, diced or shredded
- 2 stalks celery, diced
- 2 cups (220 g) prepared sliced green apples, chopped
- ⅓ cup (43 g) dried unsulfured apricots, chopped (by hand or with a few pulses in the food processor)
- ½ cup (55 g) toasted sliced almonds

From Chef Jeannette

To Complete the Meal: Serve this light salad over a bed of fresh spring greens or in a whole-grain wrap with alfalfa sprouts and shredded lettuce.

From Dr. Jonny: I love curry for two reasons. One has to do with the brain, the other with the heart (at least metaphorically). My heart loves curry because it just tastes so good—as spicy as you want it to be (you can adjust the spice levels to your own liking), always pleasing to the palate, somehow rich and light at the same time. But my brain loves it because I know what's in it—turmeric. If you read my book *The 150 Healthiest Foods on Earth*, you probably already know that turmeric is the closest thing to a superfood in the spice kingdom. The active ingredients in turmeric are called curcuminoids, and in the laboratory they've been found to have anticancer activity. Plus turmeric is one of the most anti-inflammatory foods on the planet. Curry goes beautifully with chicken, and the apricots and almonds make a perfect complement to the mix. A little apricot trivia: Apricots are one of the lowest-calorie fruits on the planet (17 calories per fruit!) and yet deliver a surprising amount of nutrition, containing potassium, magnesium, and calcium. This dish is great for picnics!

In a large bowl, whisk together the yogurt, mayo, honey, and curry powder until smooth and well incorporated. Gently stir in the chicken, celery, apples, apricots, and almonds.

Yield: 4 servings

Per Serving: 501 Calories; 26g Fat (46.0% calories from fat); 38g Protein; 32g Carbohydrate; 5g Dietary Fiber; 94mg Cholesterol; 196mg Sodium

Protein-Packed Chicken in Sun-Dried Tomato Cream over Quick Quinoa

Ingredients

1 cup (170 g) quinoa, rinsed

2¹/₂ cups (570 ml) chicken or vegetable broth, divided

2 teaspoons olive oil

2 shallots, diced fine

¹/₂ cup (230 g) silken tofu, drained and blended until smooth (quickest with immersion blender)

¹/₂ teaspoon chicken or vegetable Better Than Bouillon (or you can use ¹/₂ teaspoon salt and ¹/₂ teaspoon nutritional yeast)

¹/₂ cup (235 ml) dry white wine

¹/₂ teaspoon tarragon, optional

¹/₃ cup (37 g) sliced sun-dried tomatoes in oil, well-drained

2 cups (280 g) diced cooked chicken (use leftovers, Trader Joe's prepared diced chicken, or 1 package [8 ounces or 225 g] meatless frozen Morningstar Farms Chik'n Strips)

¹/₄ cup (10 g) fresh basil, rolled and sliced into thin strips, optional

From Dr. Jonny: Let me be perfectly clear and consistent with everything I've written in the last ten years: I am not afraid of saturated fat, which has gotten a bum rap and been unfairly blamed for a lot of things it doesn't do (such as cause heart disease, but don't get me started). Even though I'm in the minority on this issue, most people would still like to reduce their intake of saturated fats. Here's the perfect way to do it without compromising flavor. Using tofu in place of heavy cream gives you plenty of protein, a creamy texture, and zero saturated fat. (Even if you're not afraid of a little saturated fat, you'll still love it—I certainly do!) Quinoa has eight essential amino acids, is one of the highest-protein "grains" (it's technically a seed, but who cares?), and is quick-cooking and delicious.

What's not to love?

Bring the quinoa and 2 cups (475 ml) of the broth to a rolling boil in a medium saucepan over high heat. Reduce the heat, cover, and simmer for 12 minutes or until the tails have popped and the quinoa is tender.

While the quinoa is cooking, heat the oil in a large skillet over medium heat. Sauté the shallots for 2 minutes and add the tofu, remaining ¹/₂ cup (120 ml) broth, bouillon, wine, and tarragon and whisk gently until well combined. Stir in the tomatoes and chicken and bring to a simmer. Simmer for about 2 minutes or until the chicken is heated through (about 5 minutes if using frozen Chik'n Strips). Stir the basil into the cream sauce, if using.

Serve the creamed chicken over a bed of the hot quinoa.

Yield: 4 servings

Per Serving: 385 Calories; 10g Fat (25.6% calories from fat); 34g Protein; 34g Carbohydrate; 4g Dietary Fiber; 60mg Cholesterol; 715mg Sodium

From Chef Jeannette

To Complete the Meal: This also works well over 8 ounces (225 g) of whole wheat egg noodles in place of the quinoa. Talk about creamy comfort food! Enjoy it with a helping of steamed broccoli sprinkled with balsamic vinegar and a few toasted almond slices.

Using Vegan Meat Substitutes: Though they are processed foods, occasionally using "meat substitutes" is not only much faster than using real meat but also provides a tasty source of ready protein, such as the suggestion in the above dish. Use them in recognizable dishes to help ease the transition away from unhealthy (and more expensive!) factory-farmed meats. Your family won't know they aren't eating true animal meat. I once heard Dr. Walter Willett, a professor at Harvard Medical School and principal investigator on the second Nurses' Health Study, make a comment that both of his parents were vegetarians, but only one of them knew about it!

Simple, Satisfying Southwest Chicken-Pinto Bean Stew

Ingredients

4 cups (950 ml) low-sodium chicken broth

²/₃ cup (160 ml) pico de gallo sauce*

1 can (4 ounces or 115 g) green chiles, undrained

2 teaspoons prepared garlic (or 2 small cloves, minced)

½ teaspoon ground cumin

½ teaspoon salt

¼ teaspoon cracked black pepper

2 cups (280 g) leftover shredded or diced cooked chicken (or use 1 package [8 ounces] frozen faux chicken strips)

1 can (15 ounces or 425 g) pinto beans, drained and rinsed

1 cup (130 g) frozen corn

From Chef Jeannette

If You Have 5 More Minutes: Create a good-for-you garnish for the soup. While the soup simmers, in a small bowl thoroughly mix together ⅓ cup (77 g) of plain Greek yogurt; 1 large garlic clove, minced; 1½ tablespoons (25 ml) of fresh-squeezed lime juice; and ¼ cup (4 g) of chopped fresh cilantro. Serve soup with dollops of garnish.

Superspeed Garnish: Stir ⅓ cup (5 g) chopped fresh cilantro into soup just before serving.

If You Have 15 More Minutes: Make your own pico de gallo sauce for a fresh burst of nutrients and flavor. Combine 2 large, ripe tomatoes, quartered; ¼ of a red onion; ½ of a small jalapeño; 4 cloves of crushed garlic; 1 tablespoon (1 g) of fresh cilantro; and the juice of 2 limes in a food processor. Process to the consistency of relish.

From Dr. Jonny: Let me quickly share with you a concept in weight loss that's worth knowing about. It's called Volumetrics, and it was coined by Professor Barbara Rolls at Penn State University. The basic concept is that we can lose weight by eating "high-volume" foods that take up a lot of space in the tummy, have a ton of nutrients, but are low in calories, often because these foods contain a lot of water. Soups and stews are the ultimate high-volume foods, especially when they're not loaded with cream or other high-calorie ingredients. This is a great stew for long life, containing both high-fiber pinto beans and high-protein chicken, a combination that not only fills you up but keeps you feeling that way for a long time!

Pour the chicken broth into a large soup pot over high heat and stir in the pico de gallo sauce, chiles, garlic, cumin, salt, pepper, chicken, beans, and corn, and stir to combine. (If using veggie "chicken strips," add for the last 3 minutes of cooking only.) When the soup boils, reduce the heat and simmer, covered, for 10 minutes.

Yield: 4 servings

Per Serving: 567 Calories; 7g Fat (10.5% calories from fat); 57g Protein; 83g Carbohydrate; 27g Dietary Fiber; 60mg Cholesterol; 396mg Sodium

*Find prepared pico de gallo sauce in the Mexican section of your grocery store.

Lean and Light Sesame Thai Chicken and Broccoli

Ingredients

1 pound (455 g) broccoli florets, fresh or frozen

½ cup (113 g) Thai sweet chili sauce

1 tablespoon (20 g) Thai fish sauce

1 tablespoon (15 ml) low-sodium tamari

¼ cup (60 ml) lime juice (preferably fresh squeezed)

1 tablespoon (15 ml) sesame oil

1¼ pounds (567 g) chicken tenders

2 tablespoons (16 g) toasted sesame seeds

From Chef Jeannette

To Complete the Meal: Serve the chicken and broccoli over 1½ cups (247 g) of hot brown rice or quinoa (look for frozen, prepared, or parboiled quick-cooking brown rice, if you don't have leftovers).

If You Have 5 More Minutes: Thicken the sauce for better "cling" power. Dissolve 1 teaspoon of kudzu into 2 teaspoons of water and mix in well once the sauce is hot. Simmer for 1 minute or until thickened.

From Dr. Jonny: Talk to ten typical gym rats about their idea of the perfect meal and I guarantee seven of them are going to say "chicken and broccoli." (I wish I had a ten-dollar bill for every Tupperware container filled with chicken and broccoli that I've seen over the years at Gold's Gym in California!) It's kind of the ultimate weight-loss, muscle-building meal of lean protein and nutrient-rich vegetables, but Chef Jeannette has whipped up a version that tastes nothing like a "diet" meal. I think of this dish as a healthy version of General Tso's chicken. Compare this sweet and satisfying version to the breaded, syrupy, high-calorie mess at the typical Chinese takeout: It's no contest! Plus you can make this healthful, tasty alternative faster than it takes the delivery guy to get to your door!

In a large pot, steam the broccoli for 2 to 3 minutes or until just tender-crisp (you can also microwave, but steaming is healthiest).

While the broccoli is steaming, in a small bowl, whisk together the chili sauce, fish sauce, tamari, and lime juice and set aside.

Heat the oil in a large skillet or Dutch oven over medium heat. Add the tenders and sauté for 1 to 3 minutes per side until just cooked through. Add the steamed broccoli and sauce mixture to the pan, reduce heat to medium, and stir gently to coat. Cook for 1 to 2 minutes or until hot and glazed. Top with the sesame seeds and serve.

Yield: 4 servings

Per Serving: 265 Calories; 7g Fat (22.5% calories from fat); 38g Protein; 16g Carbohydrate; 4g Dietary Fiber; 70mg Cholesterol; 1475mg Sodium

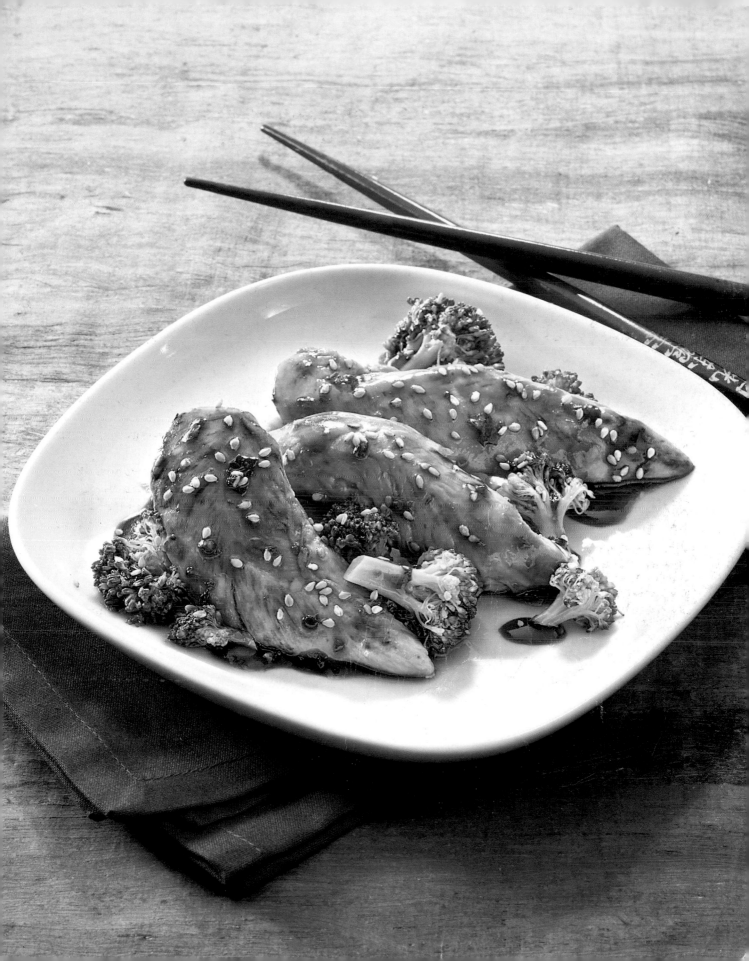

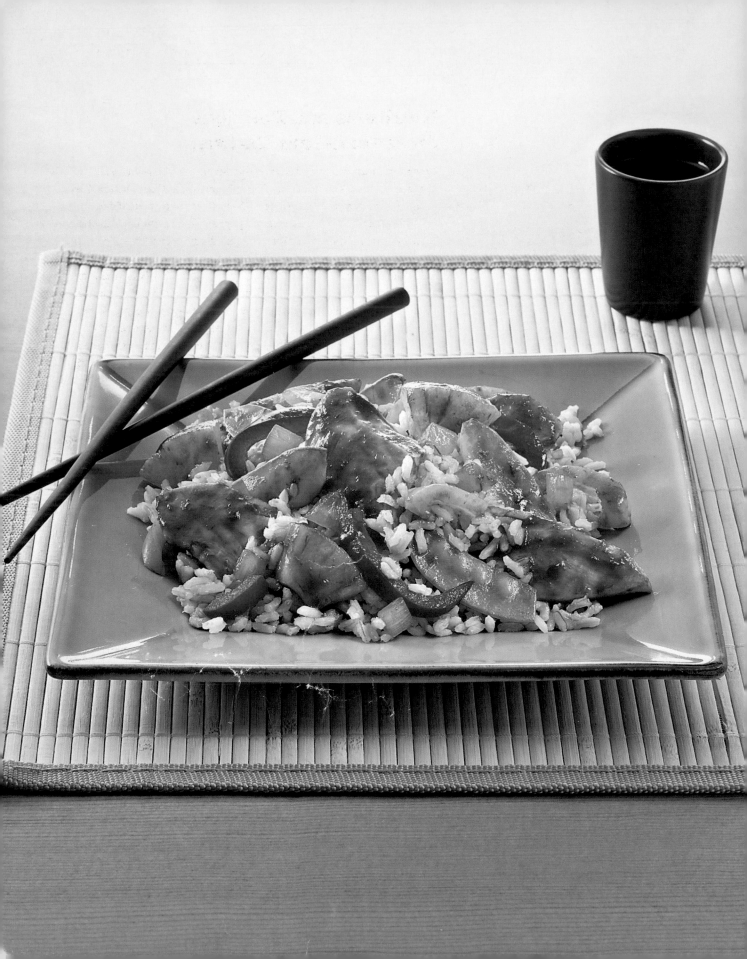

Ingredients

1 can (15 ounces or 435 g) pineapple chunks
  in water or juice (not syrup!), drained
  and liquid reserved
2 tablespoons (28 ml) low-sodium tamari
2 tablespoons (32 g) tomato paste
1 to 2 tablespoons (20 to 40 g) honey, to
  taste
1 tablespoon (15 ml) apple cider
  vinegar, or to taste
¼ teaspoon red pepper flakes
2 teaspoons peanut oil
1 pound (455 g) chicken tenders, halved
6 ounces (170 g) prepared sliced red and
  yellow bell peppers with onions
  (or use 1 large red pepper and
  ½ large onion, chopped)
1 cup (75 g) stringless snow peas
¼ cup (4 g) chopped fresh cilantro,
  optional

From Chef Jeannette

To Complete the Meal: Serve the sweet-and-sour chicken over 1½ cups (245 g) of hot cooked brown rice mixed with 1 tablespoon of toasted sesame seeds (reheat leftover, or prepare quick-cooking parboiled, or frozen cooked).

Superspeed Tip: For a cholesterol-free option, use 8 ounces (225 g) of frozen vegan "chicken strips" in place of the real chicken and skip the chicken-sautéeing step altogether. Add the frozen strips when you add the sauce and simmer for 4 minutes or until the strips are hot.

If You Have 30 More Minutes: Marinate the chicken in the sauce in glass in the fridge for 30 minutes for a stronger flavor. Remove the chicken to sauté and add the rest of the marinade as directed.

Nutritious and Delicious Sweet-and-Sour Chicken

From Dr. Jonny: If you love sweet-and-sour pork from the local Chinese restaurant, wait till you taste this much healthier version. First of all, it doesn't have MSG. Second, there are no cheap oils. Third, there's a nice vitamin boost from the peppers (high in vitamin C, which supports a healthy immune system), antioxidant support from the tomatoes, and iron and fiber from the snow peas, which also provide some vitamin K, an important nutrient for bone health. Fourth, this recipe has zero added sugar. (You'd be amazed at how much sugar is in the average Chinese take-out "sweet–and-sour" dish—how do you think they get it to taste so sweet?) Add the pineapples for still more fiber (and some natural sweetness) plus a nice dose of heart-healthy potassium (not to mention digestive enzymes) and you've got a high-protein dish that beats the pants off mass-produced restaurant fare.

In a small bowl, whisk together 3 tablespoons (45 ml) reserved pineapple juice, tamari, tomato paste, honey, cider vinegar, and red pepper flakes. Set aside.

Heat the oil in a large skillet or Dutch oven over medium-high heat. Add the chicken and cook for 1 minute on each side. Reduce the heat to medium and add the peppers, onions, and snow peas, sautéing for 2 minutes. Pour in the sauce, mix, and cook, stirring frequently, for about 3 minutes or until the veggies have started to soften. Stir in the pineapple and cook for 1 to 2 minutes or until the pineapple is hot and the chicken is cooked through. Top with fresh cilantro, if using.

Yield: 4 servings
Per Serving: 259 Calories; 3g Fat (10.5% calories from fat); 32g Protein; 32g Carbohydrate; 2g Dietary Fiber; 56mg Cholesterol; 572mg Sodium

One-Step Tangy Tarragon Chicken Salad

Ingredients

¹/₃ cup (77 g) plain low-fat yogurt

2 tablespoons (28 g) mayonnaise (we like Nayonaise or Vegenaise)

1 tablespoon (15 g) Dijon mustard

1¹/₂ tablespoons (25 ml) fresh-squeezed lemon juice

1 clove garlic, finely minced

1 teaspoon dried tarragon

¹/₄ teaspoon salt

¹/₂ cup (50 g) sliced scallions

2 cups (280 g) shredded cooked chicken

6 cups (330 g) spring greens

4 ripe heirloom tomatoes, quartered

From Dr. Jonny: Here's a little bit of interesting spice trivia for you: Tarragon has been used medicinally going back to 500 BCE. Its résumé includes helping to fight fatigue, calm the nerves, aid in digestion, and promote appetite. Not bad, huh? Replacing the mayo in a classic chicken salad with yogurt decreases the saturated fat content and adds protein and important bacteria known as probiotics, which are great for digestion and immunity. To make this work as a quick dish, all you need is a cooked chicken or cooked chicken breast. Easy to find in the grocery store—just look for organic rotisserie chicken.

In a large bowl, mix together the yogurt, mayonnaise, mustard, lemon juice, garlic, tarragon, and salt until well combined. Gently stir in the scallions and chicken.

Make four beds of spring greens and lay the tomato quarters in the center. Spoon the chicken evenly into the center of the tomatoes and serve.

Yield: 4 servings

Per Serving: 218 Calories; 10g Fat (39.1% calories from fat); 24g Protein; 9g Carbohydrate; 2g Dietary Fiber; 62mg Cholesterol; 302mg Sodium

From Chef Jeannette

Make It Ahead: If you don't wish to buy precooked chicken, you can make it easily yourself in a slow cooker. Simply wash a regular roasting chicken (or two, if your cooker is large enough), pat it dry, and place it in your slow cooker with a bay leaf and ¹/₂ cup (120 ml) of water or no-sodium chicken broth (double for two chickens). Be sure to remove any giblets from the cavities before cooking! Cook it on low for 7 to 8 hours (or 8 to 9 hours if two chickens) until cooked through. Remove the chicken from the broth and cool it enough to handle. Remove all the skin, cartilage, and bones, and you will have a few cups of tender meat, both light and dark. Freeze any extra you won't need right away in an airtight freezer bag. And don't throw away that cooking liquid! Cool it in the fridge, remove the congealed fat (from the surface) and bay leaf, and use or freeze it as sodium-free chicken stock.

In addition to being less expensive, slow-cooking your own chicken at home is also healthier than purchasing prepared. You can buy the highest-quality free-range bird and control the level of extra fat (none!) and sodium (none!) that goes into it.

Ingredients

1 tablespoon (15 ml) olive oil
1 teaspoon Dijon mustard
½ teaspoon salt
¼ teaspoon black pepper
4 skinless, boneless chicken breast halves
3 tablespoons (45 g) plain low-fat yogurt
1½ tablespoons (22 g) honey mustard
½ teaspoon mustard seeds

From Chef Jeannette

To Complete the Meal: Serve it with sweet, steamed Vidalia onions. Peel and slice two Vidalias across the middle. Place them into a microwave-safe glass dish with 2 tablespoons (28 ml) of water and cover. Cook for about 4 minutes, turning the dish once in the middle, or until soft. Garnish each half with a thin slice of butter and a sprinkling of garlic salt.

Easy Grilled Chicken with Seeded Honey-Mustard Sauce

From Dr. Jonny: In this dish, the smooth richness of the yogurt perfectly complements the grilled chicken, and the seedy, sweet mustard pulls it all together. And it's so darn easy to prepare, even I can do it. Chef Jeannette suggests a side of steamed Vidalias, so a word about Vidalia onions is in order. They're actually named for Vidalia, Georgia, where they were first grown in the 1930s. They're unusually sweet, probably because the soil in which they're grown is low in sulfur. Interesting trivia: In 1986, Georgia's state legislature passed the Vidalia Onion Act of 1986, which basically trademarked the name Vidalia onions and limited the production area to Georgia, where it has been the official state vegetable since 1990. And onions are a nutritional heavy-hitter. They're a rich source of fructooligosaccharides, which basically "feed" the healthy bacteria in your gut and suppress the growth of potentially health-robbing bacteria in the colon.

Preheat the grill to medium heat.

In a medium bowl, mix together the olive oil, Dijon mustard, salt, and pepper. Toss the four chicken breasts in the bowl to evenly coat. Lightly spray the grill with olive oil and grill the chicken for about 6 minutes per side or until cooked through.

While the chicken is cooking, in a small bowl mix together the yogurt, honey mustard, and mustard seeds until well combined. Serve the chicken with a dollop of the mustard sauce.

Yield: 4 servings
Per Serving: 174 Calories; 6g Fat (31.3% calories from fat); 28g Protein; 2g Carbohydrate; trace Dietary Fiber; 66mg Cholesterol; 445mg Sodium

Ingredients

1½ tablespoons (25 ml) olive oil, divided

2 boneless, skinless chicken breasts, cut
into 1-inch (2.5 cm) pieces (or halve
1 pound [455 g] chicken tenders; or 1
15-ounce (425 g) can of drained and
rinsed kidney beans, red or white, for
a meatless, superspeed option)

2 shallots, chopped

Salt and fresh ground black pepper, to taste

2 cups (475 ml) chicken broth

1 teaspoon crumbled sage

½ teaspoon dried thyme

1½ cups (186 g) frozen succotash (lima
beans, corn, and carrots or green beans)

¾ cup (105 g) bulgur (fine or medium grind)

2 tablespoons (28 ml) fresh-squeezed
lemon juice

1 teaspoon lemon zest, optional

From Chef Jeannette

If You Have 5 Extra Minutes: Add ¼ cup
(30 g) of toasted walnuts for a mineral
boost and crunchy finish.

Chicken Pilaf in a Pinch

From Dr. Jonny: High in protein and fiber, low in fat and calories, bulgur offers everything you need to fill up without adding inches to your waist. (FYI: A cup of bulgur has 8 grams of fiber, twice the amount in brown rice!) Bulgur is what's left after kernels of wheat have been dried, steamed, and crushed. It's a minimally processed Middle Eastern staple that actually helps keep your digestive tract healthy, largely because of its rich fiber content. Combined with chicken for protein, a symphony of healthy spices, and some crunchiness from the mineral-rich walnuts, this dish makes a perfect hearty meal for all seasons!

In a Dutch oven, heat ½ tablespoon of the olive oil over medium heat. Add the chicken and shallots to the skillet, season lightly with salt and pepper, and cook for about 1 minute, turning frequently. Add the chicken broth, sage, and thyme and increase the heat to boiling.

Add the frozen veggies and bulgur, reduce the heat, and simmer, covered, for 6 to 8 minutes (fine grind takes less time than medium) or until the chicken is cooked through and the veggies and bulgur are tender. In a large bowl, wisk together the remaining tablespoon (15 ml) of olive oil, lemon juice, and lemon zest. Add bulgar mixture, stirring gently to distribute the dressing and correct the seasonings if necessary.

Yield: 4 servings

Per Serving: 426 Calories; 13g Fat (26.6% calories from fat); 40g Protein; 41g Carbohydrate; 9g Dietary Fiber; 68mg Cholesterol; 468mg Sodium

Ingredients

2 teaspoons olive oil

2 teaspoons butter

1¼ pounds (567 g) chicken tenders

Salt and fresh ground black pepper

1 cup high-quality canned black bean soup
(we like Amy's or Muir Glen)

8 ounces (225 g) sliced mushrooms (baby
bellas, white, button, or wild mushroom
varieties all work well)

⅓ cup (80 ml) chicken broth or water

2 tablespoons (28 ml) Madeira wine (or
Marsala wine)

1 teaspoon organic Worcestershire sauce
(organic to avoid high-fructose corn
syrup—we like Annie's)

1 teaspoon Dijon mustard

From Chef Jeannette

To Complete the Meal: Steam a 12-ounce
(340 g) package of prepared broccoli
florets for 3 to 4 minutes until tender-
crisp. Remove from the heat and toss
with a vinaigrette made from 1 tablespoon
(15 ml) of olive oil, 1 tablespoon (15 ml)
of fresh-squeezed lemon juice, and 2
teaspoons Dijon mustard. Top with a
sprinkling of toasted sliced almonds, if
desired. If you are looking for a heartier
meal, this dish produces enough sauce to
serve over a small amount of whole-grain
vermicelli.

Chicken tenders, taken from the breast
meat around the ribs, are the leanest
meat on the chicken, and they cook up
much faster than whole breasts.

Quick Chicken-Mushroom Madeira

From Dr. Jonny: Here's a quick and easy dish that combines great
nutrition with terrific taste. Everyone likes chicken tenders, which are
rich in protein and relatively low in calories (assuming, of course, that
they're not deep-fried!). And the mushrooms are actually little nutritional powerhouses. Thousands of varieties are edible and hundreds
have medicinal properties, but the best known—shiitake, maitake, rei-
shi, and the plain old button mushroom—work just great. By the way,
don't discount that common white button mushroom—it's loaded with
potassium, ridiculously low in calories (15 calories per cup, if you can
believe it), and even contains a nice dose of selenium, one of the most
important minerals in our diet. But the real selling point of this recipe
is the way Chef Jeannette cleverly used the black bean soup as the
base of a sauce. It adds a richness that makes the dish taste like it was
simmered for hours—no one will know you whipped up this baby in
mere minutes!

Heat the oil and butter in a large skillet over medium-high heat. Add the
tenders and lightly season with salt and pepper. Sauté the tenders for 1 to
3 minutes per side until golden and cooked through. Set aside.

While the chicken is sautéing, blend or process the soup until silky
smooth. Once the chicken is removed from the pan, lower the heat to medium and add the mushrooms, sautéing for about 3 minutes or until they
release their juices and are just tender. You can cover for the last minute to
speed the cook time. Stir in the pureed soup, broth, wine, Worcestershire,
and mustard, mix well, and increase the heat to medium high. Pour any
juices released from the resting chicken into the sauce. Simmer for 2 to 3
minutes or until the mushrooms are tender and the sauce reaches desired
thickness. Season to taste with salt and pepper, if desired, and pour the
sauce over the tenders to serve.

Yield: 4 servings
Per Serving: 234 Calories; 6g Fat (23.7% calories from fat); 34g Protein; 9g
Carbohydrate; 2g Dietary Fiber; 76mg Cholesterol; 668mg Sodium

Super-Fast Super-Protein Salad

Ingredients

½ cup (115 g) plain low-fat yogurt

1 tablespoon (15 g) Dijon mustard

1½ cups (210 g) cooked chicken, turkey, or firm tofu, diced or shredded

1 cup (115 g) prepared cubed or shredded cheese (works well with Cheddar, Swiss, Colby, etc.)

4 hard-boiled eggs, chopped (see page 48 for how to boil eggs)

3 tablespoons (19 g) diced pimiento-stuffed green olives

3 tablespoons (45 g) diced sweet pickle

3 tablespoons (27 g) finely diced red or green bell pepper

2 tablespoons (20 g) finely diced sweet onion

From Dr. Jonny: If you've read my newsletter for a while, you've undoubtedly heard me talk about how a higher-protein diet can help with weight loss. (I also talk about that at length in my book *Living Low Carb: Controlled Carbohydrate Eating for Long-Term Weight Loss*.) But you don't have to be on a low-carb diet to enjoy the occasional high-protein dish, and this one is a doozie. Also high in flavor, this is a great way to use leftover chicken, turkey, or tofu. The yogurt adds a tangy flavor note, not to mention a dose of healthy bacteria known as probiotics, which help build immunity and aid digestion. (Note: Choose yogurt that says "contains live cultures" on the label.) Superquick, assembly-style prep answers the question, "How do I make a tasty, satisfying meal or snack in virtually no time?"

In a large bowl, mix together the yogurt and mustard until well combined. Add the poultry or tofu, cheese, eggs, olives, pickle, pepper, and onion, and stir gently to combine.

Yield: 4 servings

Per Serving: 322 Calories; 18g Fat (50.9% calories from fat); 32g Protein; 7g Carbohydrate; 1g Dietary Fiber; 287mg Cholesterol; 477mg Sodium

From Chef Jeannette

To Complete the Meal: You can also roll this salad into a whole-grain wrap with lots of lettuce, serve it on a bed of greens with salad veggies, or stuff it into a veggie "boat," such as hollowed-out tomatoes, half-cucumbers, or bell peppers. Enjoy a sliced apple or handful of veggie "straws" on the side, if desired.

Prep Speed Tip: The quickest way to dice an onion is to cut it in half from "stem to stern," so you have two equal halves, each with half the root. Peel it under water so the skin comes off cleanly in large pieces. Lay the cut side down on a cutting board designated for "pungents" such as onion, garlic, and hot peppers. Slice off the feathered top, but leave the root intact. Make several lengthwise cuts into the onion from the root side to the freshly cut top. Do not slice all the way into the root so the piece comes completely off, but leave the root end intact so it all holds together at the base. Then, holding the sliced sections together with one hand, cut widthwise across all the cuts to dice the onion into pieces. When you get to the base, discard the last root piece that's held it all together. Your onion will fall apart into a perfect dice. Make larger cuts for bigger pieces, and smaller ones for a finer dice.

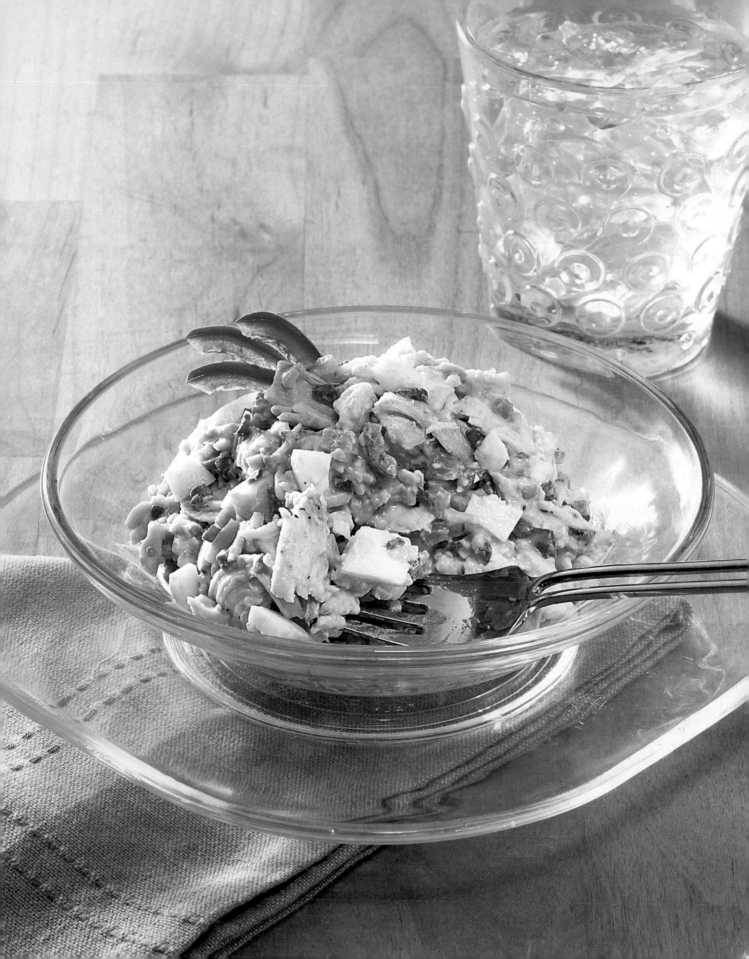

Ingredients

4 cups (950 ml) no-sodium chicken broth

2 cups (280 g) cooked chicken, shredded or
diced

1 can (14.5 ounces or 413 g) white beans,
drained and rinsed (or 2 cups [330 g]
leftover cooked grains, such as brown
rice, quinoa, or millet)

2 cups (260 g) cooked or frozen veggies
(e.g., sliced carrots, broccoli florets,
peas, zucchini, cauliflower, pearl onions, edamame, or a "stir-fry" mix—we
like Seapoint Farms Garden Blend with
Edamame)

2 to 3 (32 to 48 g) tablespoons mellow
white miso, to taste*

From Chef Jeannette

If You Have 5 More Minutes: You can
add 4 ounces (115 g) of buckwheat soba
noodles to the boiling broth for a highly
nourishing "chicken noodle" soup that
beats the pants off grandma's for fiber
and mineral content!

Easy One-Pot Chicken Miso Soup

From Dr. Jonny: Leftovers make terrific healthy meals—and if you
think outside the box, they can substitute for almost anything, including
breakfast! Here's a classic five-ingredient all-in-one meal you can make
in ten minutes that will work well with any leftovers you have in the
fridge. There's been a lot of controversy lately about soy foods, but no
matter which side of the soy fence you're on, everyone agrees that traditionally fermented soy foods are great for you, and miso is a perfect
example. Made of soybeans and koji (a culture starter from beneficial
bacteria), miso is loaded with enzymes and healthy bacteria that aid
with digestion and the assimilation of nutrients. Miso was perfected in
Japan in the seventh century and continues to be prized for its antiaging benefits in China and Japan. Add your leftovers to this basic one-
pot soup and presto! You have a tasty, healing long-life meal!

Pour the chicken broth into a large soup pot and bring to a boil over high
heat. Add the chicken, beans, and veggies and reduce the heat to a simmer
for 5 minutes or until all ingredients are hot. Stir in the miso and incorporate well (an immersion blender works perfectly for this, or you can use a
bit of hot broth to "melt" the miso in a small bowl before adding).

Yield: 4 servings

Per Serving: 499 Calories; 5g Fat (9.1% calories from fat); 48g Protein;
67g Carbohydrate; 17g Dietary Fiber; 60mg Cholesterol; 697mg Sodium

*Miso is the ultimate fast-food ingredient. It makes a flavorful and nourishing
broth for a quick soup featuring many different types of ingredients. Alkalizing
and mineralizing, it is soothing to the system, a balm for jangled nerves on a
busy day, or a simple tonic to strengthen the immune system during the cold,
dry winter months. Choose the lighter, sweet misos to accompany seafood and
light veggies and the darker varieties, such as barley miso, for root veggies and
grains. You will find miso paste in the refrigerated section of natural food stores
and whole foods grocers. Look for it near the tofu and other Asian offerings. It is
very salty, so start with less and add more to taste.

Comforting Broccolini Farfalle with Chicken Sausage

Ingredients

8 ounces (225 g) whole-grain farfalle
(we like Barilla Plus)

1 tablespoon (15 ml) olive oil, plus more,
if necessary

¾ cup (120 g) prepared diced onion
(or ½ small onion or 2 shallots,
chopped)

1 teaspoon prepared minced garlic
(or 1 clove minced), optional

4 sweet Italian chicken sausages
(3 ounces or 85 g each), sliced

1 bunch broccolini, chopped into
bite-size pieces

¼ cup (28 g) sun-dried tomato strips in oil,
barely drained

⅓ cup (50 g) crumbled feta or grated
Parmesan cheese

¼ cup (10 g) slivered fresh basil,
optional

From Dr. Jonny: Broccoli, broccoli, how many kinds of you are there? Let me count the ways! (Oh, sorry, I must have been channeling Elizabeth Barrett Browning!) Still, it's easy to see why some folks are confused. There's broccoli rabe, which actually comes from a different family and tends to be bitter; broccolini, also known as baby broccoli; and regular, garden-variety broccoli (the grown-up version of broccolini). Broccolini, used in this recipe, is sweet and tender and one of my personal favorite vegetables for grilling or stir-frying. The nutritional value is virtually the same as for its parental relative (full-grown broccoli), yet in my opinion it's a lot tastier (also much more "kid-friendly"). Just like broccoli, it's got fiber, calcium, potassium, vitamin C, and all the wonderful cancer-fighting phytochemicals that broccoli is known for. Side note: If you can get broccoli rabe just picked in spring and summertime, it tends to be much less bitter and will work well in this dish as well. The chicken Italian sausage is lower in fat and calories than regular sausage and still tastes terrific.

Cook the farfalle al dente according to the package directions. Drain quickly and return to the cooking pot.

While the pasta is cooking, heat 1 tablespoon (15 ml) olive oil in a large sauté pan or Dutch oven over medium heat. Add the onion and sauté for 2 minutes. Add the garlic, sausage, and broccolini, cover, and cook for 5 to 7 minutes, stirring frequently, or until the sausage is lightly browned and the broccolini is tender-crisp. Add the sausage mixture and sun-dried tomatoes to the hot, drained pasta, drizzling with extra olive oil if too dry, and mix gently, reheating over medium heat for a minute or so, if necessary. Finish with the cheese and basil, if using.

Yield: 4 servings
Per Serving: 484 Calories; 19g Fat (34.8% calories from fat); 32g Protein; 47g Carbohydrate; 7g Dietary Fiber; 86mg Cholesterol; 940mg Sodium

Ingredients

4 cups (950 ml) low-sodium chicken broth, divided

1 cup (235 ml) apple cider (or chicken stock or water)

¼ teaspoon salt

¼ teaspoon cracked black pepper

2 sprigs fresh rosemary, divided

1 cup (184 g) quick-cooking barley

1 red cooking apple, unpeeled, cored, and diced (McIntosh or Cortland work well, or chop 2 cups [220 g] prepared sliced apples)

1¼ pounds (567 g) chicken tenders

2 tablespoons (28 ml) balsamic vinegar

2 tablespoons (28 ml) olive oil

2 tablespoons (18 g) dried currants, optional

3 tablespoons (21 g) toasted chopped pecans

From Chef Jeannette

Poaching chicken is a quick and healthy way to cook it cleanly with no added fat. Using apple juice, fresh herbs, and chicken broth as the poaching mixture gives it a rich, full flavor while adding no extra calories and producing a juicy, tender meat.

To Complete the Meal: Serve with 4 cups (400 g) of steamed al dente haricots verts or green beans. Top them with a bit of the balsamic dressing or a small pat of butter for extra flavor.

Fast, Flavorful Fiber: Rosemary Apple-Poached Chicken and Barley

From Dr. Jonny: Sounds weird to start talking about a recipe that features delicious ingredients such as apples, currants, and pecans by discussing barley, but barley is one of those underappreciated foods that doesn't get the attention it deserves. It's a type of whole grain that originated in Southeast Asia and Ethiopia and has been cultivated for more than 10,000 years. It's high in dietary fiber, but specifically in a beneficial type of soluble fiber called beta-glucan. Two studies have shown that beta-glucan can help control the appetite by increasing the feeling of fullness, and beta-glucan has also been shown to help lower cholesterol (about 12 percent reduction in one 2000 study). This dish is rich, chewy, and warming with a hint of sweetness from the apple and currants, and bright notes from the rosemary—perfect for a cool autumn evening!

Bring 2 cups of the chicken broth in a large saucepan to a boil over high heat. Combine the remaining 2 cups of the chicken broth, the cider, salt, pepper, and 1 rosemary sprig in a large sauté pan or Dutch oven and bring to a boil over high heat.

In the saucepan, add the barley and apple to the boiling chicken broth, reduce the heat, cover, and simmer for 10 to 12 minutes or until the barley is tender and most of the liquid has been absorbed (drain extra, if necessary).

In the sauté pan, reduce the heat to medium, add the chicken tenders in one layer to the broth and cider mixture, cover, and cook for 4 to 5 minutes or until tender and cooked through, turning the pieces over if necessary for even cooking.

While the chicken and grain are cooking, strip off about a tablespoon of leaves from the remaining rosemary sprig and mince. In a small bowl, whisk together the vinegar, oil, and 1 teaspoon of the minced rosemary until emulsified.

When the chicken is done, drain it well and set aside. When the barley is done, fold in the currants, if using, and cover for about 30 seconds. Serve the chicken breast over a bed of the apple-currant barley. Drizzle the dressing over the chicken and sprinkle the pecans over all.

Yield: 4 servings

Per Serving: 530 Calories; 15g Fat (22.6% calories from fat); 49g Protein; 66g Carbohydrate; 8g Dietary Fiber; 70mg Cholesterol; 425mg Sodium

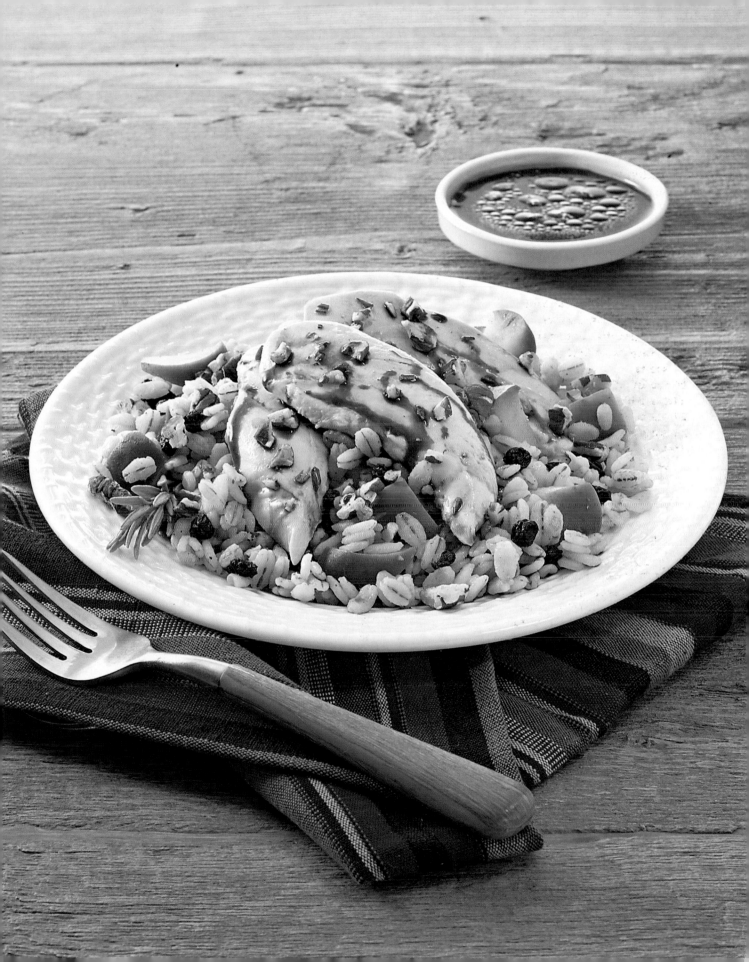

Ingredients

Quick Barbecue Sauce

1 cup (240 g) high-quality ketchup (Choose an organic variety to avoid high-fructose corn syrup—we like Annie's)

3 tablespoons (45 ml) apple cider vinegar

2 tablespoons (40 g) molasses

1 tablespoon (12 g) Sucanat, optional, to taste

2 teaspoons horseradish mustard (or Dijon)

2 teaspoons organic Worcestershire sauce (Choose organic for this, too—high-fructose corn syrup is everywhere! Try Annie's organic Worcestershire.)

1 tablespoon (15 g) prepared horseradish

½ teaspoon salt

⅛ teaspoon red pepper flakes

Wraps

3 cups (420 g) shredded cooked chicken or 3 cups (300 g) cooked beans (black-eyed peas, kidney, or pinto all work well)

4 large whole-grain wraps (sprouted wheat, sprouted corn, brown rice, etc.)

2 cups (110 g) shredded lettuce

1 cup (110 g) shredded carrots, optional

½ cup (65 g) chopped dried apricots (unsulfured), optional

Sweet, Speedy, Sinless Barbecue Roll-Ups

From Dr. Jonny: Everyone loves barbecue! But let's face it—it's really not the best dish for health, what with high-heat cooking (carcinogenic compounds form), high-sugar sauces, and factory-farmed meats. So consider the choice—a big old plate of Applebee's ribs (calorie count: ranging from 890 for the smallest portion to, are you sitting down, 1,700 calories!) or this quick, tangy barbecue made with lean chicken or, even better, high-fiber beans! This dish to me is a perfect example of how to take an old favorite comfort food and make it fabulously quick and healthy without sacrificing a drop of flavor. For even greater health impact, check out the low-carb option with a whole bunch of greens. That's a meal that's hard to beat!

Place all the sauce ingredients in a medium saucepan over medium heat and mix well. Cook for 10 minutes, lowering the heat if it sputters too much. After 10 minutes, dress the chicken or beans to your taste with the sauce and mix gently to combine well.

Lay out the wraps on a working surface and place one quarter of the lettuce and carrots on the bottom third of each wrap. Spoon equal parts of the chicken or bean mixture over the veggies and top with a sprinkle of the apricots, if using. Roll from the bottom up and place on the plate, seam side down. Store the remaining barbecue sauce in the fridge.

Yield: 4 wraps and extra sauce

Per Serving: 447 Calories; 7g Fat (13.7% calories from fat); 38g Protein; 57g Carbohydrate; 6g Dietary Fiber; 89mg Cholesterol; 1232mg Sodium

From Chef Jeannette

Low-Carb Tip: For a low-carb version, use lettuce wraps or large stemmed and cooked collard leaves (about 5 minutes in simmering water) in place of the grain wraps. You can also try scooping it onto endive spears or piling it onto a bed of cooked dark or raw salad greens with no wrap at all.

Getting the Most Out of Your Meal: You can easily double the batch of Quick Barbecue Sauce and keep it around for several quick meals. It will keep for three weeks tightly sealed in your refrigerator. Barbecue sauce makes a zippy, easy meal out of plain meats or beans. You can make wraps or salads, or try a barbecue chicken pizza with caramelized onions on a premade whole-grain crust, or even mini pizzas on sourdough English muffins with chopped apples and shredded cheddar.

Superspeed Tip: Skip making the quick BBQ sauce yourself and buy it premade. For overall taste and ingredient quality, our favorite is original Bone Suckin' Sauce.

To Complete the Meal: Add a light green salad with a cool yogurt dressing to the wraps, or a cup of tomato soup to the salad version.

Ingredients

4 large whole-grain tortillas

1½ cups (210 g) shredded or chopped cooked chicken

1 cup (110 g) grated fontina cheese

1 large peach, pitted and sliced thinly (or ripe pear, cored and sliced)

4 tablespoons (64 g) prepared chutney, or to taste

From Chef Jeannette

To Complete the Meal: Serve with a salad of spring greens, grapes, walnuts, and a fruity prepared dressing, such as a pomegranate vinaigrette.

Quickie Chicken-Chutney Quesadillas with Fontina

From Dr. Jonny: Peaches are a "low-glycemic" fruit (glycemic load is only 5 on a scale of 0 to 40+), meaning they won't play havoc with your blood sugar. And one peach contains 3 grams of fiber—that's peachy! This quesadilla is lightning fast because you use prepared chutney. It comes together in a flash, and the sweet spiciness of the chutney balances perfectly with the fontina. You'll never look at fast food quesadillas the same way!

Heat a large dry griddle over medium heat and lay out two of the tortillas. Grill until lightly toasted, about a minute, and flip. Spread one quarter of the chicken over half of each tortilla, and cover with one quarter of the cheese. Lay one quarter of the peaches over the cheese and spread 1½ tablespoons (24 g) chutney over the other half of each tortilla.

Fold the quesadilla closed and grill until hot. Flip it once, if desired, to toast more evenly.

Yield: 4 servings

Per Serving: 452 Calories; 21g Fat (41.8% calories from fat); 22g Protein; 44g Carbohydrate; 3g Dietary Fiber; 90mg Cholesterol; 646mg Sodium

Easy Asian Endive Wraps

Ingredients

1½ tablespoons (25 ml) sesame oil

4 ounces (115 g) presliced shiitake caps, chopped

1 tablespoon (10 g) prepared minced garlic (or 3 large cloves, minced)

1 pound (455 g) leanest ground turkey (or leanest ground beef)

2 tablespoons (28 ml) low-sodium tamari

2½ tablespoons (40 ml) oyster sauce

2 tablespoons (28 ml) mirin (or sake)

1 teaspoon toasted sesame oil

¾ cup (75 g) sliced scallions (greens only)

1½ cups (75 g) mung bean sprouts

2 tablespoons (16 g) toasted sesame seeds, optional

4 heads endive, cored (or use 1 head tender green lettuce leaves, such as Bibb, for a sweeter finish)

From Chef Jeannette

If You've Got 5 More Minutes: Add more low-calorie crunch with 1 stalk of celery, diced fine, and/or one drained 8-ounce (225 g) can of sliced water chestnuts, chopped. Add them at the end of the shiitake sauté time, just before the turkey.

From Dr. Jonny: In Los Angeles, where I live, one of the most perennially popular dishes at virtually all the popular chain restaurants (P.F. Chang's, the Cheesecake Factory, Elephant Bar) is the lettuce wrap. Each restaurant does its own twist on it, but the basic idea is a nice mixture of warm, Asian-spiced meat wrapped up in cool lettuce leaves, often accompanied by a variety of dipping sauces. This is our take on that classic favorite—a calorie-light version that really satisfies and that almost no one will believe you made in 15 minutes! And the ingredients are stellar: shiitake mushrooms, a classic food for building immunity, mixed with a variety of typically Asian white vegetables such as mung bean sprouts and water chestnuts (I recommend you use those!). All complement perfectly the low-fat, high-protein ground turkey. Note: If you want to try a variation, grass-fed beef works well as a substitute for the turkey. Either way, you'll love it.

In a large skillet, heat the oil over medium-high heat. Add the shiitakes and garlic and sauté for 2 minutes. Add the turkey and sauté for about 3 minutes or until almost no pink remains, draining any excess oil if necessary. Stir the tamari, oyster sauce, and mirin into the turkey to incorporate well, and continue to cook until the turkey is completely cooked, about 3 minutes.

Remove from the heat and stir in the sesame oil, scallions, bean sprouts, and sesame seeds, if using.

Divide into four portions and serve with one head endive each. To eat, separate the leaves and use as edible scoops for the turkey.

Yield: 4 servings

Per Serving: 374 Calories; 19g Fat (42.4% calories from fat); 34g Protein; 24g Carbohydrate; 18g Dietary Fiber; 90mg Cholesterol; 598mg Sodium

Ingredients

1 bag (6 ounces or 170 g) chopped romaine
   lettuce
1 smoked turkey breast (³⁄₄ pound [340 g],
   nitrate-free: we like Applegate Farms
   Smoked Turkey Breast), sliced thick
4 hard boiled eggs, peeled and quartered
   lengthwise
1 bag (14 ounces or 400 g) prepared sliced
   green apples, about 4 cups (440 g),
   or 2 apples, sliced
1 cup (115 g) cubed or 4 ounces (115 g) sliced
   cheese, diced, such as Muenster, Colby,
   Gruyère, or Cheddar
2 medium ripe Hass avocados, halved and
   pitted
¹⁄₃ cup (40 g) walnut pieces

Dressing

3 tablespoons (45 ml) walnut oil (or almond
   or olive oil)
1¹⁄₂ tablespoons (25 ml) apple cider vinegar
1 teaspoon honey
1 tablespoon (15 ml) frozen apple juice concentrate, melted
Pinches salt and black pepper

Smoked Turkey-Apple Cobb Salad in Seconds

From Dr. Jonny: Whenever I teach my course for weight-loss coaches or give a seminar for the public on healthy eating and weight management, I talk about the ideal diet: high in protein, healthy fat, and fiber. The Smoked Turkey-Apple Cobb Salad is a textbook example of combining those three ingredients. Protein from the turkey and eggs; healthy fat from the avocados, egg yolks, walnut oil, and cheese; and fiber from the apples and—surprise, surprise, the avocado! (Little-known secret: Avocados are actually high in fiber, providing more than 13 grams per single fruit!) This Cobb salad is particularly good for the heart with its nice complement of apples, walnuts, and turkey. Not to mention that it goes together in a flash and tastes great—fresh, light, and perfect for a summer afternoon.

In a large salad bowl make a bed of the chopped romaine. Roll the turkey slices (double up if sliced thin) and lay across one end of the salad. Lay the egg quarters, if using, out in a row beside the turkey. Lay the apples across the middle of the bowl in a row next to the eggs. Lay the cheese out in a row next to the apples.

Peel the avocado halves (try scooping intact halves out of their skins with a spoon), and slice each half lengthwise into four slices. Lay the slices out in a row next to the cheese.

In a small bowl, whisk together the walnut oil, cider vinegar, honey, apple juice concentrate, salt, and pepper until lightly emulsified. Drizzle the dressing over the salad to taste and sprinkle the salad evenly with the walnut pieces.

Yield: 4 servings
Per Serving: 563 Calories; 42g Fat (64.8% calories from fat); 28g Protein; 23g Carbohydrate; 5g Dietary Fiber; 262mg Cholesterol; 131mg Sodium

From Chef Jeannette

Keep boiled eggs on hand for quick, balanced protein anytime. To boil them in a pan sized to fit their number, cover generously with cold water, cover, set the timer for 15 minutes, and bring to a boil over high heat. Once they are boiling, reduce the heat to medium high and cover partially. When the timer goes off, drain the water and place the eggs in the fridge for later, or, if you want them right away, cover with cold water to cool for peeling.

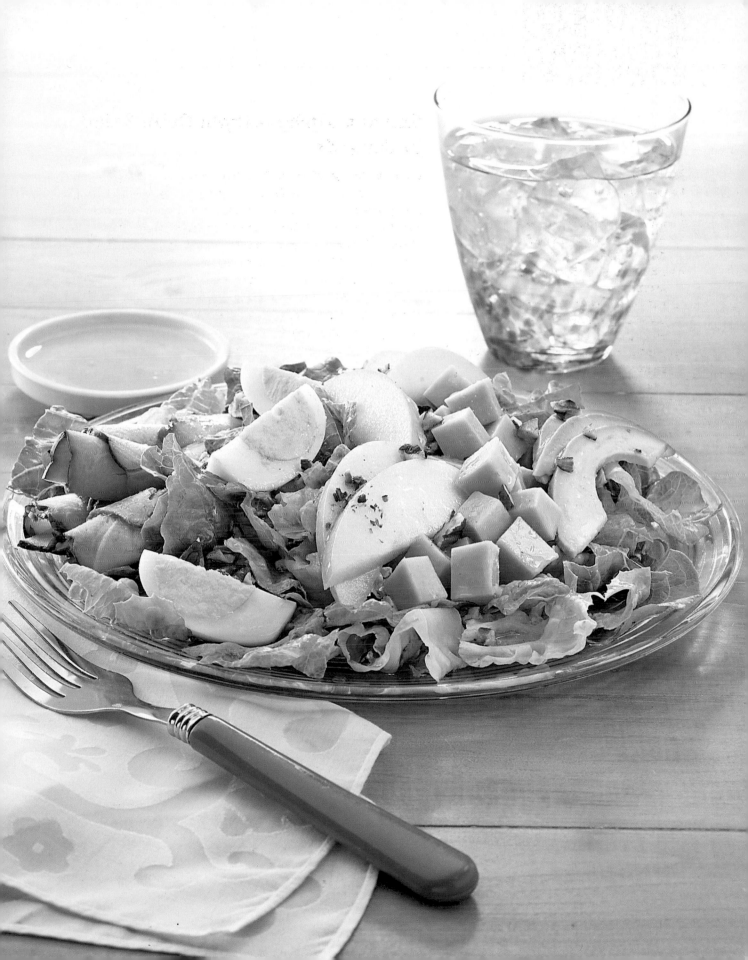

Ingredients

1 cup (160 g) prepared diced onion
    (or 1 small yellow onion, diced)

1 teaspoon prepared minced garlic
    (or 2 large cloves, minced)

8 ounces (225 g) presliced cremini mush-
    rooms, optional

1 pound (455 g) leanest ground turkey

1/2 teaspoon salt

1/4 teaspoon fresh ground pepper

4 cups (950 ml) chicken broth

2 tablespoons (28 ml) red wine vinegar

2 teaspoons dried thyme (or 2 tablespoons
    [4.8 g] chopped fresh)

1/4 teaspoon red pepper flakes, optional

1 can (15 ounces or 425 g) navy beans,
    drained and rinsed

1 bunch Swiss chard, stemmed and chopped

From Chef Jeannette

If You Have 5 Extra Minutes: Top the soup with 1/4 cup (30 g) grated Gruyère cheese for extra calcium and/or 2 tablespoons (18 g) of toasted pine nuts.

One-Pot Pleasure:
Swiss Chard and Turkey Soup

From Dr. Jonny: If you're interested in keeping your weight down, here's a tip for you. Have some soup. Studies by Barbara Rolls at Penn State University have shown that when people eat soup, they tend to eat fewer calories during the meal. Something about the mix of liquid and food eaten together, which, by the way, does not apply when you simply drink water as an accompaniment to solid food. For some reason it has to be actual soup. And this particular soup is a dandy. High in protein and fiber and absolutely loaded with antioxidants from the Swiss chard, this is a simple one-pot meal that's not only completely satisfying but remarkably low in calories.

In a large soup pot, heat the olive oil over medium-high heat. Add the onion, garlic, mushrooms, if using, turkey, salt, and pepper, and sauté for 3 to 5 minutes until the turkey is cooked almost all the way through. Drain any excess fat. Add the broth, vinegar, thyme, red pepper flakes, if using, beans, and chard, and increase the heat to a boil. Reduce the heat, cover, and simmer for about 7 minutes or until the chard is tender.

Yield: 4 servings

Per Serving: 616 Calories; 15g Fat (21.3% calories from fat); 50g Protein; 72g Carbohydrate; 28g Dietary Fiber; 90mg Cholesterol; 1168mg Sodium

Ingredients

½ teaspoon salt

¾ teaspoon curry powder

¼ teaspoon ground cumin

4 turkey cutlets (6 ounces or 170 g each)

1 teaspoon almond or coconut oil

¼ cup (80 g) juice-sweetened apricot spread (we like Polaner's All Fruit with Fiber)

⅓ to ½ cup (80 to 160 ml) prepared orange juice (or fresh squeezed)

½ teaspoon dried ginger

Small pinch ground cardamom, optional

1 teaspoon orange zest, optional

From Chef Jeannette

To Complete the Meal: Serve the glazed cutlets over orange brown rice on a bed of dark salad greens. To make orange brown rice: Prepare 2 cups (330 g) of frozen cooked (or parboiled) brown rice (we like Trader Joe's) according to the package directions, and stir 1 teaspoon butter, ¼ teaspoon salt, 1 tablespoon (15 ml) melted frozen orange juice concentrate, and ¾ teaspoon orange zest into the hot rice until well incorporated. Sprinkle the turkey and rice with a small amount of toasted, sliced almonds, if desired.

Variation Tip: For a reduced-cholesterol, vegetarian version of this dish, substitute four ⅓-inch (0.7 cm) slices of pressed and drained extra-firm tofu for the turkey. Just increase the coconut or almond oil to 1 tablespoon (15 ml) and reduce the heat to medium when you cook the tofu "cutlets." Follow the rest of the directions as indicated.

Ginger-Apricot Turkey Fillets in a Jiffy

From Dr. Jonny: One of the reasons we all love cranberry sauce with our turkey dinner is that turkey just tastes better with a hint of sweet fruit. Chef Jeannette captured the taste of that winning combo perfectly by creatively substituting apricots and oranges for the usual cranberry fare, and then adding a taste of ginger to the mix. The resultant sauce is simply divine, a perfect accompaniment to this healthy, low-fat source of protein, and proof positive that turkey doesn't have to be just for holidays. In addition to vitamin C, oranges contain both calcium and 3.4 grams of fiber. The taste of this dish is warm and sweet with an exotic hint of Indian spices from the curry and cumin. Note: These fillets travel well; take a couple in a lunchbox or wrap one in a big lettuce leaf for a delicious, flavorful low-carb "sandwich."

In a small cup, mix together the salt, curry powder, and cumin, and sprinkle evenly over the turkey cutlets with your fingers, rubbing to distribute if necessary. Heat the oil in a large skillet over medium-high heat. Add the turkey cutlets in a single layer and cook for 1 to 3 minutes per side or until just cooked through. Remove the turkey cutlets, set aside, and reduce the heat to medium.

Add the jam, orange juice, ginger, and cardamom, if using, and whisk together, deglazing the pan for 1 to 2 minutes or until smooth, stirring in any juices produced by the resting turkey cutlets. Stir in the zest, if using, and spoon over the warm fillets.

Yield: 4 servings

Per Serving: 286 Calories; 12g Fat (39.0% calories from fat); 28g Protein; 15g Carbohydrate; trace Dietary Fiber; 91mg Cholesterol; 355mg Sodium

Terrific Teriyaki Turkey and Glass Noodles in No Time

From Dr. Jonny: You can use either ground beef or turkey for this recipe, but choose grass-fed beef or organic turkey! Both taste great and go beautifully with the light glass noodles, flavored with ginger and garlic and sweetened with maple syrup. This delicious dish satisfies on so many levels. The clear glass noodles give you something to chew on without knocking your blood sugar through the roof. The beef (or turkey) mixed with edamame beans gives you a ton of protein; the garlic, red peppers, and ginger inject just the right degree of spice; and just for good measure, the carrots provide a rich helping of vitamin A, potassium, beta-carotene, and the eye-supporting nutrients lutein and zeaxanthin. Strongly recommended: Follow Chef's Jeannette's advice and pair with her mineral-rich salad for the perfect meal!

Ingredients

4 ounces (115 g) glass noodles (also called cellophane noodles or clear bean threads)*

1 pound (455 g) lean ground turkey (or leanest ground beef)

2 teaspoons prepared garlic (or 4 cloves, minced)

1 cup (110 g) prepared shredded carrots (or prepared diced red peppers)

¼ cup (60 ml) low-salt tamari

2 tablespoons (28 ml) sherry

2 tablespoons (40 g) maple syrup

2 tablespoons (28 ml) water

1½ teaspoons ground ginger (or 1½ tablespoons [9 g] prepared minced ginger)

¼ teaspoon red pepper flakes, or to taste, optional

2 cups (236 g) shelled, precooked edamame beans (prepared fresh or frozen, thawed)

Prepare the bean threads according to the package directions (usually soaking for 5 minutes in water that's been boiled and removed from the heat, then draining and rinsing).

While the bean threads are soaking, place the turkey, garlic, and carrots, breaking up the meat to mix, in a large nonstick skillet over medium-high heat. Cook, stirring frequently, for 4 to 6 minutes until the pink is almost gone from the meat. Drain any excess fat.

While the meat is cooking, in a small bowl, whisk together the tamari, sherry, syrup, water, ground ginger, and red pepper flakes, if using. Pour the sauce over the meat and increase the heat to bring to a simmer. When the meat is cooked through and no pink remains (1 to 2 minutes), stir in the edamame and remove from the heat. Toss with the prepared glass noodles to serve.

Yield: 4 servings

Per Serving: 388 Calories; 11g Fat (26.8% calories from fat); 26g Protein; 42g Carbohydrate; 3g Dietary Fiber; 90mg Cholesterol; 1271mg Sodium

*Look for bean threads in Asian markets or the ethnic sections of natural grocers.

From Chef Jeannette

To Complete the Meal: Add a cucumber salad garnished with a few tablespoons of soaked hijiki and dressed with a simple vinaigrette of equal parts rice vinegar, tamari, and sesame oil. Hijiki is an alkalizing, brown sea vegetable that's rich in minerals, especially calcium. Look for it (dried) in Asian markets or the macrobiotic section of natural food stores. You can also use arame, its milder cousin.

If You Have 5 Extra Minutes: To boost the nutrients even more, add 1 cup of frozen corn when you add the sauce and garnish with 1½ tablespoons (12 g) of toasted sesame seeds.

A Healthier Sandwich: Turkey-Apple De-Light

From Dr. Jonny: Okay, I'll be the first to admit I'm not a huge fan of the sandwich as a go-to meal. Why? Because your basic deli sandwich uses junky, low-quality, high-carb bread and meats that are filled with nitrate and sodium, not to mention sauces loaded with sugar. But there's no doubt that a sandwich can make an excellent quick (and healthy!) meal, providing you build it with the right materials. We use sprouted-grain wraps and pockets, but you can also use whole-grain options. Sprouted grains retain their natural plant enzymes, which are beneficial for digestion and are also nutrient rich. Some argue that the nutrients in sprouted-grain breads are easier to absorb, but others argue that the effect is minor. No matter. Sprouted, and whole-grain, wraps are preferable to the bulky rolls made with refined white flour that come with the average deli sandwich. Whole grains are fine, but make sure the first ingredient is whole-wheat or whole oats, and look for at least 2 grams of fiber per slice, preferably 3. Turkey is a great source of protein (as is Cheddar cheese), and the apples add phytochemicals, fiber, and a crunchy sweet taste that perfectly complements the meat.

Ingredients

1 teaspoon honey mustard

1 sprouted-grain wrap (8 inches or 20 cm diameter)

2 ounces (55 g) sliced turkey breast (also tastes great with smoked!)

½ crisp apple (Granny Smith or Honeycrisp work well), unpeeled, cored, and sliced thin (or buy prepared sliced in the refrigerator section)

1 ounce (28 g) grated or sliced Cheddar cheese

Spread the honey mustard evenly over one side of the wrap and place it in a dry skillet over medium heat, mustard side up. Toast the wrap for 1 minute. Layer the turkey and apple evenly over one half of the wrap, leaving a ½-inch (1 cm) edge. Sprinkle or lay the cheese evenly over the apple and fold the wrap in half, pressing down with a large spatula to "glue" the sandwich together. Once the bottom half of the wrap is a golden brown, carefully flip it, pressing down evenly again, and allow the other side to toast.

When the cheese is melted and the sandwich is toasted on both sides, it's ready to serve.

Yield: 1 sandwich

Per Serving: 386 Calories; 17g Fat (39.0% calories from fat); 24g Protein; 35g Carbohydrate; 7g Dietary Fiber; 62mg Cholesterol; 411mg Sodium

Ingredients

1 pound (455 g) low-fat ground turkey

1 small apple, peeled, cored, and grated

½ cup (120 ml) chicken broth (or apple cider or water)

1 teaspoon ground coriander

½ teaspoon ground ginger

½ teaspoon ground fennel

½ teaspoon ground nutmeg

½ teaspoon ground thyme

¼ teaspoon dried basil

½ teaspoon salt

¼ teaspoon black pepper

¼ teaspoon cayenne pepper

From Chef Jeannette

To Complete the Meal: These patties make a balancing, high-protein accompaniment to many of the typical quick, higher-carb breakfast options that aren't great for your blood sugar level on their own. While the patties cook, prepare a bowl of quick-cooking oatmeal, muesli, or high-protein granola to complete a balanced breakfast. I like this sausage with a bowl of fresh mixed fruit, especially in the summertime.

If You Have 10 More Minutes: Let the mixture rest in the fridge for 10 minutes or so before sautéing to give the flavors more time to develop and combine.

Slimming, Sweet, and Savory Turkey-Apple Sausage

From Dr. Jonny: This is a great no-grease answer to a sausage craving, and it's especially good at breakfast. Low-fat ground turkey takes the place of factory-farmed pork, the apple gives it a terrific sweetness (not to mention an infusion of nutrients such as vitamin C), a plethora of great spices such as thyme and basil give it a nice mouthfeel, and best of all it's got zero additives (translation: no nitrates!). Low cal and low sugar, this is one sausage you can enjoy without having to worry about how it was made!

In a large mixing bowl, combine all the ingredients and mix with your hands until well combined. Form into eight thin patties. Spray a griddle or large skillet lightly with olive oil and heat over medium heat. Cook the patties for about 4 minutes per side or until cooked through.

Yield: 4 servings

Per Serving: 175 Calories; 8g Fat (40.6% calories from fat); 19g Protein; 6g Carbohydrate; 1g Dietary Fiber; 61mg Cholesterol; 422mg Sodium

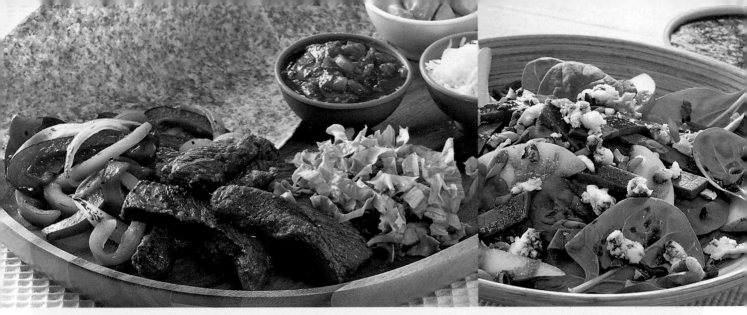

Meat

Meat is beginning to lose its undeserved reputation as a "bad" food; but, there's an important "but"—make sure it's not the processed kind. Recent research shows that health issues with meat have more to do with the processing, sodium, and nitrates than with the meat itself. To avoid eating meat that contains hormones, steroids, and antibiotics, choose grass-fed meat whenever possible.

Gorgonzola Beef with Spinach, Super-Fast

Body-Building Broiled Steak with Mushrooms

Healthy Peanut-Hoisin Beef and Bean Sprouts in Seconds

Iron-Rich Blackstrap Balsamic Steak

Quick-Sizzle Beef Satay Shish Kebab

Cheater Fajiters

Game Time Five-Layer Salad, Lightened

15-Minute Middle Eastern Lamb Chops

Protein Powerhouse Lamb with Figs in a Flash

Luscious Moroccan Lamb Burgers in Less Time

Easy Grilled Lamb Chops Dijon

Gorgonzola Beef with Spinach, Super-Fast

Ingredients

2 tablespoons (28 ml) pear or orange vinegar (we like Cuisine Perel's D'Anjou Pear
Vinegar or Trader Joe's Orange Muscat
Champagne Vinegar, or substitute balsamic)

2 teaspoons Dijon mustard

1 to 2 teaspoons honey, to taste

⅛ teaspoon fresh ground black pepper

2 tablespoons (28 ml) walnut oil

6 cups (180 g) baby spinach

10 ounces (280 g) sliced low-sodium roast
beef, deli style, diagonally sliced

2 ounces (55 g) Gorgonzola cheese, finely
crumbled

½ cup (50 g) sliced scallions

2 small ripe pears (red Anjou or Bosc work
well), cored and sliced

¼ cup (30 g) toasted walnut pieces

From Dr. Jonny: A cursory glance through this book reveals that we have only one red-meat dish in our no-cook section, for obvious reasons. If you want red meat and no-cook together, you're going to have to use deli meats, which, honestly, we're not huge fans of. But truth be told, it's fine to use them occasionally as long as you choose an organic, and nitrate-free, variety. Chef Jeannette also suggests they be low sodium, which I wholly endorse, as most of the excess sodium in our diet doesn't come from the saltshaker but from processed foods (such as canned foods and deli meats). Dump the nitrates and lower the sodium, opt for organic, and you're good to go. Spinach, Gorgonzola, and pears have become the new trifecta for perfect salads—they mix and match tastes and textures in a way that is just short of heavenly. Add the protein from the—did I happen to mention nitrate-free?—beef, and the fiber, minerals, and omega-3s from the walnuts, and you've got a flavorful, fruity, easy, no-cook meal!

In a small bowl, whisk together the vinegar, mustard, honey, pepper, and walnut oil.

In a large salad bowl, make a bed of spinach and top with the beef, Gorgonzola, scallions, and pears. Dress to taste and garnish with the walnuts.

Yield: 4 servings
Per Serving: 382 Calories; 24g Fat (53.7% calories from fat); 26g Protein; 20g Carbohydrate; 4g Dietary Fiber; 68mg Cholesterol; 305mg Sodium

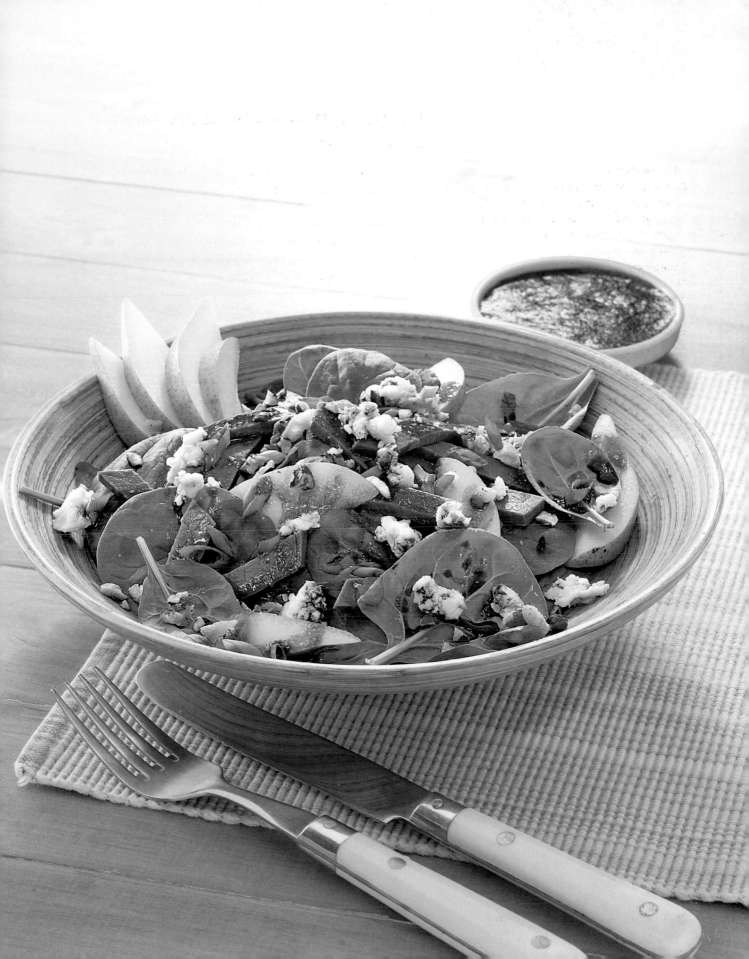

Body-Building Broiled Steak with Mushrooms

From Dr. Jonny: When people come up to me at book signings, workshops, and lectures, they frequently ask me whether I'm a vegetarian, as if being healthy is synonymous with a vegetarian lifestyle. They're often surprised (and often delighted!) to find that I'm not. It's absolutely possible, even desirable, to include animal products in our diet, as long as they're the right kind of animal products (see Nutritional Note opposite). And as long as those animal products are balanced with plenty of vegetables and fiber. So for you beef eaters, here's a terrific dish that's quick and easy. Steak goes beautifully with mushrooms, which are among the most healing foods on the planet. Even the common white button mushroom has a ton of potassium (a cup of sliced mushrooms beats the pants off a banana on the potassium scale), not to mention 18 mcg of selenium, an important mineral that is a powerful antioxidant and also has anticancer activity. And watercress (in the suggested side), despite the fact that it has almost no calories, is packed with vitamin A and two superstar nutrients for eye health, lutein and zeaxanthin. This dish comes together quickly and tastes as good as beef can taste!

Ingredients

1 sirloin steak (1 to 1½ pounds [455 to 710 g], 1-inch thickness)
½ teaspoon salt + 1 pinch more
½ teaspoon black pepper
1 tablespoon (15 ml) olive oil
2 teaspoons butter
2 shallots, chopped
8 ounces (225 g) sliced mushrooms (white, button, cremini, and shiitake all work well)
1 tablespoon (2.4 g) minced fresh thyme (or ¾ teaspoon dried)

Preheat the broiler and lightly oil a broiler pan. Set aside.

Pat the steak dry and season lightly with ½ teaspoon salt and pepper on both sides. Broil the steak 3 to 4 inches (7.5 to 20 cm) from the heating element for 4 to 5 minutes and turn. Broil for 4 to 5 minutes more for medium rare. Remove from the heat and tent with foil to keep warm until the mushrooms are ready.

Heat the oil and butter in a large sauté pan over medium heat. Add the shallots, mushrooms, and pinch of salt, and sauté for 3 to 5 minutes until the mushrooms are just tender.

Stir in the thyme and sauté for 1 more minute or until the mushrooms reach desired tenderness. Remove from the heat.

Spoon the mushrooms over the steak and serve.

Yield: 4 servings
Per Serving: 298 Calories; 21g Fat (64.3% calories from fat); 22g Protein; 4g Carbohydrate; 1g Dietary Fiber; 76mg Cholesterol; 381mg Sodium

From Chef Jeannette

To Complete the Meal: Slice the steak into thick strips and serve over dressed greens. Dress watercress (2 large bunches) or baby arugula (4 cups or 80 g) with 2 tablespoons (28 ml) of olive oil, 1 tablespoon (15 ml) of red wine vinegar, a teaspoon of mustard, and pinches of salt and fresh ground pepper, to taste.

The Goodness of Grass-Fed Beef

I've been an outspoken advocate for grass-fed beef almost from the day I became a nutritionist. (I wrote about it at length in my previous books). Yes, it's expensive, but here's why it's totally worth it: Factory-farmed meat, the kind you get in most supermarkets and at all fast-food places, is filled with antibiotics, steroids, and hormones.

In addition, feedlot-farmed meat is fed nothing but grain, which is the most unnatural food in the world for cows. It makes them sick, which is one of the reasons they have to be fed copious doses of antibiotics. Grain-feeding—even organic grain—changes the quality of the animals' fat. Grain-fed meat from feedlot farms is high in inflammatory omega-6 fats and has almost no omega-3 fats.

A quick look at the documentary film *Food, Inc.* will show you all you need to know about how the animals on feedlot farms are treated and the conditions under which they're raised, which is enough to turn you off meat completely—but remember, that documentary is about animals on feedlot farms. Animals raised on pasture, in addition to having far more tranquil and happy lives, eat their natural diet of grass. Studies show that grass-fed meat has much higher amounts of the highly beneficial, anti-inflammatory omega-3 fats, as well as a particular kind of cancer-fighting fat called CLA (conjugated linolenic acid), which is conspicuously absent from the meat of feedlot-farmed animals.

Nearly all farms that raise grass-fed meat are concerned about the health and welfare of their animals, and the farmers rarely if ever use chemicals, steroids, or antibiotics. The bottom line is that it costs a lot more to raise grass-fed meat, but you are getting a healthy food as opposed to the junk that has been associated with higher rates of cancer and disease. If you can't find grass-fed meat in your local store, you can order online and get the best quality shipped to your door. Two sources I recommend highly are U.S. Wellness Meats (which you can find through a link on my website, www.jonnybowden .com, under Online Store/Healthy Foods) or the wonderful Novy Ranches (www.novyranches.com), owned by a health-conscious veterinarian named Lowell Novy, who raises grass-fed Angus beef that tastes amazing—rich, flavorful, juicy, and decidedly more healthy for you than "commercial" meat. I'd rather eat one serving of (admittedly more expensive) grass-fed meat once a week than seven burgers from a fast-food restaurant, and that's exactly what I do. I recommend you do the same.

Healthy Peanut-Hoisin Beef and Bean Sprouts in Seconds

Ingredients

2 teaspoons peanut oil, divided
1 boneless top sirloin or flank steak (1 to 1¼
    pounds [455 to 567 g]), fat trimmed and
    cut into ¼-inch (0.5 cm)-thick slices,
    2 to 3 inches (5 to 7.5 cm) long
Salt and fresh ground black pepper
1½ tablespoons [9 g] prepared minced
    ginger
1 teaspoon prepared garlic
2½ tablespoons hoisin sauce
2½ tablespoons (40 ml) low-sodium tamari
3 cups (150 g) mung bean sprouts (or
    prepared cabbage and carrot slaw mix)
2 tablespoons (18 g) crushed roasted
    peanuts (or ¼ cup [35 g] whole,
    to save time)

From Chef Jeannette

To Complete the Meal: Serve with Thai
cucumber salad. Using a mandoline or
food processor, julienne or shred 1 small
peeled English cucumber. Dress with
2 tablespoons (28 ml) of unseasoned rice
vinegar or fresh lime juice, 1 teaspoon
of Sucanat, 2 teaspoons of low-sodium
tamari, 1 teaspoon of toasted sesame
oil, 1 teaspoon of Thai sweet chili sauce
(optional), ½ cup (50 g) of sliced
scallions, and 2 tablespoons (18 g) of
crushed peanuts. Optional addition: ¼
cup (4 g) of chopped fresh cilantro.

From Dr. Jonny: Sprouts got a touchy-feely reputation when they became associated with all of us "granola-eating, tree-hugging" types who used to be called—amazingly—health nuts. (Now the tides have shifted, and those who don't care about their health could reasonably be called "nuts"!) Anyway, bean sprouts (or mung bean sprouts) contain a plethora of plant chemicals known to be valuable for health. Saponins, for example, protect plants against disease, bacteria, and predators and offer a similar kind of protection to your cells. Sprouts combine beautifully with a high-protein dish such as steak. The juicy lightness of the plump, water-based sprouts mixed with the slightly sweet hoisin sauce creates the deliciously satisfying feel of Asian food with a light touch. Highly recommended: Make the Thai cucumber salad at the end to perfectly round off the meal's flavors!

In a large skillet, heat 1 teaspoon of the oil over medium-high heat for 1 minute. Add the steak strips, season lightly with salt and pepper, and sauté, turning frequently, for 3 to 5 minutes or until cooked to desired doneness. Remove the steak and set aside.

Drain the pan and lower the heat to medium. Add the remaining teaspoon of oil, ginger, and garlic and sauté for 1 minute. Stir in the hoisin and tamari sauces and cook for 1 minute. Add the steak to the pan and cook for 1 minute. Serve the steak and sauce over the mung bean sprouts (or slaw mix) garnished with the peanuts.

Yield: 4 servings
Per Serving: 254 Calories; 12g Fat (38.3% calories from fat); 33g Protein; 9g Carbohydrate; 2g Dietary Fiber; 66mg Cholesterol; 609mg Sodium

Iron-Rich Blackstrap Balsamic Steak

Ingredients

1 sirloin steak (12 to 14 ounces [340 to 400 g], 1 to 1½ inches [2.5 to 3.5 cm] thick), trimmed

Salt and fresh ground black pepper

2 tablespoons (40 g) blackstrap molasses

2 tablespoons (28 ml) balsamic vinegar

Pinch dried thyme

Pinch ground nutmeg

From Chef Jeannette

To Complete the Meal: Slice the steak into thick strips and serve it over a chunky salad. Combine 4 cups (120 g) of baby spinach (or chopped red lettuce), four quartered plum tomatoes, half a red onion sliced into rings, and chunky slices of peeled cucumber to make a bed for the steak.

If You Have 10 More Minutes: Slice a whole yellow onion into rings and sauté until soft in 1 tablespoon (15 ml) of olive oil with pinches of salt and pepper over medium heat (cooked onion will replace the raw red onion in the suggested side).

From Dr. Jonny: Once you taste what blackstrap molasses does to food, you'll want to find more ways to use this healthy sweetener. Molasses is actually the byproduct of sugar refining. It contains all of the nutrients found in the raw sugarcane plant, which are completely lost in processed white sugar. Blackstrap molasses, though still technically a sweetener, actually has a fairly high amount of nutrients. You might even call it the anti-sugar. A good source of iron, calcium, magnesium, potassium, manganese, and copper, it makes a sweet glaze, which Chef Jeannette used to liven up this simple steak. Note: Pan-frying is a simple way to get some good lean protein on your plate and save some grill-heating time. (And beef is still, after all, one of the best sources of absorbable iron in the diet, with each serving of steak providing 3 or 4 milligrams' worth.) Don't forget to choose high-quality beef!

Season the sirloin with salt and pepper to taste.

Spray a large skillet (or grill pan) with olive oil to lightly coat. Heat the pan over medium-high heat (the pan is ready when you touch a fatty edge of the steak to the center and it sizzles quickly). Lay the sirloin in the pan and cook for 4 to 6 minutes per side for medium rare, slicing the steak open to check for desired doneness.

When the steak is finished, remove from the pan and reduce heat to low.

Add molasses, vinegar, thyme, and nutmeg to the cooled pan and stir quickly for a minute or so until hot. Drizzle it lightly over the steak to serve.

Yield: 4 servings

Per Serving: 197 Calories; 12g Fat (54.2% calories from fat); 16g Protein; 7g Carbohydrate; 0g Dietary Fiber; 53mg Cholesterol; 49mg Sodium

Quick-Sizzle Beef Satay Shish Kebab

From Dr. Jonny: Satay is a type of shish kebab dish that is wildly popular in Indonesia and Thailand. Usually it's associated with Thai food and made of cubes of meat (beef, chicken, lamb), which are usually dipped in a traditional peanut sauce. Delish. Shish kebab in general is actually a quick and healthy way to grill both meats and veggies and is adaptable to the seasons. Just skewer whatever's in season and grill 'em up. This version uses lean beef (please buy grass-fed if at all possible) and nutrient-rich zucchini, mushrooms, and cherry tomatoes, all of which lend themselves to skewering quite well. If you're feeling adventurous and ambitious, try whipping up your own peanut sauce or buy ready-made. (If you do make your own peanut sauce, why not use peanut butter that comes right out of the grinder? You can get that at a lot of supermarkets these days, and it has zero trans fats and zero added sugar, something that's not always true of commercial peanut butters.) If not, no worries—the dish tastes fabulous either way. The minced garlic adds a nice touch—don't forget to check out the Nutritional Note about it!

Ingredients

Beef Satay

2 shallots, peeled

¼ cup (4 g) coarsely chopped fresh cilantro

1 tablespoon (6 g) prepared minced ginger (or chopped fresh)

1 teaspoon prepared minced garlic (or 2 cloves, crushed and chopped)

1 tablespoon (15 ml) low-sodium tamari

1 tablespoon (15 ml) peanut oil

1 pound (455 g) sirloin steak, cut into 1 × ½-inch (2.5 × 1 cm) slices

High-heat cooking oil spray

Veggies

2 teaspoons olive oil

Salt and fresh ground black pepper, to taste

12 cherry tomatoes

1 small zucchini, stemmed and cut into 8 equal-sized chunks

8 white mushrooms, whole if small or halved if large (zucchini and mushroom should be about the same size)

From Chef Jeannette

If You Have 30 More Minutes: Let the beef marinate in the paste for a richer flavor.

Preheat the grill to medium heat.*

Using an immersion blender or food processor, process the shallots, cilantro, ginger, garlic, tamari, and peanut oil into a moist paste, adding a teaspoon or two of water to thin slightly, if necessary. Toss the beef strips in the paste, coating well, and set aside.

In a large bowl, combine the olive oil, salt, pepper, tomatoes, zucchini, and mushrooms, and toss gently to coat. Thread alternating zucchini chunks and mushrooms onto one metal skewer and place on the grill for 7 to 10 minutes or until softened, turning once or twice.

Thread the meat (scraping off the excessive paste) evenly onto two metal skewers, spacing the pieces apart, lightly spray the grill with high-heat cooking oil spray, and place the skewers on the grill for 6 to 7 minutes for medium rare or to desired doneness, turning once or twice.

Thread the tomatoes onto one skewer and place on the grill for 3 to 4 minutes or until soft, but not falling off the skewer. Divide all the skewers into four equal portions and serve.

Yield: 4 servings

Per Serving: 319 Calories; 22g Fat (59.6% calories from fat); 26g Protein; 7g Carbohydrate; 2g Dietary Fiber; 71mg Cholesterol; 221mg Sodium

*These can be broiled as well if you don't have a grill. Keep them about 6 inches (15 cm) from the heating element.

Garlic: The Secret Is in the Allicin

The key to the astonishingly wide range of health benefits in garlic—documented in more than 1,200 published studies—is a compound called *allicin*. But this is the good part: Allicin isn't actually in garlic.

So here's a brain teaser for you: If allicin is the key to garlic's benefits, and it isn't technically in garlic, what's the connection?

Here's the answer. Garlic cloves contain an amino acid called *allin*. They also contain an enzyme called *allinase*. Allin and allinase live in completely different compartments in the garlic plant, much like Siamese fighting fish have to be kept in separate parts of a fish tank. When you crush garlic, it's like lifting the barrier between the Siamese fighting fish. The enzyme allinase reacts with the amino acid allin, and presto bingo, the interaction produces allicin!

Mystery solved.

Now the reason this is important to cooks is this: How you prepare garlic is critical. It's got to be chopped, crushed, or otherwise broken up in some way (the finer, the better) so that those two components—allin and allinase—get to interact. (If you were to swallow a whole clove of garlic on a dare, you would probably not get the full health benefits of this terrific edible herb.)

Allicin starts to degrade shortly after it's produced, so the fresher the garlic is when you use it, the better. Garlic experts advise crushing a little raw garlic and combining it with the cooked food shortly before serving.

Full disclosure: We used prepared minced garlic in many places in this book, but we did it to save time. It was a tradeoff. Crushing it fresh may take a bit longer, but it has way more nutritional impact.

If you'd like to read a more thorough discussion of the health benefits of garlic and the research that supports those benefits, please check out the subject in my book *The 150 Healthiest Foods on Earth*.

Ingredients

³/₄ teaspoon chili powder

¹/₂ teaspoon ground cumin

¹/₂ teaspoon dried oregano

¹/₂ teaspoon salt

¹/₄ teaspoon cracked black pepper

1¹/₄ pounds (567 g) beef tenderloin, top
   sirloin, or top round, trimmed and thinly
   sliced across the grain (¹/₄ × 1-inch
   [0.5 × 2.5 cm] strips)

1 tablespoon (25 ml) peanut oil

2 cups (320 g) prepared sliced onions and
   bell peppers (in the refrigerated section
   or frozen, thawed)

2 tablespoons (28 ml) fresh-squeezed lime
   juice

1 tablespoon (15 ml) low-sodium tamari

8 small whole-grain or sprouted wraps
   or tortillas (about 6 inches [15 cm]
   in diameter)

From Chef Jeannette

To Complete the Meal: Serve the fajitas
with prepared salsa, shredded lettuce,
chopped avocado, and/or shredded Jack
cheese, to taste.

Superspeed Tip: In a pinch, save time by
substituting a premade fajita seasoning
pack for the homemade seasonings. Just
make sure it's 100 percent natural, low
sodium, and sugar free! We like Simply
Organic Fajita Seasonings.

Cheater Fajiters

From Dr. Jonny: When I first arrived in Southern California ten years
ago, I did not know the difference between a taco, a fajita, and a bur-
rito. Considering there are more Mexican restaurants per square foot
here than anywhere else I know north of the border, this was a serious
cultural drawback. It didn't last long—with fabulous Mexican food everywhere I came to love the fajita, but the challenge is to come up with
one that isn't 2,500 calories! Interested? Look no further. You've got
your lean beef; tons of low-calorie, high-nutrient peppers and onions;
a whole-grain sprouted wrap; and a taste of Tex-Mex inspired by
Los Angeles!

In a medium bowl, mix the chili powder, cumin, oregano, salt, and pepper.
Toss the sliced beef with the spices to coat. Heat the oil in a Dutch oven
over medium-high heat. Add the beef, onions, and peppers, and cook until
the meat has reached desired doneness and onions and peppers are soft,
5 to 7 minutes. Stir in the lime juice and tamari for the last minute of cook
time. Serve one quarter of the hot meat and two wraps per serving with the
optional condiments, if using.

Yield: 4 servings

Per Serving: 562 Calories; 19g Fat (29.8% calories from fat); 44g Protein;
56g Carbohydrate; 12g Dietary Fiber; 82mg Cholesterol; 786mg Sodium

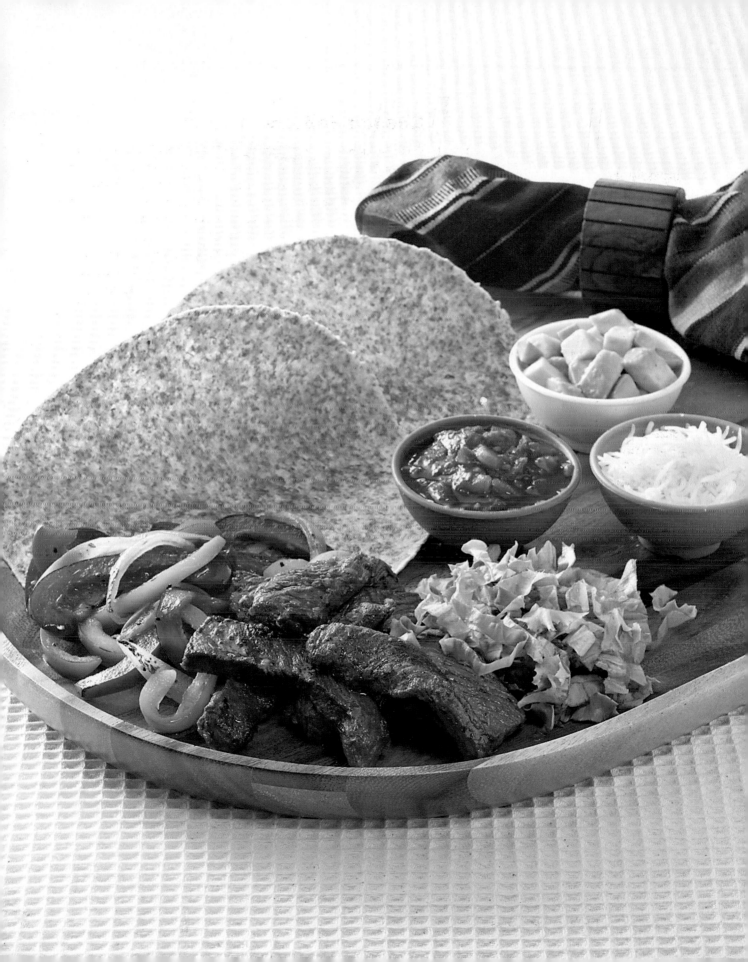

Game Time Five-Layer Salad, Lightened

Ingredients

1 pound (455 g) leanest ground beef or turkey

½ teaspoon salt

¼ teaspoon ground black pepper

1 tablespoon (15 ml) lime juice (preferably fresh squeezed)

1 jar (16 ounces or 455 g) spicy salsa

¼ cup (4 g) chopped fresh cilantro, optional

4 cups (220 g) chopped lettuce

2 large heirloom tomatoes, chopped

1 avocado, peeled, pitted, and sliced

½ lime, optional

1 can (15 ounces or 425 g) beans (kidney, black, or pinto), drained and rinsed

½ cup (58 g) prepared grated Jack cheese

¼ cup (35 g) toasted pepitas, optional

From Dr. Jonny: For most of my life I have managed to resist the appeal of spectator sports (except for tennis), but I recently succumbed to Laker fever in Los Angeles and am now a confirmed fan. Which means I, like just about everyone else in America, apparently, need to find myself some game-night food. But I'd like to find some that won't bankrupt my health. Enter the five-layer salad. These layered Mexi-salads are fun to fix and serve and are a great compromise for game-night food. There's a ton of volume and taste in this salad, but it's way light on calories. Unlike any other typical television snack food, this nibbly salad has protein, tons of fiber, and high-antioxidant veggies. And you won't have to apologize for serving "healthy" food once the Laker fans start digging in.

Place the ground meat in a large skillet over medium-high heat and stir in the salt and pepper. Cook, stirring frequently to break up the meat, for 5 to 7 minutes or until completely cooked, no pink remaining. Remove from the heat, drain any excess fat, and stir in the lime juice, salsa, and cilantro, if using.

While the meat is cooking, arrange the salad in a large salad bowl (clear glass if possible, to see the pretty layers!): lettuce, tomatoes, and avocado. Squeeze the lime juice over the avocado, if using (this tastes great and will also help prevent it from browning). Layer the avocado with the beans, and top with the hot ground meat. Sprinkle the cheese over all and garnish with the pepitas, if using.

Yield: 4 servings

Per Serving: 605 Calories; 37g Fat (54.5% calories from fat); 34g Protein; 36g Carbohydrate; 12g Dietary Fiber; 98mg Cholesterol; 1298mg Sodium

Ingredients

Orange Carrots

1 tablespoon (14 g) butter

1/2 cup (235 ml) orange juice (preferably fresh squeezed)

1 teaspoon orange zest, optional

1/4 teaspoon salt

1/4 teaspoon ground allspice or ginger, optional

2 cups (220 g) prepared grated carrots

Lamb Chops

1/2 teaspoon ground cumin

1/2 teaspoon sweet paprika

1/2 teaspoon ground coriander

1/4 teaspoon ground cinnamon

1/2 teaspoon salt

1/2 teaspoon cracked black pepper

8 loin lamb chops

1/3 cup (5 g) chopped fresh cilantro, optional, for garnish

From Chef Jeannette

Using dry rubs is a healthy way to add a lot of flavor to meats without adding a lot of calories. Purchase a few high-quality prepared dry-rub combos you like to keep on hand. With a selection of great rubs and a grill (or broiler), you can prepare a variety of lean cuts of meat in minutes.

If You Have 15 Extra Minutes: Make your own rub from whole spices for more nutrient and flavor impact. Try toasting equal amounts of whole cumin seeds and peppercorns with a couple of allspice berries in a dry skillet for 3 to 5 minutes until they are fragrant. Grind them to a powder and mix with an equal part of sweet paprika and a half part of ground cinnamon. Tightly sealed in a glass jar, this will keep for months, though potency reduces over time.

15-Minute Middle Eastern Lamb Chops

From Dr. Jonny: Some of the things that make lamb such a good food source can't be seen by just reading the nutrition facts labels. The U.S. Department of Agriculture database will tell you, for example, that a single lamb chop has only a couple of hundred calories, 16 grams of protein, about half the potassium of a banana, and about 18 mg of selenium, an important mineral that happens to be associated with lower rates of cancer. But what the database won't tell you is that lamb is rarely if ever factory farmed, that Australian and New Zealand lamb is always grass fed, and that lamb meat rarely if ever comes with a side helping of antibiotics, steroids, and hormones, the way factory-farmed meat does. In this hearty offering, the spicy chops are perfectly complemented by orange carrots, all pulled together nicely by the crisp bite of fresh cilantro.

Preheat the grill to medium heat.

Melt the butter in a large skillet over medium heat. Stir in the orange juice, zest, if using, salt, allspice, if using, and carrots. Cover and cook, stirring occasionally, for 5 to 7 minutes or until tender-crisp.

While the carrots are cooking, in a small bowl, combine the cumin, paprika, coriander, cinnamon, salt, and pepper. Sprinkle evenly over the lamb chops and gently rub in. Lightly spray the grill with olive oil and grill the chops for 4 minutes, flip, and grill for about 4 minutes more for medium rare or to desired doneness. Serve two lamb chops with one quarter of the cooked carrots and garnish all with the cilantro, if using.

Yield: 4 servings

Per Serving: 670 Calories; 54g Fat (72.8% calories from fat); 32g Protein; 13g Carbohydrate; 2g Dietary Fiber; 148mg Cholesterol; 423mg Sodium

Protein Powerhouse Lamb with Figs in a Flash

Ingredients

1¼ pounds (567 g) thin, boneless lamb loin medallions (have the butcher cut the meat from the bone of loin chops to save time, or slice lean lamb fillets)

Salt and fresh ground black pepper

1 tablespoon (15 ml) macadamia nut oil (or other neutral high-heat oil)

¼ cup (80 g) black fig preserves (or 3 table-spoons [60 g] fig jam)

½ cup (235 ml) red wine

4 cups (120 g) baby spinach

¼ cup crumbled (30 g) blue cheese (or chèvre or feta), or more, to taste

2 tablespoons (220 g) toasted slivered almonds, optional

From Chef Jeannette

To Complete the Meal: Serve with whole wheat couscous and sweet peas. Bring 1 cup (235 ml) of water or broth to a boil. Add ½ cup (75 g) of baby sweet peas for the last minute of cook time. Reduce the heat to low, stir in just under 1 cup (175 g) of whole wheat couscous, and cook for 1 minute or until most of the liquid is absorbed. Season to taste with salt and freshly ground pepper, cover, and set aside for 5 minutes. Fluff with a fork before serving.

From Dr. Jonny: This warm, sweet flavor combo will delight your taste buds with only a few carefully chosen ingredients. It's classic Chef Jeannette: amazing flavors and textures combined in delightful and surprising ways. In this case she's put lamb—almost always a healthy dish as it is not factory farmed and rarely contains antibiotics, steroids, or hormones—together with figs(!) and blue cheese. Talk about an unusual and delicious combo! The spinach adds color and texture, not to mention a boatload of nutrients such as calcium, iron, phosphorus, magnesium, and potassium. Bonus points for using macadamia oil, an excellent substitute for virgin olive oil, high in heart-healthy monoun-saturated fats!

Trim the fat from the chops and sprinkle with salt and fresh ground pepper to taste.

Heat the oil in a skillet over high heat. Add the lamb and cook for 1 to 2 minutes per side until nicely browned. Remove from the pan and set aside.

Reduce the heat to medium, add the preserves and wine, whisk together, and cook, stirring occasionally, for 2 to 3 minutes until the sauce has started to thicken a bit.

Add the chops and their juices back to the pan and cook the lamb to desired doneness (about 1 minute per side for medium rare).

Serve the lamb over the spinach, topped with blue cheese and a drizzle of the fig sauce, to taste. Garnish with the almonds, if using.

Yield: 4 servings
Per Serving: 838 Calories; 63g Fat (69.8% calories from fat); 32g Protein; 30g Carbohydrate; 7g Dietary Fiber; 89mg Cholesterol; 235mg Sodium

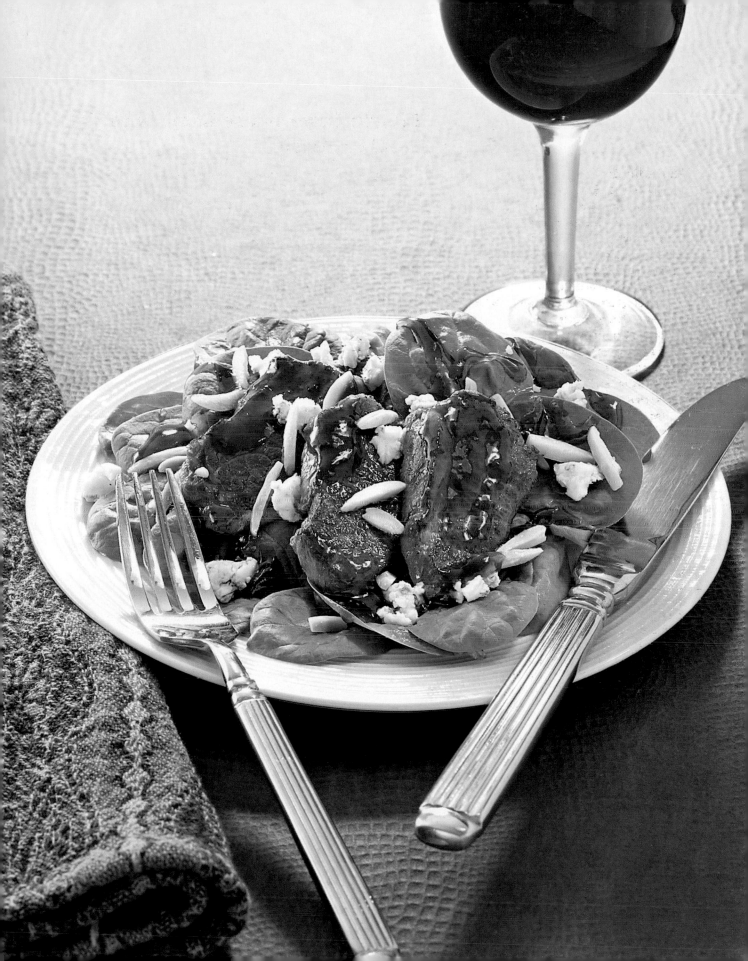

Luscious Moroccan Lamb Burgers in Less Time

Ingredients

1 pound (455 g) lean ground lamb
⅓ cup (82 g) tomato sauce
¼ cup (20 g) quick-cooking oats
⅓ cup (50 g) raisins, optional
1 teaspoon prepared minced garlic
   (or 1 large clove, minced)
½ teaspoon ground coriander
½ teaspoon ground cumin
½ teaspoon salt
⅛ teaspoon cayenne, optional
¼ teaspoon black pepper
¼ cup (38 g) chèvre or feta
Red onion rings, to taste
4 slices ripe tomato, optional

From Chef Jeannette

To Complete the Meal: Serve the burgers over lots of torn, crisp lettuce and extra sliced tomatoes with a squeeze of lemon or a sprinkle of salt.

If You Have 15 More Minutes: Slow-cook the carrots for a richer taste (and to avoid microwave use, which we think flattens the flavor and life energy of fresh foods).

1 pound (455 g) baby carrots
2 teaspoons prepared minced garlic
  (or 2 cloves crushed and chopped)
2 teaspoons ghee
½ teaspoon smoked paprika
½ teaspoon cumin seeds
¼ teaspoon salt, or to taste
¼ teaspoon cracked black pepper
¼ teaspoon red pepper flakes

From Dr. Jonny: One person who sampled these babies put it this way: "These are freaky good." You could almost expect that, given that this is one of those dishes where just reading the ingredients can make your mouth water. (At least it did mine.) Chèvre, the generic name for goat cheese, is just luscious, and mixed with lamb and raisins it becomes nothing short of divine. And though you may have some feeling about eating creatures as sweet as lambs (I share those feelings), the fact is that lamb is one of the healthiest of meats. Being young, it doesn't accumulate as many toxins as older animals, and it is almost never "factory farmed" (though many Colorado lambs are "finished" at feedlots, and there are a few other isolated exceptions). This means lamb meat is unlikely to contain antibiotics, steroids, or hormones. Most of the fat in lamb is monounsaturated (the same kind found in olive oil), and it's a wonderful source of high-quality protein. P.S.: A friend made these for a dinner party one night, and everyone was dueling over the last one! Worth mentioning is the benefit of cumin for the digestive system—it's traditionally been used for all kinds of digestive ailments from gas to indigestion.

Preheat the grill to medium-low heat.

   In a large bowl, mix together the lamb, sauce, oats, raisins, if using, garlic, coriander, cumin, salt, cayenne, if using, and black pepper well with your hands. Form into 4½-inch (11 cm) patties and grill for 4 to 5 minutes per side or until desired doneness. Garnish with a spread of cheese, red onion, and a slice of tomato, if using.

Yield: 4 servings

Per Serving: 412 Calories; 28g Fat (59.5% calories from fat); 21g Protein; 21g Carbohydrate; 3g Dietary Fiber; 83mg Cholesterol; 473mg Sodium

While the burgers are grilling, place the carrots and garlic into a large saucepan and add water to just cover. Bring to a boil over high heat for about 3 minutes or until the carrots are tender-crisp (boil longer for softer carrots). When the carrots reach desired tenderness, drain the cooking water and return them to the pan over medium-low heat (drain through a fine-mesh sieve to retain all the garlic, if desired). Add the ghee, paprika, cumin seeds, salt, and peppers and stir well. Cook for 2 minutes or until very fragrant.

Ingredients

2½ tablespoons (38 g) Dijon mustard

1½ tablespoons (6 g) herbes de Provence

2 teaspoons finely minced shallots (or
   1 teaspoon onion powder, for a
   superspeed option)

½ teaspoon salt

¼ teaspoon fresh ground black pepper

8 lean lamb loin chops

Olive oil, for grilling

From Chef Jeannette

To Complete the Meal: Add a healthy side that you can whip up while the lamb is grilling.

2 cups (300 g) cooked grain (such as
   quinoa, brown rice, or barley)

1 can (14.5 ounces or 413 g) diced
   tomatoes, in their juice (or use 1½
   cups (270 g) chopped fresh with a
   tablespoon or two of chicken broth or
   water, if needed for moisture)

2 cups (60 g) baby spinach

1 tablespoon (15 ml) lemon juice

½ teaspoon salt

¼ teaspoon fresh ground black pepper

⅓ cup (50 g) crumbled feta cheese
   (optional)

Combine the cooked grain, tomatoes, spinach, lemon juice, salt, and pepper in a medium saucepan over medium heat. Cook for about 5 minutes or until hot throughout. Garnish with crumbled feta, if using, to serve.

Easy Grilled Lamb Chops Dijon

From Dr. Jonny: If you're going to eat meat, it's hard to think of a better choice than lamb. It's almost never factory farmed, it's by definition a young animal (so it hasn't had time to accumulate a ton of toxins), and it's almost always grass fed. This deliciously scented and flavored dish will make you feel like you're in the French countryside. With a healthy grain (such as high-protein quinoa or fiber-rich barley) and a nutrient-rich green vegetable such as spinach, you've got the makings of a perfect meal. The dish features ease of preparation, speed, and, best of all, the fragrant herbes de Provence. Your family will think you've been secretly taking classes in French cooking.

Preheat the grill to medium heat.

In a small bowl, mix together the mustard, herbes de Provence, shallots, salt, and pepper. Spread the mixture evenly over the lamb chops. Lightly oil the grill with olive oil.

Oil the grill well with olive oil. (Mustard can stick.) Grill the chops for 4 minutes, flip, and grill for about 4 minutes more for medium rare or to desired doneness.

Yield: 4 servings

Per Serving: 593 Calories; 51g Fat (70.2% calories from fat); 31g Protein; 1g Carbohydrate; trace Dietary Fiber; 141mg Cholesterol; 397mg Sodium

Seafood

Fish is the ultimate high-protein, low-calorie dish. And cold water fish, such as wild Alaskan salmon, has the added advantage of providing tons of long-chain omega-3 fats, universally recognized as one of the most healthful components of the human diet. Even a basic whitefish such as flounder provides a surprising array of minerals (including more than 100 percent of the daily value for selenium), as well as nice amounts of vitamin B_{12}. There's no limit to the extraordinary quick dishes you can prepare using fish. It's endlessly adaptable.

Thyme-Saving, Fiber-Fantastic Grilled Bass over Fennel

Fortified Fish Soup with Sweet Onion

Antioxidant Paradise: Teriyaki Salmon with Pineapple

Jonny's Mega Omega Salmon in a Snap

Heart-Healthy Smoked Salmon with Whole-Wheat Orzo

Simple and Sweet Chili Salmon Cakes

A Healthier Sandwich: Ginger-Salmon Pocket on the Go

Hasty and Tasty Shrimp Cilantro Soup

Shrimp Stir-Fry Salad in No Time

Flavor in a Flash: Shrimp-Fried Rice

Swift and Savory Shrimp Sauté with Chèvre and Roasted Reds

15-Minute Low-Cal Shrimp and Citrus Ceviche

Tasty, Time-Saving Thai Shrimp and Rice Noodle Salad

Nutrient-Filled Chilled Shrimp Salad

Speedy, Spicy Shrimp over Low-Carb Zucchini "Pasta"

Light and Sassy Caribbean Seafood Salad

Quick Energy Coconut-Lime Salmon and Couscous

Fresh and Fast Lemon-Pesto Crabmeat Quinoa

Crab-Acados

One-Pot Sherried Scallops and Collards without the Calories

Busy Day Whole-Grain Linguine with Clam Sauce

No-Fuss Mussels in Spicy Beer Broth

Tone Up with 10-Minute Tilapia over Lemony Tomatoes

Light and Breezy Wasabi Tuna Boats

Power-Up with Quick and Healthy Curried Halibut

Simple and Energizing Salad Niçoise

Tuna Sashimi with Edamame Daikon Rice Threads

Super-Selenium Bluefish in a Snap

Light and Lemony 10-Minute Flounder

Fast and Fiery Smoked Trout Wraps

Ingredients

$^1/_2$ teaspoon olive oil

1 fresh skinless striped bass fillet (1$^1/_4$ to 1 $^1/_2$ pounds [567 to 710 g])

Salt and fresh ground black pepper

1 tablespoon (15 ml) almond oil (or macadamia nut or olive oil)

2 medium fennel bulbs, fronds removed, sliced

1 cup (235 ml) dry white wine

1 tablespoon (2.4 g) fresh minced thyme (or $^3/_4$ teaspoon dried)

$^1/_2$ lemon

From Chef Jeannette

To Complete the Meal: Serve with minted oranges. Peel, segment, and slice 2 to 3 large oranges and toss in a bowl with 3 tablespoons (18 g) of chopped mint.

If You Have 10 More Minutes: Bake the bass instead of grilling it. Preheat the oven to 250°F (120°C, gas mark $^1/_2$). Cut the bass into four equal pieces. Lightly oil a baking dish with olive oil, lightly season the bass all over with salt and pepper, and lay the pieces in the dish in a single layer. Bake for 15 to 20 minutes or until the bass turns white and soft when pierced by a fork.

Thyme-Saving, Fiber-Fantastic Grilled Bass over Fennel

From Dr. Jonny: I wasn't that much of a fisherman growing up, but my father used to take my brother and me to a little lake near Saugerties, New York, where we would fish for striped bass (usually unsuccessfully). These fish are prized for their rich taste and beauty—they have bright silver skin accented by striking lateral black stripes and a mild, sweet flavor with a firm, flaky texture. Truly delicious. They're also high in protein (more than 20 grams per 3-ounce [85 g] serving), and have almost as much potassium as a banana! Fennel and thyme are the perfect spices to bring out the natural flavor of this lovely fish.

Preheat the grill to medium-low heat.

Lightly oil the fish and season to taste with salt and pepper. Lay the fillet on the grill and cook for 7 minutes. Carefully turn the fish over and grill for 5 to 7 more minutes until it is cooked through (white and soft when pierced with a fork).

While the fish is grilling, heat the almond oil in a large skillet over medium heat.

Add the fennel and sauté for 2 minutes. Add the wine and thyme and simmer 10 to 12 minutes until the fennel is tender-crisp and the wine is nearly cooked off. Make a bed of the fennel, lay the fillet on top, and squeeze the lemon over all to serve.

Yield: 4 servings

Per Serving: 275 Calories; 10g Fat (35.9% calories from fat); 28g Protein; 10g Carbohydrate; 4g Dietary Fiber; 96mg Cholesterol; 163mg Sodium

Ingredients

2 tablespoons (28 ml) sesame oil

4 ounces (115 g) sliced shiitake caps

1 large Vidalia onion, halved and sliced
thinly (or 2½ cups [400 g] prepared
sliced onion)

1 tablespoon (15 ml) low-sodium tamari

¼ cup (60 ml) sake (or mirin, sherry, or
a combination)

4 cups (950 ml) vegetable broth

1 pound (455 g) boneless, skinless Pacific
cod, cut into 1½-inch (3.5 cm) pieces
(or haddock, for a milder flavor)

3 tablespoons (30 g) shredded wakame,
optional

¼ cup (25 g) sliced scallions for garnish,
optional

From Chef Jeannette

To Complete the Meal: Serve crudités,
such as celery sticks, lemon-cucumber
quarters, red bell pepper sticks, carrot
sticks, blanched green beans, or broccoli
florets, with a prepared ginger dressing.

Fortified Fish Soup with Sweet Onion

From Dr. Jonny: Truth be told, the first time Vidalia onions got on my radar was when one of my experts listed them as a "top-ten" food for health (in my book *The 150 Healthiest Foods on Earth*). The expert, Andrew Rubman, N.D., called Vidalia onions "a low-glycemic, sweet-tasting, sulfur-rich delight," which, translated, means that they're sugar sweet but are low in carbs and don't raise your blood sugar. In addition, they provide sulfur, the little known (but smelly!) mineral that is so critical for healthy hair, skin, and nails (not to mention liver supportive). Pacific cod, one of my favorite fish, is a protein heavyweight, containing a whopping 20 grams per fillet for a ridiculously low number of calories (89); that same fillet also contains more potassium than a banana. Here's a tip: If cod's light "fishiness" is too strong for you, mix in a tablespoon of sweet or mellow white miso when you remove the soup from the heat for a dose of healing probiotics and a saltier finish.

Heat the oil over medium heat in a heavy-bottomed soup pot. Add the shiitakes and onions and sauté for 4 minutes. Add the tamari and sake, increase the heat to medium high, and sauté for 3 to 4 minutes or until the mushrooms and onion are tender (it's preferable if not all the sake is cooked off). Add the vegetable broth, increase the heat to high, and bring just to a boil.

Reduce the heat to a simmer, add the fish and wakame, if using, and cook for about 2 minutes or until the fish is just cooked through—do not overcook or the fish will become tough.

Remove from the heat and top the soup with the scallions, if using, to serve.

Yield: 4 servings

Per Serving: 437 Calories; 11g Fat (23.0% calories from fat); 32g Protein; 53g Carbohydrate; 7g Dietary Fiber; 45mg Cholesterol; 1931mg Sodium

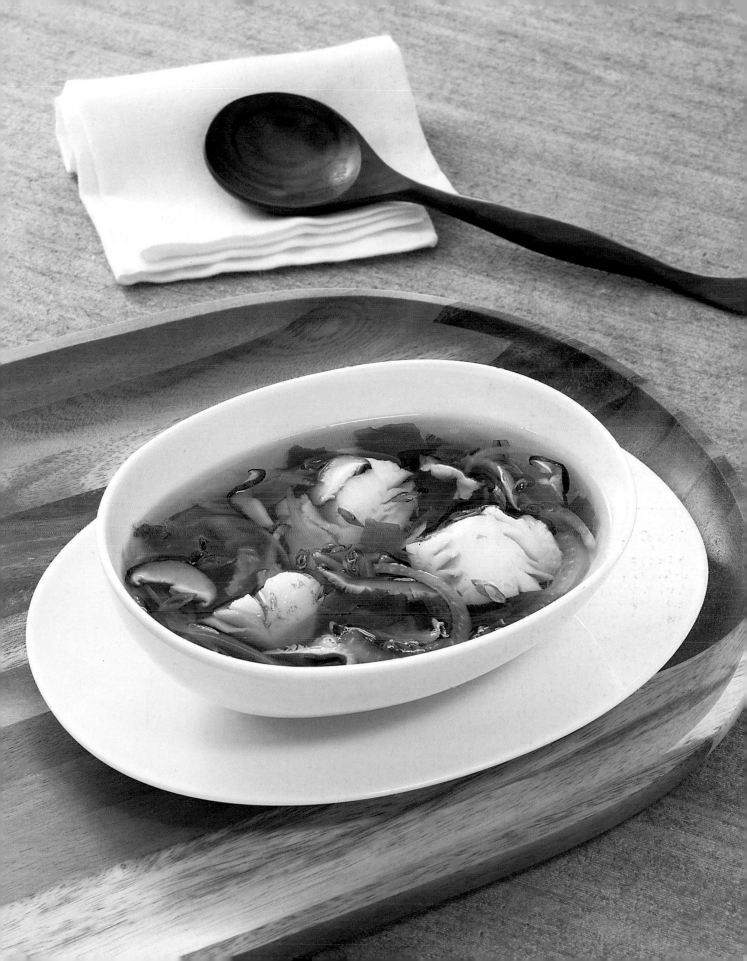

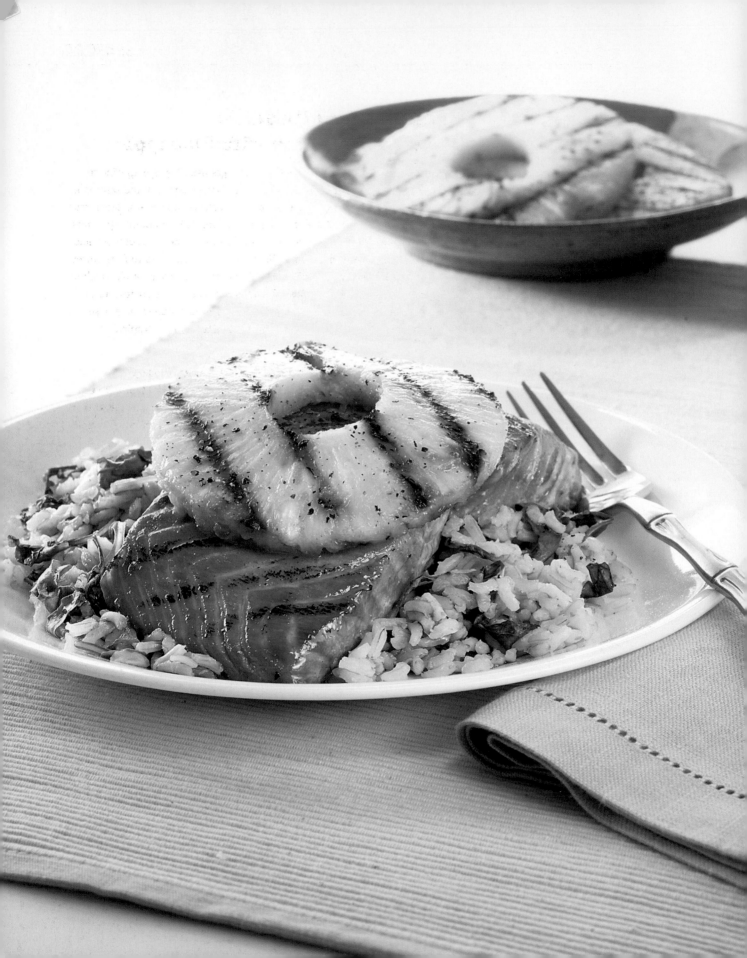

Antioxidant Paradise: Teriyaki Salmon with Pineapple

Ingredients

⅓ cup (80 ml) pineapple juice (if there is enough, use the juice from the prepared pineapple rings)

¼ cup (60 ml) low-sodium tamari

1 tablespoon (15 ml) mirin (or honey)

2 tablespoons (12 g) prepared minced ginger (or minced fresh)

¼ teaspoon garlic powder, optional

4 skinless salmon fillets (6 ounces or 170 g each; we recommend Vital Choice Alaskan wild salmon, which you can find in the Online Store/Healthy Foods section at www.jonnybowden.com)

6 fresh pineapple rings (prepared, in the refrigerator case)

Salt and cracked black pepper, to taste

2 cups (330 g) precooked frozen brown rice (e.g., Trader Joe's Frozen Organic Brown Rice)

2 cups (40 g) loosely packed baby arugula or baby spinach

From Dr. Jonny: About once a week I get asked by a magazine to offer a top-ten list of superfoods, and I always start with the same one: wild salmon. Not only is it a terrific, low-calorie source of protein, but it's one of the richest sources of the two most important omega-3 fats on the planet: eicosapentaenoic acid (EPA) and docosahexaenoic acid (DHA). But wait, there's more! Wild salmon, as opposed to farm raised, gets its red color from dining on little crustaceans called krill, which in turn are loaded with a powerful (red) antioxidant called astaxanthin. It's a winner on all counts, and you can't do much better taste-wise than pairing it with pineapple. This dish tastes like the tropics!

Preheat the grill to medium heat (or preheat the oven broiler).

To make the teriyaki sauce, in a small bowl, whisk together the juice, tamari, mirin, ginger, and garlic powder, if using. Set ⅓ of the teriyaki sauce aside. Pour the remaining ⅔ of the teriyaki sauce over the salmon to coat and use it to baste the salmon several times while grilling.

Sprinkle the pineapple with pepper, if desired. Grill the salmon and pineapple rings for 2 to 3 minutes per side (depending on thickness), or until the fish reaches desired doneness and the pineapple rings have light grill marks.

Prepare the frozen rice as directed on the package and stir in the arugula, if using, while it's piping hot, letting it rest for a minute or two to wilt. Serve the fish over the rice and greens and dress to taste with the remaining third of the teriyaki dressing.

Yield: 4 servings

Per Serving: 561 Calories; 7g Fat (10.3% calories from fat); 48g Protein; 87g Carbohydrate; 4g Dietary Fiber; 88mg Cholesterol; 745mg Sodium

From Chef Jeannette

To Complete the Meal: Toss 1 pound (455 g) of asparagus spears (the larger, Rubenesque "female" asparagus works better for roasting than the thin spears) in a tablespoon or two of olive oil with a little salt and pepper to taste for about 10 minutes in a 400°F (200°C, gas mark 6) oven. Finish them with a squeeze of fresh lemon and a sprinkle of sliced toasted almonds, if desired.

If You Have 5 More Minutes: If you want to thicken the teriyaki dressing, heat it to a simmer over medium-high heat in a small saucepan and stir in 2 teaspoons of kudzu dissolved in 2 teaspoons of pineapple juice or water, continuing to simmer for about 2 more minutes or until it thickens slightly.

If You Have 30 More Minutes: Marinate the fillets in two thirds of the teriyaki sauce before grilling, and use the remaining third to dress the dish as directed. You can also leave the fish to marinate overnight.

Jonny's Mega Omega Salmon in a Snap

Ingredients

1 1/2 tablespoons (25 ml) Barlean's coconut oil

4 Vital Choice Wild Alaskan skinless salmon fillets (6 ounces or 170 g each), thawed

2 Vital Choice organic spice packs (included with the salmon order, or use salt and black pepper, to taste)

1 bag (6 ounces or 170 g) triple-washed baby spinach

1 teaspoon turmeric

3/4 teaspoon lemon pepper

2 tablespoons (28 ml) water

2 teaspoons butter

From Dr. Jonny: This is one of the few recipes in the several books Chef Jeannette and I have done together that I can actually take credit for inventing—hence the title! Although I'm no gourmet cook, I've learned to throw a few things together over the years that taste good, are easy as pie to make, and are nutritionally fabulous. I gave the outline of my very unscientific recipe to Chef Jeannette—"throw in a handful of spinach"—she worked out the delicious details, and came up with this much better version! The thing of it is, wild salmon blends beautifully with sautéed spinach, and when both are lightly cooked in the best coconut oil on the planet, the resulting taste is superb. We love the organic spice pack that comes with the salmon we get from Vital Choice (see www.jonnybowden.com, under Online Store/Healthy Foods), but you can make your own spice mix or use salt and pepper—just don't forget the turmeric. Turmeric is the superspice of all time, having both serious anti-inflammatory properties and some anticancer activity as well. You can knock this dish out in less than 10 minutes. Full of flavor, it satisfies without stuffing, and best of all, it has minimal impact on blood sugar, ensuring that you won't experience cravings and hunger ten minutes after the meal! Note: I sometimes sprinkle a few slivered almonds on the dish right before it finishes cooking.

Heat the coconut oil in a large Dutch oven over medium-high heat. Add the salmon fillets to the pan and sprinkle the Vital Choice spice packs to taste over the surface of the fillets. Sear for 1 minute or until lightly browned. Flip and sear the uncooked side for 1 minute, sprinkling the spice packs on the seared sides, to taste. Reduce the heat to medium low and add the spinach.

Sprinkle the turmeric and lemon pepper over the spinach and add the water. Cover for 2 minutes. Remove the cover, add the butter, stir, and re-cover for about 1 to 3 minutes or until the salmon is cooked to your liking. Do not overcook!

Yield: 4 servings

Per Serving: 276 Calories; 14g Fat (45.3% calories from fat); 35g Protein; 2g Carbohydrate; 1g Dietary Fiber; 94mg Cholesterol; 231mg Sodium

Heart-Healthy Smoked Salmon with Whole Wheat Orzo

Ingredients

1 cup (195 g) uncooked whole wheat orzo

1 tablespoon (15 ml) olive oil

1½ cups (240 g) prepared diced onion (or 1 yellow or Vidalia onion, diced)

1 cup (460 g) soft silken tofu

¾ cup (175 ml) milk (cow's, unsweetened plain, soy, or almond)

3 tablespoons (45 g) Dijon mustard

1 tablespoon (15 ml) brandy or cognac

1 tablespoon (11 g) mustard seeds

2 cups (300 g) peas (or use 1 can [14 ounces or 400 g] quartered artichoke hearts, well drained)

1 package (8 ounces or 225 g) sliced smoked salmon, in 1-inch (2.5 cm) strips

From Chef Jeannette

To Complete the Meal: Serve with sautéed asparagus (see page 174) or green beans amandine (see page 105).

If You Have 5 More Minutes: Garnish with ¼ cup (15 g) chopped fresh parsley for a touch of fresh green.

From Dr. Jonny: A reader wrote in to my "Ask the Doc" column in *Clean Eating* magazine and asked whether smoking (or drying) salmon affects its omega-3 fat content. The answer is kind of a cool math problem. The omega-3 content remains exactly the same—unaffected by smoking or drying. But because there is less moisture in the fish, the omega-3 is now more concentrated. So an ounce of regular salmon (part of which is water) has less omega-3 by *percentage* than an ounce of dried salmon (none of which is water). Get it? Don't worry if you didn't—the point is, smoked salmon is still a great source of omega-3 fats, and this particular hearty and satisfying dish is especially rich and slightly smoky!

Prepare the orzo according to the package directions.

Heat the oil in a skillet over medium heat. Add the onion and sauté for 5 minutes. While the onion is sautéing, blend together the tofu, milk, mustard, and brandy, using an immersion blender or food processor. Stir in the mustard seeds.

When the onion is tender, add the cream sauce, peas, and salmon, and mix gently to combine. Reduce the heat to medium-low and cook for 2 to 3 minutes until hot throughout. Serve over the hot orzo.

Yield: 4 servings

Per Serving: 503 Calories; 15g Fat (26.6% calories from fat); 34g Protein; 58g Carbohydrate; 8g Dietary Fiber; 35mg Cholesterol; 218mg Sodium

Simple and Sweet Chili Salmon Cakes

Ingredients

1 large egg

2 tablespoons (28 g) sweet chili sauce, plus extra for topping

2 tablespoons (5 g) minced fresh basil or cilantro, optional

1 can (14¾ ounces or 420 g) wild Alaskan salmon (or 2 cans [7.5 ounces or 210 g each] Vital Choice Wild Red), drained and flaked

2 tablespoons (10 g) quick-cooking oats

2 teaspoons sesame oil

From Chef Jeannette

To Complete the Meal: Serve over a bed of lettuce with seasoned cucumber. To prepare the cucumber salad, peel and grate or thinly slice 1 English cucumber and dress with 3 tablespoons (45 ml) of unseasoned rice vinegar, 1 teaspoon of agave nectar or Sucanat, 1 teaspoon of low-sodium tamari, and 1 teaspoon of toasted sesame oil. The longer it sits, the stronger the flavor.

From Dr. Jonny: Chef Jeannette and I were talking the other day, and we both have noticed the explosion of "limited-ingredient" products that are hitting the supermarket shelves. Seems there's a premium on simplicity these days—one of my favorite brands of dog food even has a limited-ingredient version. The appeal of five-ingredient recipes is that you know exactly what's in them, and they're generally really easy to make. Here's Chef Jeannette's version of a five-ingredient nutritional powerhouse. (Okay, I'm fudging slightly. There's a sixth optional ingredient herb.) By now you've heard me talk about the benefits of salmon so many times, you're probably sick of hearing about it, but in case you missed it the first 100 times, salmon is high in omega-3 fats, which contribute to the health of your brain and heart; high in protein; and high in a powerful antioxidant called astaxanthin. All the ingredients in this dish are easy to find—look for the sweet chili sauce in the Asian or ethnic section of any large grocery store.

In a medium bowl, mix together the egg, 2 tablespoons (28 g) of the chili sauce, and fresh herb, if using. Add the salmon and oats and mix until well combined. Form into four 1-inch (2.5 cm) patties. Heat the oil in a large skillet over medium. Add the patties and cook until lightly browned and cooked through, about 4 minutes per side. Serve the salmon cakes with extra chili sauce for topping, if desired.

Yield: 4 servings

Per Serving: 172 Calories; 7g Fat (39.5% calories from fat); 23g Protein; 2g Carbohydrate; trace Dietary Fiber; 108mg Cholesterol; 90mg Sodium

A Healthier Sandwich: Ginger-Salmon Pocket on the Go

Ingredients

½ can (6 ounces or 170 g) wild salmon, drained (we like Vital Choice)

1 ½ to 2 tablespoons (25 to 28 ml) prepared ginger dressing, to taste

2 tablespoons (20 g) diced red onion

¼ cup (35 g) grated English cucumber (or seeded regular cucumber)

Sprouted-grain pita pocket

½ cup (10 g) spring or mesclun mix

2 slices heirloom tomato

From Dr. Jonny: Okay, I'll be the first to admit I'm not a huge fan of the sandwich as a go-to meal. Why? Because your basic deli sandwich uses junky, low-quality, high-carb bread and meats that are filled with nitrate and sodium, not to mention sauces loaded with sugar. But there's no doubt that a sandwich can make an excellent quick (and healthy!) meal, providing you build it with the right materials.

We use sprouted-grain wraps and pockets, but you can also use whole-grain options. Sprouted grains retain their natural plant enzymes, which are beneficial for digestion and are also nutrient rich. Some argue that the nutrients in sprouted-grain breads are easier to absorb, but others argue that the effect is minor. No matter. Sprouted, and whole-grain, wraps are preferable to the bulky rolls made with refined white flour that come with the average deli sandwich. Whole grains are fine, but make sure the first ingredient is whole wheat or whole oats, and look for at least 2 grams of fiber per slice, preferably 3. For protein and omega-3 fats you can't do better than salmon. Heirloom tomatoes taste like tomatoes are supposed to taste, plus they offer a nice helping of the antioxidant lycopene.

In a small bowl, mix together the salmon, dressing, red onion, and cucumber until well combined.

Slice the pita open, leaving one section connected so it holds together. Open it and lay the greens and tomato slices over one half. Pile the salmon mixture on top and close the top over all to cover.

Yield: 1 sandwich

Per Serving: 480 Calories; 16g Fat (30.4% calories from fat); 43g Protein; 40g Carbohydrate; 9g Dietary Fiber; 88mg Cholesterol; 650mg Sodium

Hasty and Tasty Shrimp Cilantro Soup

From Dr. Jonny: Honestly, I don't make soup very often because, let's face it, it's a big project. So tell me about a healthy, delicious soup that tastes of cilantro and can go from conception to table in 15 minutes, and you've got my attention. Cilantro is an underappreciated herb that has a long and honorable medicinal history. It's a terrific detoxifying agent. It contains components, such as borneol and linalool, that help cleanse the liver, as well as many natural anti-inflammatories and antioxidants. It also tastes phenomenal, and in the high concentrations used in this soup, is a power pack of vitamins K, A, and C. The shrimp and coconut are a match made in culinary heaven. The two combine to make a light, mild soup deliciously suffused with the sweet, citrusy tang of fresh cilantro. Can't beat that!

Ingredients

4 cups (950 ml) vegetable broth, divided

1 bag (1 pound or 455 g) frozen chopped red and green bell peppers and onions (or colored bell pepper strips)

10 ounces (280 g) fresh cilantro (about 2 bunches)

1 can (14 ounces or 400 g) light coconut milk

½ teaspoon salt

1 ¼ pounds (567 g) small shrimp, shelled and deveined

1 tablespoon (15 ml) lime juice, preferably fresh squeezed, or to taste

1 cup (180 g) chopped tomatoes (grape or plum work well)

Combine 2 cups (475 ml) of the broth with the frozen vegetables in a large soup pot and bring to a boil over high heat. Let it boil for about a minute or until the vegetables are just tender.

While the soup is cooking, lay the cilantro bunches side by side, chop off the stems, and discard. Make two more cuts across the bunches and submerge the roughly chopped cilantro in cold water to rinse well, and spin or shake to remove excess water.

Place it in a blender with the remaining 2 cups (475 ml) of the veggie broth, and blend until the cilantro is well pureed, 1 to 3 minutes (just over a minute in my Vita-Mix). Pour the mixture back through a double-mesh sieve into a large bowl, swirling the fibers around to drain out all the liquids. Discard the fibers.

Add the cilantro broth, coconut milk, salt, and shrimp to the boiling soup and cook for about 2 minutes or until the shrimp are cooked through. (Do not overcook! See Superspeed Tip.)

Stir in the lime juice and top with the tomatoes to serve.

Yield: 4 servings

Per Serving: 603 Calories; 15g Fat (20.8% calories from fat); 52g Protein; 76g Carbohydrate; 12g Dietary Fiber; 218mg Cholesterol; 2289mg Sodium

From Chef Jeannette

To Complete the Meal: Serve this soup with a hearty fruit salad. Try a mix of orange segments, pineapple chunks, shredded coconut (unsweetened), and julienned jicama or drained, canned water chestnuts, garnished with cilantro or crushed macadamia nuts.

Superspeed Tip: To save time shelling fresh raw shrimp yourself, use frozen, preshelled shrimp, precooked or raw. For frozen shrimp, simply add to the simmering soup and cook for about 2 minutes (for precooked), or 3 to 4 minutes (for raw) until just cooked—be careful not to overcook or shrimp will get tough.

If You Have 15 More Minutes: You can seed and chop three medium colored bell peppers to use in place of the frozen. You will need to increase initial simmering time by 5 to 10 minutes to soften them.

Shrimp Stir-Fry Salad in No Time

From Dr. Jonny: Cabbage and broccoli are both vegetable royalty. As members of the brassica family, they contain valuable chemicals called indoles, which are known as cancer fighters because of the positive effect they have on the metabolism of hormones. If that sounds a little technical, don't worry about it. These foods are really good for you, and best of all, the whole process of putting together this superlight stir-fry takes all of about 10 minutes. And you can't beat shrimp for low-calorie protein! The seeds offer a nice crunchy note to this already delicious dish!

Ingredients

1½ (25 ml) tablespoons peanut oil
2 cloves garlic, minced
1 tablespoon (8 g) fresh grated ginger (or ¾ teaspoon powdered)
1 pound (455 g) medium shrimp, peeled and deveined (fresh or frozen, thawed)
1 bag (12 ounces or 340 g) fresh slaw mix (shredded cabbage, carrots, and broccoli)
1 tablespoon (15 ml) mirin
2 tablespoons (28 ml) low-sodium tamari
1 teaspoon toasted sesame oil
1 tablespoon (8 g) toasted sesame seeds

Heat the oil in a large sauté pan over medium heat. Add the garlic and ginger and sauté 2 for minutes. Add the shrimp and sauté for 1 minute. Add the slaw veggies, mirin, and tamari, stirring well to coat, and sauté for 1 to 2 minutes until the shrimp are cooked through and the veggies are hot and just wilted, but still crunchy. Remove from the heat, add the sesame oil and seeds, and toss to coat.

Yield: 4 servings
Per Serving: 224 Calories; 10g Fat (37.7% calories from fat); 30g Protein; 7g Carbohydrate; 2g Dietary Fiber; 173mg Cholesterol; 475mg Sodium

From Chef Jeannette

Stir-frying is an excellent quick and healthy cooking technique. The short cooking time in a small amount of high-quality oil both enriches the flavors and retains the nutrients of the meats and veggies. I like to stir-fry as an end-of-the-week technique for using up whatever leftover vegetables I still have in the crisper.

Ingredients

1½ tablespoons (25 ml) sesame or peanut oil

1 teaspoon prepared minced garlic (or 1 large clove, minced)

2 tablespoons (12 g) prepared minced ginger (or finely chopped fresh)

2 cups (140 g) prepared shredded broccoli slaw mix (or use 2 cups [140 g] shredded Napa cabbage)

1 cup (130 g) frozen peas

2 cups (330 g) cooked brown rice (prepare frozen cooked or parboiled brown rice if you don't have leftovers on hand)

1 egg

3 tablespoons (45 ml) low-sodium tamari

⅔ cup (110 g) sliced scallions, optional

¾ pound (340 g) cooked medium shrimp, peeled and deveined

2 tablespoons (16 g) toasted sesame seeds, optional

From Chef Jeannette

To Complete the Meal: Serve this dish with a prepared seaweed salad, which you can find in the refrigerated Japanese or sushi section of larger or whole foods grocers.

Variation Tip: For a cholesterol-free vegetarian option, replace the shrimp with diced, preseasoned tofu (e.g., Wildwood Organics). Just add the tofu when you would add the shrimp and proceed as directed.

Flavor in a Flash: Shrimp-Fried Rice

From Dr. Jonny: Sure you love fried rice at the local Chinese joint— who doesn't? But healthy? Come on. What if you could have that same delicious taste in a dish that wasn't a nutritional nightmare? Well, you can. Our version is light, made with healthy oils, and seasoned with all sorts of things that are good for you, such as garlic! And the dish is pretty complete: You get protein from the shrimp and eggs; a great assortment of health-packed vegetables such as cabbage, peas, and onions; and a healthy whole grain in the brown rice. No MSG added! And as a bonus, you can use low-sodium tamari and not lose an eyedropper of taste!

Heat the oil in a large nonstick sauté pan or Dutch oven over medium heat. Add the garlic, ginger, and slaw mix and sauté for 3 minutes or until the cabbage is slightly wilted and reduced. Add the peas and rice, stirring to combine well, cover, reduce heat to medium-low, and cook for 3 to 4 minutes until hot, stirring occasionally.

While the rice is heating, whisk the egg and tamari together in a small bowl.

Increase the heat to medium, pour the egg mixture over all, mixing well and stirring rapidly to distribute the egg as it cooks. Fold in the scallions, if using, and shrimp. Cover and remove from the heat. Let it rest for a couple of minutes or until the shrimp are heated through.

Stir in the sesame seeds, if using, and serve.

Yield: 4 servings
Per Serving: 328 Calories; 11g Fat (28.9% calories from fat); 32g Protein; 30g Carbohydrate; 5g Dietary Fiber; 182mg Cholesterol; 621mg Sodium

Swift and Savory Shrimp Sauté with Chèvre and Roasted Reds

Ingredients

1½ tablespoons (25 ml) olive oil

1¼ pounds (567 g) medium shrimp, shelled and deveined

½ teaspoon ground fennel

¼ teaspoon cracked black pepper

Salt, to taste

1 bag (6 ounces or 170 g) baby spinach

¼ teaspoon white pepper

3 prepared roasted red peppers, drained and sliced

⅓ cup (50 g) chèvre (or feta)

2 tablespoons (28 ml) lemon juice (fresh squeezed is best)

From Chef Jeannette

To Complete the Meal: Serve with Sesame Brown Rice (see page 33 for instructions) or lemon sesame stir-fried veggies (page 134) for a "carb-light" side.

From Dr. Jonny: One of the best pieces of nutritional advice I ever heard was also one of the simplest: Shop for color. When that conveyer belt at the supermarket checkout looks like a postcard of one of those big, overflowing French vegetable markets, you know you've hit pay dirt. And the reason is simple: The pigments that give fruits and vegetables their color belong to a family of plant chemicals called anthocyanins, and they contain powerful antioxidants and anti-inflammatory properties that help protect the plants from predators. These plant chemicals offer the same kind of protection inside your body. There are thousands of them, and different ones are found in red, yellow, orange, and green plants, making a combination of colors (such as the red peppers and green spinach) an ideal mix for longevity. The only thing you need to add is protein—oh, wait, there it is in the shrimp! Bon appétit!

Heat the oil in a large sauté pan over medium heat. Add the shrimp and sprinkle with fennel, black pepper, and a few pinches of salt. Sauté for 30 seconds and add the spinach. Sprinkle with salt, to taste, and white pepper, and cover for 1 minute. Remove the cover and stir in the red peppers. Cover for 30 seconds or until the shrimp is just cooked through and the spinach is mostly wilted. Remove from the heat, stir in the chèvre, and sprinkle lemon juice over all.

Yield: 4 servings

Per Serving: 257 Calories; 11g Fat (39.1% calories from fat); 32g Protein; 7g Carbohydrate; 2g Dietary Fiber; 227mg Cholesterol; 384mg Sodium

15-Minute Low-Cal Shrimp and Citrus Ceviche

Ingredients

1 pound (455 g) peeled, deveined, cooked small shrimp
1/3 cup (80 ml) fresh-squeezed lime juice
1/4 teaspoon salt
1 small jalapeño, seeded
1/4 small red onion
1 small cucumber, peeled and cut into chunks
1 navel orange, peeled and diced
1 large, ripe heirloom tomato, diced (if you have time, seed and dice 2 medium tomatoes for a tidier presentation)
3 tablespoons (3 g) chopped fresh cilantro
1 ripe avocado, peeled, pitted, and thickly sliced (8 slices)
16 endive spears (or 8 lettuce leaves)

From Chef Jeannette

To Complete the Meal: Serve it with a modest portion of baked corn tortilla chips.

If You Can Prepare the Night Before: You can make a more traditional ceviche. Use raw shrimp, scallops, or a pound (455 g) of thin white fish fillets (such as tilapia or flounder—should be wild caught and very fresh!) and finely dice it. Add the lime juice and salt, stir well to combine, and store it in glass in the refrigerator overnight. As noted above, long-term marinating in fresh citrus juice "cooks" the fish without heat so it can be eaten. This is a superfresh and healthy way to prepare shrimp or tilapia!

From Dr. Jonny: The definition of *ceviche*, in case you're wondering, is "a citrus-marinated seafood." The acid in the citrus actually "cooks" the seafood. If you think that sounds fresh, light, and healthy, you're right. Ceviche was believed to have originated in Polynesia, but its true birthplace remains a subject of controversy. Many countries claim to have invented the idea of light seafood seasoned with limes or lemons, and no wonder—it tastes great. This version is made with precooked shrimp, so it's not technically traditional ceviche—but on the plus side it takes only 15 minutes to get it to the table. That's a compromise we're willing to make, and you will be, too, once you serve it. The cucumber and orange are a brilliant touch. They fit in perfectly, adding extra juiciness and crunchiness to an already-light dish packed with nutrition. The cucumber has almost zero calories—okay, 19, I mean really!—and a fair amount of nutrition: half the potassium of a banana, 22 mg of calcium, 19 mg of magnesium, and 1 mg of fiber. Overall this high-protein, low-calorie dish is a winner in every way.

Put the shrimp into a medium glass container and add the lime juice and salt, tossing to coat. Cover and set aside for 10 minutes while you prepare the vegetables.

Put the jalapeño and onion in a food processor and pulse a few times to chop.

Add the cucumber and pulse a few times to chop, turning the contents between pulses to chop evenly. You should have what looks like a chunky relish. Add the cucumber mix to a medium bowl and stir in the orange, tomato, and cilantro. Pour the veggie mix over the shrimp and mix gently to combine. Arrange four endive leaves and two avocado slices on each of four plates. Scoop about 1/4 cup of the mix into each endive leaf and serve.

Yield: 4 servings
Per Serving: 244 Calories; 10g Fat (35.7% calories from fat); 25g Protein; 15g Carbohydrate; 3g Dietary Fiber; 173mg Cholesterol; 314mg Sodium

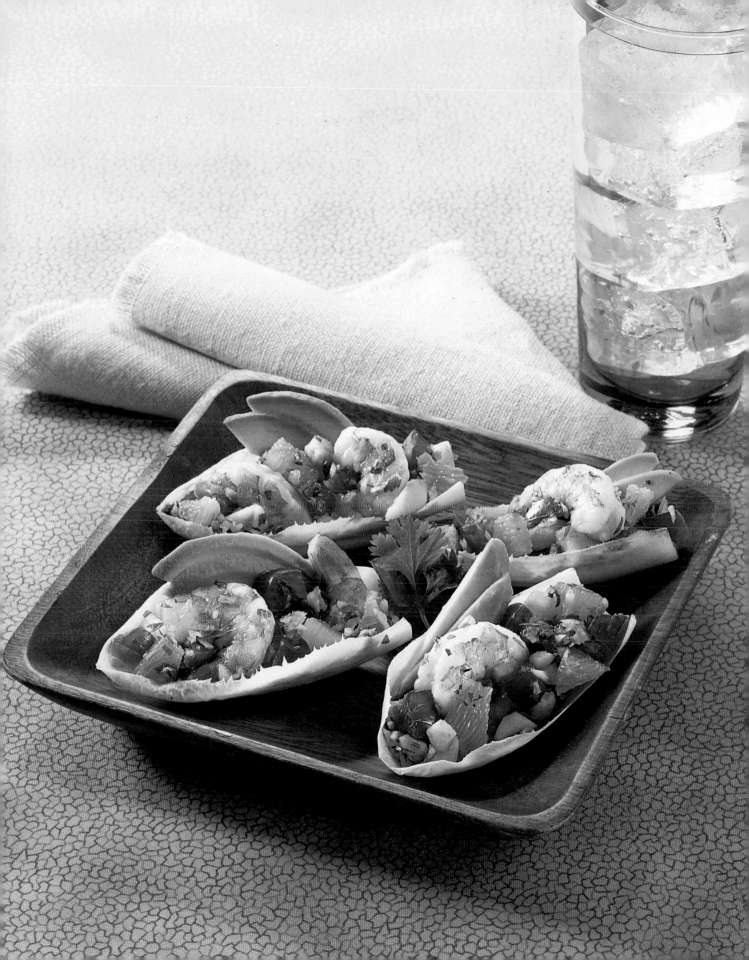

Tasty, Time-Saving Thai Shrimp and Rice Noodle Salad

Ingredients

8 ounces (225 g) rice noodles, fettuccine-
    style (we like Thai Kitchen Stir-Fry Rice
    Noodles)

3 tablespoons (45 ml) low-sodium tamari

¼ cup (65 g) natural peanut butter

1 tablespoon (20 g) honey

1 tablespoon (15 ml) rice wine vinegar

1 tablespoon (15 ml) lime juice (fresh
    squeezed is best)

1 teaspoon ground ginger

1 bunch fresh cilantro, divided

1 pound (455 g) frozen cooked shelled me-
    dium shrimp, thawed

1 bag (12 ounces or 340 g) slaw veggies
    (broccoli, cabbage, and carrots)

2 cups (100 g) mung bean sprouts

⅔ cup (97 g) roasted peanuts

From Chef Jeannette

Variation Tip: For a low-cholesterol,
vegan option, swap out the shrimp
for diced, preseasoned tofu. We like
Wildwood Organics Teriyaki Baked Tofu.

From Dr. Jonny: Ever wonder what to make for a hot summer night? Something light and nourishing yet easy to throw together? Look no further. Shrimp is one of those great go-to ingredients, easy to make, high in protein, low in calories—and shrimp fits easily into all kinds of dishes. In this case, Chef Jeannette has taken the delicious step of adding peanut butter to the mixture, giving the dish a kind of traditional Thai peanut-sauce flavor that blends just perfectly with the light rice noodles that serve as a base. Just for good measure: a whole bunch of cruciferous vegetables complete with their cancer-fighting indoles and a host of vitamins and minerals. It tastes so good, your family will never even suspect it's healthy!

Follow the package directions for preparing the rice noodles (usually soaking for 5 to 7 minutes in a large pot of water that's been boiled and removed from heat, rinsing in cold water, and draining well).

While the noodles are soaking, prepare the dressing. Place the tamari, peanut butter, honey, rice wine vinegar, lime juice, ginger, and ⅓ cup (5 g) cilantro in a food processor and process until smooth, scraping down the sides as necessary.

In a large bowl, combine the shrimp, slaw veggies, bean sprouts, rice noodles, and remaining cilantro. Add the dressing to taste and toss well to combine. Garnish with the peanuts.

Yield: 4 servings
Per Serving: 620 Calories; 22g Fat (31.0% calories from fat); 43g Protein; 68g Carbohydrate; 6g Dietary Fiber; 173mg Cholesterol; 721mg Sodium

Nutrient-Filled Chilled Shrimp Salad

Ingredients

Salad

4 cups (220 g) spring greens mix

1 small zucchini, unpeeled, diced

1 red, yellow, or orange bell pepper, seeded and diced (or $^{2}/_{3}$ cup [100 g] prepared diced tricolor peppers)

1 cup (130 g) corn (fresh, cooked, or frozen, thawed)

1 small cucumber, peeled and sliced

1 pint (300 g) cherry tomatoes

1 pound (455 g) chilled medium cooked shrimp, peeled (frozen, thawed are fine)

$^{1}/_{2}$ avocado, peeled and roughly chopped

$^{1}/_{2}$ cup (80 g) sliced scallions

4 tablespoons (60 ml) high-quality prepared herb vinaigrette, or to taste (we like Seeds of Change Organic Italian Herb Vinaigrette or Organicville Tarragon Dijon Organic Vinaigrette)

From Dr. Jonny: I frequently hear complaints from readers about how frustrating it is for them that nutritionists can't seem to agree on anything. I share their pain. But actually, it's not 100 percent true that we don't agree on anything—certain principles we all agree on (more vegetables!) and certain dishes would get a five-star rating from any of us, no matter how much we might disagree on nutritional philosophy. This is one of those dishes. High in protein, low in fat, and absolutely loaded with a wide range of plant antioxidants and anti-inflammatory properties courtesy of multicolored vegetables such as zucchini, bell peppers, and cukes, this is a salad everyone will love. The bright, fresh flavors of the herbs bring this crowd-pleaser to life! It's remarkably low in calories too!

In a large salad bowl, combine greens mix, zucchini, peppers, corn, cucumber, tomatoes, shrimp, avocado, and scallions. Dress to taste, toss to mix, and adjust the seasonings if necessary.

Yield: 4 servings

Per Serving: 297 Calories; 14g Fat (42.4% calories from fat); 27g Protein; 17g Carbohydrate; 5g Dietary Fiber; 173mg Cholesterol; 190mg Sodium

From Chef Jeannette

Superspeed Tip: With all the fresh raw veggies, there is a large amount of chopping in this recipe. To save time, you can feed the zucchini and cucumber (halved lengthwise to fit) through the grater attachment on the food processor to shred in seconds.

If You Have 5 More Minutes: Make your own herbed vinaigrette for a burst of fresh, vital flavor and nutrients:

Vinaigrette

$2^{1}/_{2}$ tablespoons (40 ml) champagne vinegar (or white wine vinegar)

1 tablespoon (15 ml) lemon juice (preferably fresh squeezed)

2 teaspoons Dijon mustard

2 $^{1}/_{2}$ tablespoons (40 ml) olive oil

1 small shallot, minced*

2 teaspoons chopped fresh thyme (or 1 teaspoon dried)

2 tablespoons (8 g) chopped fresh parsley (or $^{3}/_{4}$ teaspoon dried)

$^{1}/_{4}$ teaspoon salt

$^{1}/_{4}$ teaspoon white pepper

In a small bowl, whisk together the vinegar, lemon juice, mustard, and olive oil. Mix in the shallot, thyme, parsley, salt, and pepper.

*To quickly mince the shallot, slice it in half, add it to the whisking ingredients, and use an immersion wand for just a few pulses.

Speedy, Spicy Shrimp over Low-Carb Zucchini "Pasta"

Ingredients

2 medium zucchini, stemmed

1 tablespoon (15 ml) plus 2 teaspoons olive oil, divided

2 teaspoons prepared minced garlic (or 2 small cloves, minced)

Salt and fresh ground pepper, to taste

1 teaspoon ground cumin

1 teaspoon turmeric

1 teaspoon ground coriander

½ teaspoon salt

¾ teaspoon cracked black pepper

¼ teaspoon ground cardamom

1 can (14.5 ounces or 413 g) diced tomatoes, undrained

1½ pounds (710 g) raw medium shrimp, peeled and deveined (fresh or frozen, thawed)

From Chef Jeannette

To Complete the Meal: Serve with a light, cooling salad of a large grated, peeled cucumber and 2 medium chopped fresh tomatoes dressed with 1 cup (230 g) of plain low-fat yogurt mixed 2 tablespoons (28 ml) of lemon juice, ½ teaspoon of cumin, and a pinch of salt.

If You Have 5 Extra Minutes: Chop ⅓ cup (5 g) of fresh parsley or cilantro and stir it into the shrimp just before serving.

From Dr. Jonny: You know that old expression about having your cake and eating it, too? That's how I feel about pasta. I want to control my blood sugar, which I generally do by keeping my carb intake reasonably low, but I want my pasta, too. Solution? Come up with pasta "substitutes" that are lower in carbs and just as satisfying in the taste and texture department. (Or use Barilla Plus pasta with lots of vegetables, another solution we've used in this book.) Here Chef Jeannette has devised a "faux" pasta made of low-calorie, high-nutrient zucchini and combined it with antioxidant-rich tomatoes and high-protein shrimp in a relatively low-calorie dish that satisfies. Bonus points for the fabulous superspice turmeric, one of the most anti-inflammatory compounds on the planet!

Using the grating attachment on your food processor, shred the zucchini (this is easiest if you slice them in half lengthwise and feed the halves through the opening). Heat 1 tablespoon of the oil in a large sauté pan over medium heat and add the shredded zucchini. Season with salt and fresh ground pepper, cover, and cook for about 6 minutes, stirring occasionally. Remove the lid, stir, and test for tenderness. If the zucchini is very juicy, drain and discard extra liquids. Continue cooking for another minute or so until tender, if required.

While the zucchini is cooking, heat the remaining 2 teaspoons of oil in a large skillet over medium. Add all the spices from cumin through cardamom and sauté for 1 minute or until very fragrant.

Stir in the tomatoes and shrimp, and cook until the shrimp are just cooked through. Serve the shrimp over the squash "pasta."

Yield: 4 servings

Per Serving: 279 Calories; 9g Fat (30.3% calories from fat); 38g Protein; 10g Carbohydrate; 3g Dietary Fiber; 270mg Cholesterol; 542mg Sodium

The Real Benefit of Olive Oil

You might expect this nutritional note to extol the benefits of the heart-healthy fat found in olive oil (technically called monounsaturated fat, and even more technically called oleic acid). Well, I'll get to that part. But first let me give you my own personal opinion about why olive oil is so darn good for you, and, big surprise, my opinion is just a little different from the conventional wisdom.

Monounsaturated fat, the kind found in olive oil, macadamia nut oil, avocados, and so on, is a fat that causes you no harm whatsoever. Diets high in this fat, including the Mediterranean diet—have been associated with lower blood pressure, lower rates of heart disease, and even lower risks for dementia and Alzheimer's.

My good friend Mark Houston, M.D., director of the Hypertension Institute at St. Thomas Hospital, Nashville, says that monounsaturated fats (like that found in olive oil) help make available to the body a miracle molecule called nitric oxide, which helps keep your arteries open. Houston even recommends 4 tablespoons a day of olive oil for his patients!

But here's my not-so-secret theory, and it's beginning to be shared by more and more of us on the cutting edge of nutrition. The real health benefits of olive oil have more to do with polyphenols, the class of plant chemicals found in olives and the oil that's made from them. These olive polyphenols have been found to be effective against a host of microbes, and they are powerful antioxidants as well.

But the question of whether it's the polyphenols or the monounsaturated fat is a moot point. You get both when you use extra-virgin olive oil, so who cares? Either way you win, and your health benefits.

And if you happen to be wondering what the heck *extra virgin* means, here's the deal: Olive oil is one of the very few oils in the world that you can consume in its crude form, without a drop of processing. You could literally stomp around in a barrel of olives, gather up the liquid from the bottom of the barrel, and pour it on your salad. Not refining the oil conserves all the amazing antioxidants and other nutrients found in the plant.

But once you start machine harvesting, and processing the oil with heat, you start damaging a lot of those delicate compounds that are responsible for the health benefits. *Extra virgin* simply means it's as close to the "stomp on the olives" type of oil as you can get—minimal or no processing, very low heat, and as rich in the health-giving properties of olives as you can get without going to Australia or Greece and plucking the olives yourself!

Ingredients

12 ounces (340 g) lump crabmeat, such as
blue crab (drain if using canned)
½ pound (225 g) chilled cooked medium
or small shrimp, shelled and deveined
(okay to use thawed, frozen)
1 cup (175 g) prepared diced mango
(or grapes or grape tomatoes)
1 small serrano pepper, stemmed and
chopped (remove seeds for less heat)
¼ cup (20 g) unsweetened shredded coconut
½ cup (80 g) sliced scallions
¼ cup (60 ml) lime juice (preferably fresh
squeezed)
1 teaspoon macadamia nut oil
(or olive oil)
1 teaspoon honey, optional
Pinches salt
¼ cup (34 g) toasted macadamia nuts,
lightly crushed, optional
1 head red lettuce, cored, leaves
separated

Light and Sassy Caribbean Seafood Salad

From Dr. Jonny: For some reason, this salad reminds me of sitting in my favorite beach bar about thirty feet from the ocean's edge in my favorite place in the world, the French side of St. Martin in the Caribbean. Maybe it's the lightness of the fish with the fresh taste of coconut mixed with lime and the hint of crunchiness from nuts that somehow seem like they were just gathered this very morning. The whole thing just feels and looks so healthy you feel you should be eating it in a bathing suit under a beach umbrella in the afternoon sun. But maybe that's just me. High in protein and low in calories, this salad is light and fresh no matter where you eat it. The zippy bite from the jalapeño is a delightful counterpart to the gentle sweetness of the coconut.

In a large bowl, gently mix together the crab, shrimp, mango, pepper, coconut, and scallions. In a small bowl, whisk together the lime juice, nut oil, honey, if using, and salt to taste and drizzle over the salad. Stir gently to coat. Lay out the lettuce leaves, spoon the seafood mixture over all, and garnish with the macadamia nuts, if using.

Yield: 4 servings
Per Serving: 259 Calories; 11g Fat (38.0% calories from fat); 28g Protein; 12g Carbohydrate; 3g Dietary Fiber; 152mg Cholesterol; 339mg Sodium

From Chef Jeannette

To Complete the Meal: Serve with wedges of fresh, ripe melon, such as honeydew or cantaloupe, for added potassium and vitamin A.

If You Have 5 More Minutes: Peel and dice half a medium cucumber for added low-calorie crunch. To brighten the flavor and add a little fresh herb punch, add ¼ cup (7 g) of chopped fresh cilantro or mint.

Ingredients

Salmon

4 boneless, skinless wild Alaskan salmon
  fillets (6 ounces or 170 g each; we like
  Vital Choice)
½ teaspoon salt
½ teaspoon black pepper

Couscous

1 cup (235 ml) light coconut milk
¾ cup (132 g) whole wheat couscous
1 teaspoon honey, optional
2 tablespoons (15 g) dried, unsweetened
  coconut, optional
Zest of 1 lime

Sauce

¾ teaspoon prepared garlic (or 1 clove
  minced)
2 tablespoons (28 ml) lime juice (fresh
  squeezed is best)
¼ teaspoon salt
¼ teaspoon cayenne pepper
¼ cup (60 ml) coconut oil, mostly melted

From Chef Jeannette

To Complete the Meal: Steam-sauté 4
large fresh baby bok choys (separated
into stalks) in 2 teaspoons of coconut oil
with 2 tablespoons (28 ml) of water and
sprinkles of salt and pepper until tender.

Superspeed Tip: To juice a lime or lemon
in no time flat, microwave the whole,
unpeeled fruit for 10 seconds, then roll
it under the heel of your palm for 5
seconds. Halve it, and use a reamer or
press to extract the juice. It will burst
right out of the fruit

Quick Energy Coconut-Lime Salmon and Couscous

From Dr. Jonny: Couscous in coconut milk? You betcha. Coconut
milk is used as a cooking base liquid in many cultures, especially in
Thailand, but also in Africa, the West Indies, and Hawaii. And with
good reason. First of all it tastes great. Second of all, it's really healthy.
The main fat in coconut milk (and coconut oil) is lauric acid, which
has been shown to contain antimicrobial and antiviral properties, and
the fat in coconut tends to be used by the body for energy rather than
stored as fat. Best of all, coconut milk imparts a delicious, rich taste
to anything you cook in it, such as, for example, couscous! Wait till
you taste this surprisingly refreshing, light, nutty couscous with a hint
of lime. Paired with high-protein, high-omega-3 wild salmon, this dish
makes a stunning main course; for total perfection, add a vegetable
side dish or salad. The whole thing comes together in minutes.

To cook the salmon: Preheat the grill to medium heat. Lightly season the
fillets evenly with salt and pepper and grill for about 4 minutes per side or
until desired doneness.

To cook the couscous: While the salmon is cooking, bring the coconut
milk to a boil over medium-high heat. Reduce the temperature to medium
low and stir in the honey, if using, couscous, and dried coconut, if using.
Stir well to combine and cover for 1 to 2 minutes or until the couscous has
absorbed most of the liquid. Stir in the zest, cover, and set aside.

To prepare the sauce: In a small bowl whisk together the garlic, lime
juice, salt, pepper, and coconut oil until well combined and lightly emulsified. (Or you can use an immersion blender.)

Serve the salmon over the couscous with a dollop of the coconut-lime
sauce, to taste, on the fish.

Yield: 4 servings
Per Serving: 476 Calories; 26g Fat (47.9% calories from fat); 38g Protein;
24g Carbohydrate; 4g Dietary Fiber; 88mg Cholesterol; 532mg Sodium

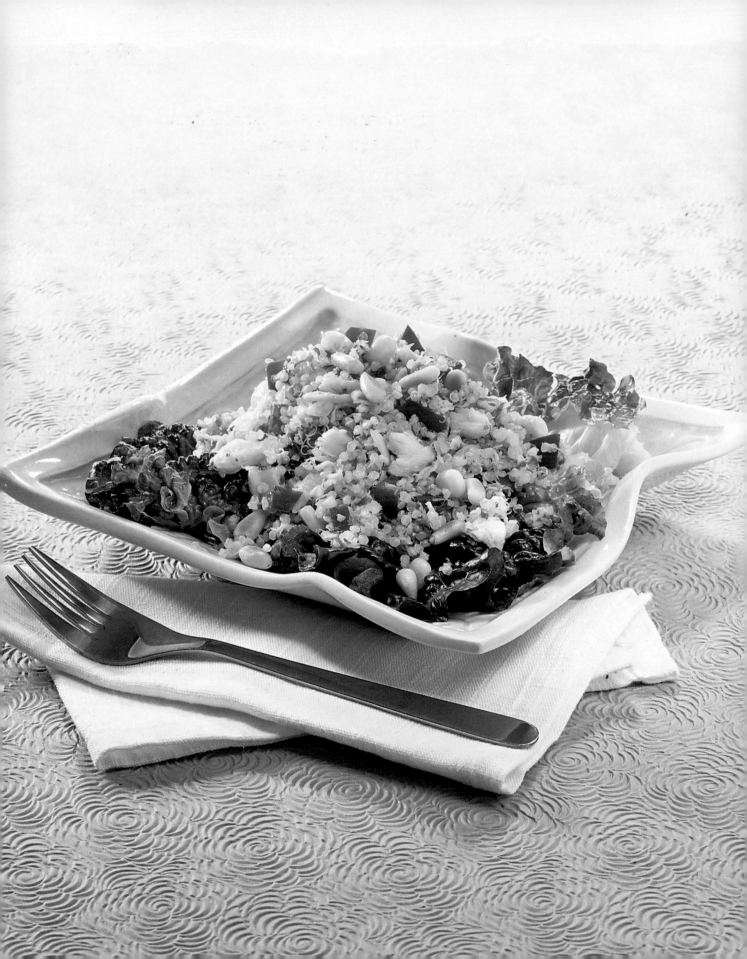

Ingredients

2½ cups (570 ml) chicken or vegetable broth
1¼ cups (213 g) quinoa, rinsed
1 cup (130 g) frozen corn, optional
¾ cup (30 g) tightly packed fresh basil
¼ cup (25 g) shaved or grated Parmesan cheese
3 tablespoons (45 ml) olive oil
2 cloves garlic, crushed
½ cup (70 g) toasted pine nuts, divided
Zest of 1 lemon plus 1 tablespoon (15 ml) fresh-squeezed lemon juice plus more, to taste
2 cans (6 ounces or 170 g each) white crabmeat, rinsed and well drained
2 large zebra tomatoes, diced
Salt and fresh ground black pepper, to taste
1 head red leaf lettuce, washed and leaves separated

From Chef Jeannette

Superspeed Version: To make this one-pot meal even quicker, use an equal amount of whole wheat couscous in place of the quinoa: It cooks up in less than 5 minutes, and the whole-grain version has a little more fiber than regular couscous.

Fresh and Fast Lemon-Pesto Crabmeat Quinoa

From Dr. Jonny: Here's a riddle for you: What looks like a grain, tastes like a grain, cooks up like a grain, but is really a seed? Answer: quinoa! Considered a superfood by the Incas as far back as 6,000 years ago, it originated in the Andean region of South America and remains a staple food for the American Indians of South America. It's the highest protein of the "cereal" grains (remember it's really not a cereal or a grain), and way healthier than a straight pasta dish but just as filling. Real crabmeat (not the fake stuff used in California rolls) has a ton of protein—a mere 3 ounces (85 g) of canned blue crabmeat has more than 17 grams! This is a true "one-pot" dish, with the lemony tang uniting multiple flavors in this light-but-hearty and truly delicious meal.

Bring the broth to a boil over high heat in a large saucepan. Add the quinoa, reduce the heat to a simmer, cover, and cook until tender and the tails have popped, about 12 minutes. Stir in the corn, if using, and let it sit covered for 1 to 2 minutes.

While the quinoa is cooking, make the pesto. Combine the basil, Parmesan, olive oil, garlic, ¼ cup (35 g) of the pine nuts, zest, and lemon juice in a food processor and process until well minced but not completely smooth.

In a large bowl, combine the hot quinoa, crabmeat, and pesto, to taste, and stir gently to combine well. Adjust the flavors with additional lemon juice, salt, or pepper, if necessary. Gently fold in the tomatoes and garnish with the remaining ¼ cup (35 g) pine nuts.

Serve the quinoa over individual beds of red lettuce leaves.

Yield: 4 servings
Per Serving: 522 Calories; 24g Fat (41.0% calories from fat); 32g Protein; 46g Carbohydrate; 5g Dietary Fiber; 71mg Cholesterol; 840mg Sodium

Ingredients

3 tablespoons (45 g) plain Greek yogurt

1 tablespoon (14 g) natural or vegan mayonnaise (we like Nayonaise or Vegenaise), or use more yogurt

1 tablespoon (15 ml) fresh-squeezed lemon juice plus extra

Pinch salt

1 tablespoon (4 g) chopped fresh dill, tarragon, or cilantro, or to taste

2 scallions, sliced thin

12 ounces (340 g) lump crabmeat (or use three quarters of a 16-ounce [455 g] can blue-crab claw meat, drained)

2 large ripe avocados, carefully peeled, pitted, and halved

From Chef Jeannette

To Complete the Meal: Try a refreshing grapefruit and tomato salad. Combine 2 cups (340 g) of fresh prepared grapefruit sections (in the refrigerated section) with 1 pint (300 g) of grape tomatoes and toss with a simple tangy dressing: Whisk together 2 teaspoons each of olive oil and fresh-squeezed lemon juice, 1 teaspoon of honey, pinches of salt and pepper, and, if desired, a teaspoon of fresh minced tarragon or mint.

Crab-Acados

From Dr. Jonny: Every so often Chef Jeannette comes up with ways to put some of my favorite foods together in a way you'd never think of doing, and the sheer magic of the result blows your mind. This is one of those times. Avocados are one of the greatest foods on the planet—most people know that they're rich in healthy monounsaturated fat, but less well-known is that they are also fiber heavyweights (between 9 and 17 grams, depending on size and origin). The crab is high protein and low calorie, and the creamy avocado goes surprisingly well with the tart flavor of grapefruit (in the suggested side). Couple that with the slightly acidic taste of antioxidant-rich tomatoes and you've got a winning combo! Cold, fresh, and delicious, this dish requires zero cooking. It comes together in a flash and is perfect for a busy summer evening!

In a large bowl, whisk together the yogurt, mayonnaise, 1 tablespoon (15 ml) lemon juice, salt, and herb until well combined. Gently stir in the scallions and crabmeat.

Sprinkle the extra lemon juice on the avocado halves and lightly coat using your fingers—lemon juice will slow the browning of the avocado flesh. Mound the crab salad evenly onto the four avocado halves.

Yield 4 servings
Per Serving: 272 Calories; 19g Fat (61.9% calories from fat); 18g Protein; 9g Carbohydrate; 3g Dietary Fiber; 70mg Cholesterol; 267mg Sodium

Ingredients

1 pound (455 g) fresh sea scallops

⅓ (80 ml) cup sherry

1 tablespoon (15 ml) olive oil

½ cup (80 g) prepared diced onion

1 bag (1 pound or 455 g) prepared chopped collard greens (or 1 pound [455 g] fresh leaves, stemmed and chiffonade cut, which steam-sauté quicker)

¼ cup (60 ml) vegetable broth or water

2 tablespoons (28 ml) mirin

1 tablespoon (15 ml) organic Worcestershire sauce (we like Annie's)

2 teaspoons butter (or nonhydrogenated vegetable spread, such as Earth Balance)

Salt and fresh ground black pepper, to taste

½ fresh lemon, optional

From Chef Jeannette

To Complete the Meal: Serve over lemon brown rice if you'd like a heartier meal (this tastes great with brown basmati rice, so next time you cook a batch, try it with lemon!). Prepare 2 cups (330 g) of frozen cooked brown rice (or parboiled brown rice) according to the package directions, and stir in 1½ tablespoons (25 ml) of lemon juice, 1 teaspoon of lemon zest, ½ teaspoon of salt, and ½ teaspoon of butter, nonhydrogenated vegetable spread, or olive oil. Mix well to combine and serve.

One-Pot Sherried Scallops and Collards without the Calories

From Dr. Jonny: Most of my weight-loss philosophy could be summed up in two words: *protein* and *vegetables*. Case in point: scallops and collards. The scallops are a great source of protein mixed with a superstar vegetable that's vanishingly low in calories (49 per cup!), relatively high in vegetable protein (4 grams), high in fiber (5 grams), and comes with a nice helping of both calcium and folate too. The quick sherry marinade helps to boost the buttery flavor of the dish and actually makes it taste much richer without globs of actual butter!

Rinse and drain the scallops and pour the sherry over all, mixing well to cover, if possible. Let them marinate while the collards are cooking (they can marinate for up to overnight if you purchased them the day before).

Heat the oil in a large sauté pan (or Dutch oven) over medium heat. Add the onion and sauté for 3 minutes. Add the collards, broth, mirin, and Worcestershire sauce, mixing well to combine. Cover and simmer for 8 to 10 minutes until tender. Remove the cover and push the collards to the outer edge of the pan, forming a ring around an empty space in the middle. Add the butter to the middle of the pan and quickly drain the marinating scallops. Add the scallops to the butter and sauté, turning occasionally, until just cooked through, about 1 to 2 minutes (30 to 45 seconds per side to seal). Do not overcook or the scallops will be tough. Leave a little pink in the centers. While the scallops are cooking, sprinkle salt and pepper to taste over all. Squeeze the lemon, if using, over all just before serving.

Yield: 4 servings

Serving: 232 Calories; 7g Fat (29.0% calories from fat); 23g Protein; 16g Carbohydrate; 5g Dietary Fiber; 43mg Cholesterol; 388mg Sodium

Busy Day Whole-Grain Linguine with Clam Sauce

Ingredients

8 ounces (225 g) whole-grain linguine or
  fettuccine (we like Barilla Plus)
1 tablespoon (15 ml) olive oil
2 shallots, chopped
1½ teaspoons prepared garlic (or 3 large
  cloves, minced)
1 can (10 ounces or 280 g) baby clams,
  undrained (high quality, stored in their
  own broth)
¼ cup (60 ml) dry white wine (great with a
  sauvignon blanc)
1 can (14.5 ounces or 413 g) diced tomatoes,
  drained
½ teaspoon fresh ground black pepper, or
  to taste
¼ teaspoon red pepper flakes, optional
2 tablespoons (5 g) chopped fresh thyme or
  slivered fresh basil (or ½ teaspoon dried
  thyme or dried basil)
¼ cup (15 g) chopped flat-leaf parsley

From Dr. Jonny: Barilla is a huge European food company that was founded in 1877 in Parma, Italy. You may have noticed that we're very fond of Barilla Plus pasta. Why? Because as pasta goes, it's high in protein and fiber, extremely high quality, and it tastes fantastic. This tomato sauce is easy to make (and awfully good), but I personally recommend that you check out the longer-cooking version with fresh littlenecks for a luxurious Saturday afternoon. Also recommended: the side dish of artichokes. Artichokes are a nutritional bargain. One cup provides an impressive 8 grams of fiber, 5 grams of protein, and a measly 1 gram of sugar, all for a caloric cost of—are you sitting down?—76 calories. Can't beat that!

Cook the pasta al dente according to the package directions.

While the pasta is cooking, heat the olive oil in a large skillet over medium heat. Add the shallots and cook for 3 minutes. Add the garlic and cook for 1 minute. Add the clams and their broth and wine, increase the heat to medium-high, and simmer for 3 minutes. Add the tomatoes, black pepper, and red pepper, if using, and simmer for 2 to 3 more minutes. (If using dried herbs, add them now.) Stir in the fresh herbs and toss with the hot pasta to serve.

Yield: 4 servings
Per Serving: 318 Calories; 5g Fat (14.6% calories from fat); 18g Protein; 51g Carbohydrate; 6g Dietary Fiber; 24mg Cholesterol; 56mg Sodium

From Chef Jeannette

To Complete the Meal: Serve with steamed artichokes. Clean two medium artichokes and trim the stems close. Place them, stems down, in a microwave-safe glass container and fill to ½ inch (1 cm) with water. Seal with microwave-safe plastic. Microwave on high for 10 to 12 minutes or until a leaf at the base pulls away easily. Use caution when removing the plastic wrap—that steam will burn! Serve with a few tablespoons of balsamic vinegar for dipping.

If You Have an Extra 45 Minutes: Prepare the fresh-fest version of this dish. Swap the canned tomatoes for 4 to 5 chopped fresh plum tomatoes, and swap the canned clams for fresh. Scrub 24 littlenecks clean and steam in a large stockpot with ¾ cup (175 ml) of white wine for 2 to 4 minutes or until they open (discard the ones that don't open). Clean the clams and chop them roughly. Use ¼ cup (60 ml) of the liquid in the pan for broth, but it will be sandy, so strain it before using (a double-mesh sieve lined with a damp paper towel works well for this).

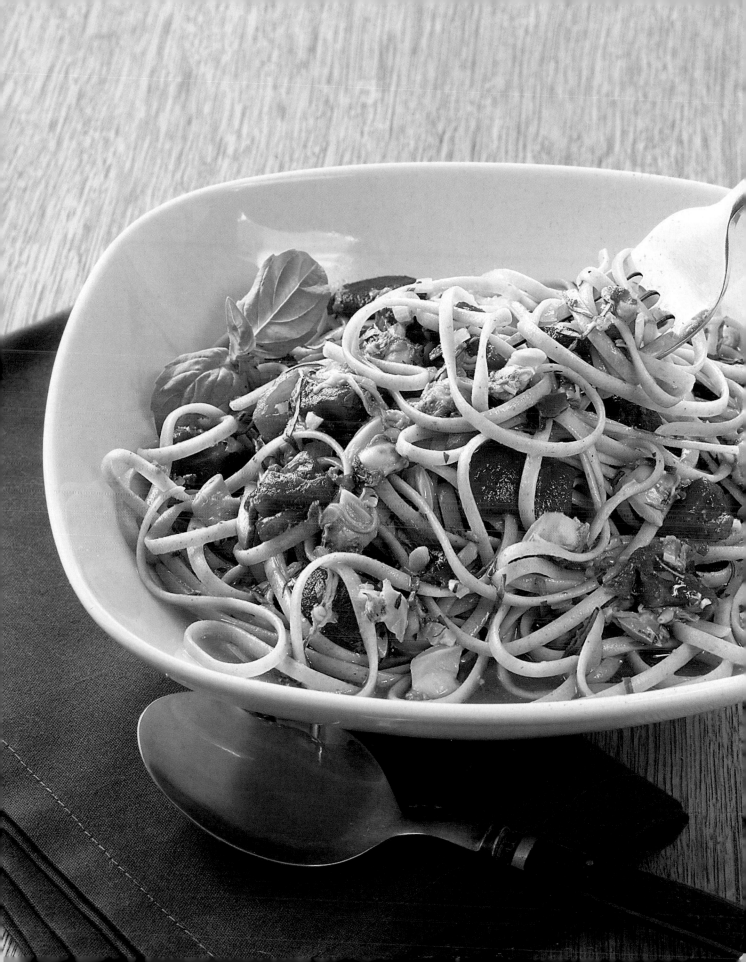

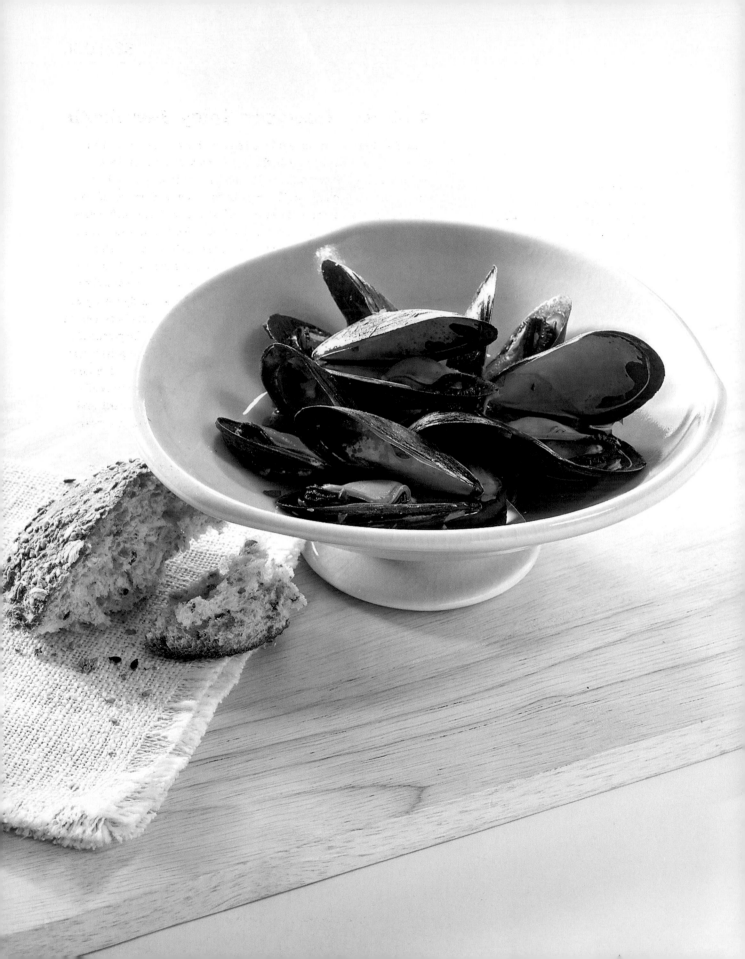

No-Fuss Mussels in Spicy Beer Broth

From Dr. Jonny: I'm not a drinker, so dark beer, or any other kind of beer, doesn't speak to me in the same way it does to my drinking friends, but I can tell you this: When you use it to cook with, it's a whole different experience. The alcohol cooks out and you're left with a hearty flavor that works incredibly well with any of several families of *Bivalvia Mollusca* (the fancy name for mussels). Mussels are a high-protein dish that is also an excellent source of selenium, as well as vitamin B$_{12}$. They also contain a few milligrams of zinc. Oysters, mussels, and clams don't have a strong taste, so the sauce is what makes eating them a taste sensation, and in this case that's exactly what it is. The anchovy powder lends a smoky, spicy bite to the dark beer and the bright tang of the cilantro. Highly recommended: Make the portobello mushrooms to complete the meal. This highly nutritious vegetable has almost no calories (35 per cup!), a surprisingly high amount of protein (nearly 4 grams!), and almost half the recommended minimum daily intake of selenium, one of the most important minerals on earth and one that has been consistently associated with lower rates of cancer.

Ingredients

2 teaspoons butter

1 teaspoon prepared, minced garlic

1½ cups (355 ml) high-quality dark beer

¼ to ½ teaspoon ancho chile pepper, to taste (or cayenne pepper, or 1 small whole dried chile variety)

2 pounds (900 g) mussels (about 40), scrubbed

⅓ cup (5 g) chopped fresh cilantro

Heat the butter in a large soup or stockpot over medium heat. Add the garlic and sauté for 1 minute. Add the beer, stir in the pepper, and bring to a simmer. Add the mussels, cover, and steam until just opened, 4 to 5 minutes.* Remove from the heat, stir in the cilantro, and serve with some of the beer broth poured over the mussels.

Yield: 4 servings

Per Serving: 252 Calories; 7g Fat (28.0% calories from fat); 27g Protein; 12g Carbohydrate; trace Dietary Fiber; 68mg Cholesterol; 670mg Sodium

*Discard any mussels that do not open with the others.

From Chef Jeannette

To Complete the Meal: Sauté 2 prepared sliced portobello caps over medium heat in 1 tablespoon (15 ml) of olive oil and 1 teaspoon of butter with a teaspoon of prepared minced garlic and a pinch of salt for 5 to 7 minutes or until soft. The rich mussels and beefy portobellos virtually cry out for a dark, sprouted-grain bread to sop with—just keep the portions moderate.

Tone Up with 10-Minute Tilapia over Lemony Tomatoes

Ingredients

1 tablespoon (15 ml) macadamia nut oil (or rice bran oil)

1¼ pounds (567 g) boneless, skinless tilapia fillets

Salt and cracked black pepper

2 tablespoons (28 ml) olive oil

1 teaspoon prepared garlic (or 1 large clove, crushed and sliced)

1 large lemon, peel and pith cut away, and roughly chopped (seeds removed, if possible)

1 pound (455 g) Campari tomatoes, halved (or use 2 pints [600 g] whole cherry tomatoes to save chopping time)

½ cup (50 g) whole pitted Kalamata or green olives, drained

2 tablespoons (18 g) capers

½ lemon, optional

¼ cup (15 g) chopped parsley, for garnish, optional

From Chef Jeannette

To Complete the Meal: Serve with a salad with curly endive, grated carrots, a sprinkle of feta cheese, and a drizzle of high-quality prepared Italian vinaigrette.

From Dr. Jonny: I live in Los Angeles, supposedly one of the trendiest cities in the nation, and as I write these words there's hardly a restaurant in the City of Angels that doesn't feature tilapia. If fish were starlets, tilapia would be on the cover of *People* magazine! It's a light white fish, high in protein, ridiculously low in calories, and much like Forrest Gump, it seems to be able to take on the flavor of anything it's paired with. In this case, the chunky rustic Italian vegetables combine beautifully with this flaky fish to give it a salty tang that sings on your tongue! (Good to note: This is one of Chef Jeannette's favorites!)

Heat the macadamia nut oil in a large skillet or Dutch oven over medium-high heat.

Evenly season the tilapia fillets to taste with salt and pepper. Add the fillets in a single layer to the skillet and allow them to cook, undisturbed, three-quarters of the way through, 3 to 4 minutes depending on the thickness of the fillets. Gently flip the fish and sear the other sides for 1 to 2 minutes or until just cooked though. (Try to flip the fish only once to prevent breakage.)

While the fish is cooking, heat the olive oil in large sauté pan at just below medium-high heat. Add the garlic, lemon, and tomatoes, and sauté for 3 to 4 minutes until the tomatoes start to soften. Add the olives and capers and sauté for 2 minutes more (bursting some of the cherry tomatoes, if using), until everything is hot and tender.

Make a bed in the hot lemon tomatoes and olives, and arrange the fillets on top.

Squeeze the lemon over all and garnish with the parsley, if using.

Yield: 4 servings

Per Serving: 247 Calories; 13g Fat (44.6% calories from fat); 27g Protein; 8g Carbohydrate; 2g Dietary Fiber; 61mg Cholesterol; 296mg Sodium

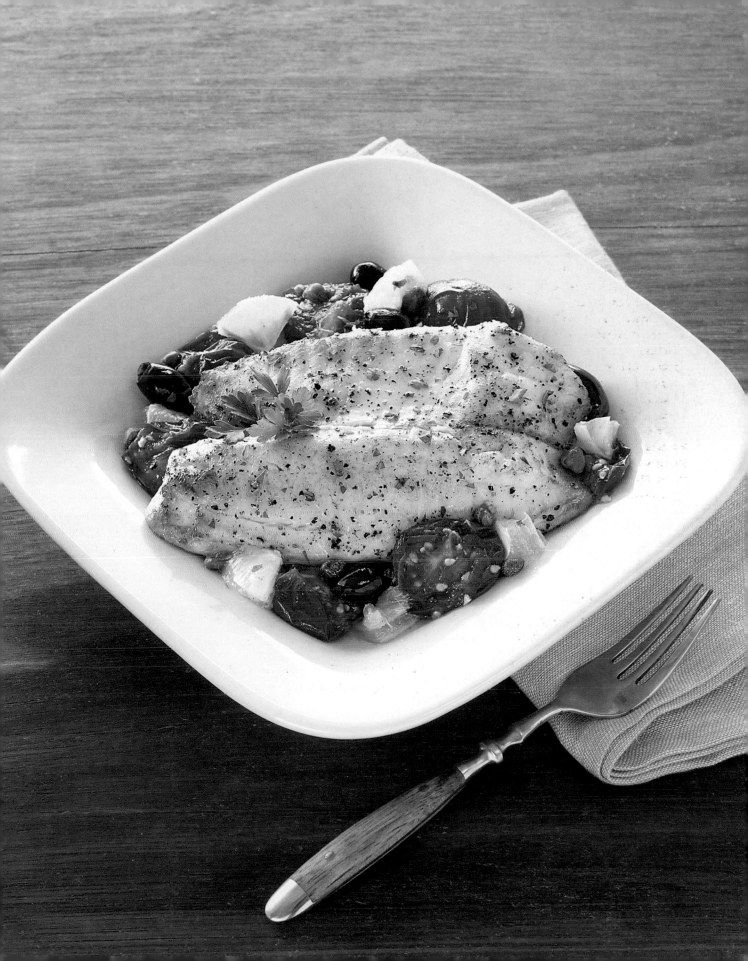

Light and Breezy Wasabi Tuna Boats

From Dr. Jonny: If you eat at sushi restaurants, you've undoubtedly encountered wasabi, even if you didn't know its name. It's a root vegetable that's ground into that little green paste served with sushi and sashimi and, if you're not careful, will make your mouth feel like it's on fire. But the fact is that wasabi has some surprising health benefits. It's rich in chemicals called isothiocyanates, which are anticancer compounds also found in the brassica family of vegetables (broccoli, cabbage, and the like). These compounds activate detoxification enzymes in the liver and actually have an anticancer effect. I love the mix of hot wasabi with sweet honey, tart lemon, and smooth yogurt—an incredible dressing! This dish is high on flavor and low on calories—and it makes a great meal for the hot weather of high summer!

Ingredients

Dressing

⅓ cup (77 g) plain low-fat yogurt

2 tablespoons (28 ml) fresh-squeezed lemon or lime juice

1 to 2 tablespoons (20 to 40 g) honey, to taste

2 teaspoons wasabi powder

Salad Boats

4 smallish cucumbers, peeled

2 cans (5 ounces or 140 g each) water-packed tuna, drained and flaked (we like Vital Choice)

½ cup (80 g) sliced scallions

1 tablespoon (8 g) toasted sesame seeds

1 head red oak lettuce, cored and torn, optional

In a small bowl, whisk together the yogurt, juice, honey, and wasabi powder until well combined. Set it aside to rest for a few minutes so the wasabi's flavor can develop.

Slice the cucumbers lengthwise, scoop out the seeds, and discard (or better yet, eat them!). Slice a thin strip from the bottom of each cucumber "boat" so it will sit flat without rolling over.

In a medium bowl, mix the tuna and scallions with the prepared dressing, to taste, until well combined.

Scoop equal portions of tuna salad into each cucumber boat and sprinkle with the sesame seeds. Serve on a bed of lettuce, if using.

Yield: 4 servings

Per Serving: 184 Calories; 2g Fat (9.7% calories from fat); 22g Protein; 21g Carbohydrate; 3g Dietary Fiber; 21mg Cholesterol; 262mg Sodium

From Chef Jeannette

Variation Tip: Substitute canned salmon for the tuna in this recipe if you prefer a higher concentration of omega-3s. You can also make the boats out of cored and halved red, yellow, or orange bell peppers instead of the cucumbers for a higher concentration of antioxidants.

Power-Up with Quick and Healthy Curried Halibut

Ingredients

2 teaspoons coconut oil

2 teaspoons prepared minced ginger
(or fresh, grated)

2 teaspoons prepared minced garlic
(or 3 cloves, minced)

2 teaspoons high-quality curry powder

1/2 teaspoon ground coriander

1/2 teaspoon salt

1/4 teaspoon cayenne pepper

1 can (14 ounces or 400 g) light coconut
milk

3 tablespoons (45 ml) lemon juice
(preferably fresh squeezed)

4 boneless, skinless halibut fillets
(4 ounces or 115 g each)

From Chef Jeannette

To Complete the Meal: While the fish is cooking, microwave 12 ounces (340 g) of prepared fresh or frozen green beans for 3 to 4 minutes in a sealed glass container until tender-crisp (or boil for 5 minutes in a large pot of unsalted water). While the beans are cooking, in a small bowl whisk together 1 1/2 tablespoons (24 g) of mellow white miso, 2 tablespoons (28 ml) of warm water, 2 tablespoons (6 g) of almond meal (e.g., Bob's Red Mill, or finely grind toasted almonds in a food processor), and 1 teaspoon of ginger juice (e.g., The Ginger People, or grate and squeeze a few tablespoons of fresh ginger), until well incorporated. Add the miso mixture to the hot beans and toss to coat.

From Dr. Jonny: Personally, I can't get enough of curry. If Ben and Jerry's came up with a curry-flavor ice cream, I'd probably be the first to buy it. (Then again, I was at the head of the line to buy the buggy first-edition iPhone, and look how that turned out.) The stuff that makes curry yellow is a spice called turmeric, which I consider a superfood of the spice kingdom. It contains active ingredients called curcuminoids, which have been found to have anticancer activity and are also one of the most anti-inflammatory plant compounds on the planet. Warm coconut curry is an absolutely great treatment for a tender fish such as halibut. And the nutty, salty gingered beans are the perfect finisher!

Heat the oil in a large skillet over medium heat. Add the ginger, garlic, curry powder, coriander, salt, and cayenne, and sauté for 1 minute until fragrant. Add the coconut milk, increase the heat, and bring to a boil, stirring to mix well. Stir in the lemon juice and add the fish, decreasing the heat to a simmer. Cook, flipping once, for 7 to 8 minutes or until the fish is cooked through (should flake with a fork).

Yield: 4 servings

Per Serving: 201 Calories, 10g Fat (43.8% calories from fat); 23g Protein; 6g Carbohydrate; trace Dietary Fiber; 33mg Cholesterol; 349mg Sodium

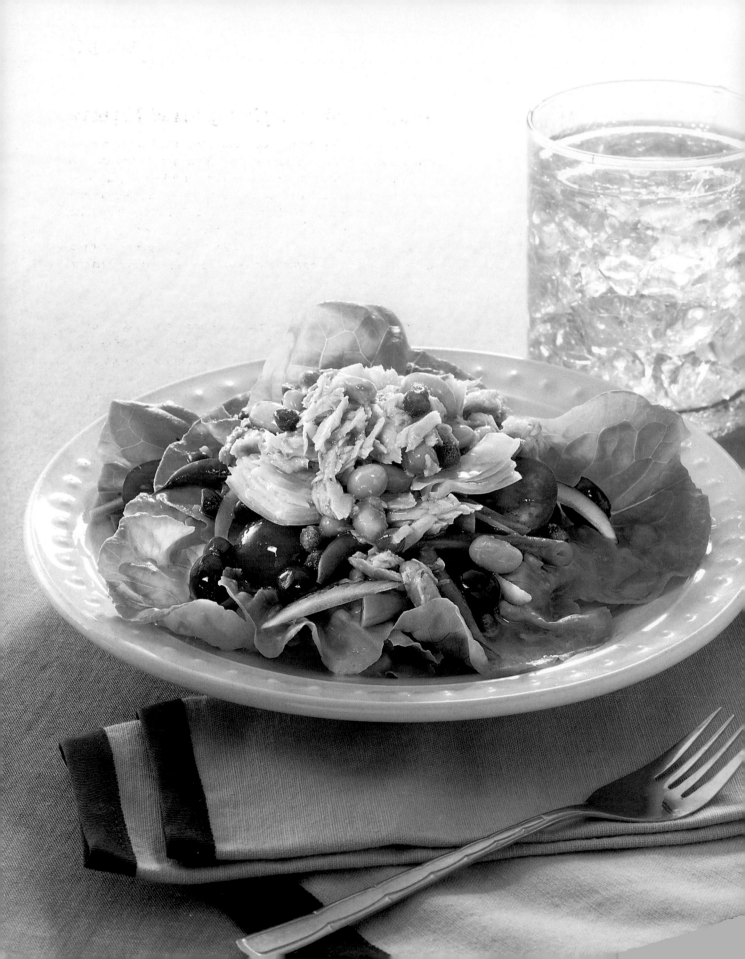

Simple and Energizing Salad Niçoise

From Dr. Jonny: It's hard to think of too many better basic sources of protein than good old-fashioned tuna fish. Rich in tyrosine, a precursor of the "alert" neurotransmitter dopamine, tuna can wake you up and energize you, not to mention fill you up and satisfy. It's just an all-around great food, and there are few better ways to eat it than in salad niçoise. In our version, canned Great Northern white beans take the place of the more traditional (and way less nutritious) white potatoes. That substitution alone has the double advantage of adding extra fiber and saving extra cooking time!

Ingredients

2 cups (248 g) frozen cut green beans (or prepared fresh)

½ red onion, very thinly sliced

2 cans (6 ounces or 170 g each) tuna packed in extra-virgin olive oil (we like Vital Choice albacore packed in organic extra-virgin olive oil), well drained

1 can (15 ounces or 425 g) Great Northern beans (or other white bean), drained and rinsed

7 ounces (195 g) quartered artichoke hearts in water (about 1½ cups or 355 ml), drained

1 bag (6.5 ounces or 185 g) butter lettuce

1 cup (100 g) niçoise olives, pitted and drained (or Kalamata)

1 pint (300 g) heirloom cherry or teardrop tomatoes

Dressing

¼ cup (60 ml) olive oil

1 tablespoon (28 ml) champagne vinegar (or white wine vinegar)

1 tablespoon (28 ml) lemon juice

¾ teaspoon prepared garlic (or 1 large clove garlic, minced)

1 teaspoon Dijon mustard

¼ teaspoon salt

¼ teaspoon fresh ground black pepper

1½ tablespoons (13.5 g) capers, drained, or to taste

Steam the frozen beans in the microwave in a tempered glass container with a vented rubber lid (we like Pyrex) for 2 to 3 minutes or until tender-crisp (or steam on the stovetop as directed on the package). Set aside to cool slightly.

Submerge the onion slices in a bowl of cold water while you assemble the rest of the salad (cold-water soaking removes some of the "bite" of raw onion).

In a medium bowl, whisk together the olive oil, vinegar, lemon juice, garlic, mustard, salt, and pepper. Stir in the capers and pour half the dressing into a cup and set aside. Add the tuna, beans, and artichoke hearts and gently stir to evenly combine and coat.

Drain the onions and pat dry. In a large salad bowl, make a bed of lettuce, add the olives, tomatoes, onions, and green beans, and spoon the tuna evenly over the top.

Pour the remaining dressing evenly over the salad.

Yield: 4 servings

Per Serving: 681 Calories; 20g Fat (25.5% calories from fat); 47g Protein; 83g Carbohydrate; 27g Dietary Fiber; 43mg Cholesterol; 831mg Sodium

From Chef Jeannette

To Complete the Meal: Serve with a medium-bodied white wine with a touch of fruitiness, such as a Côtes du Rhône, or try Santa Carolina Pinot Noir from Chile for a red option.

Superspeed Tip: No time to make a dressing from scratch? Try Newman's Own Organic Tuscan Italian, or Annie's Naturals Artichoke Parmesan for something with a little bite.

If You Have 5 More Minutes: Add a teaspoon of lemon zest and a sprinkle of dried basil to the dressing to brighten the flavor.

Ingredients

Edamame Daikon Rice Threads

2 cups (236 g) frozen shelled edamame,
unsalted

8 ounces (225 g) stir-fry rice noodles (vermicelli style; we like Thai House)

½ cup (58 g) grated, peeled daikon radish,
optional

⅓ cup (5 g) chopped fresh cilantro

½ cup (120 g) pickled ginger*

2 cups (110 g) curly endive lettuce, stemmed
and pulled apart

1 tablespoon (8 g) gomasio** (or black sesame seeds or toasted regular sesame
seeds), optional

Dressing

2 tablespoons (28 ml) low-sodium tamari

2 tablespoons (28 ml) sake (or rice wine or
mirin)

1 teaspoon toasted sesame oil

Sashimi and Condiments

1 pound (455 g) sushi-grade tuna (e.g., Vital
Choice Tataki or albacore medallions),
thinly sliced***

4 teaspoons wasabi paste, or to taste

¼ cup (60 ml) low-sodium tamari, or to
taste

From Chef Jeannette

To Complete the Meal: Serve with small glasses of warmed sake.

Tuna Sashimi with Edamame Daikon Rice Threads

From Dr. Jonny: In the late '80s, when I was a traveling musician, I conducted a production of *Blues in the Night* in Japan, and not surprisingly, I spent an awful lot of time in Japanese restaurants. I learned that sushi making is such a respected art that chefs apprentice for two years just learning how to make the little plastic models of the sushi that are on display in every restaurant window. Picking out the right cuts of fish takes an even longer internship. Fortunately, better fish markets can do the work for you by choosing cuts of tuna that are suitable for eating raw, a practice that is perfectly healthy when the fish is properly chosen and prepared. This tuna sashimi dish uses the finest-quality raw tuna, loaded with protein and omega-3 fatty acids, plus edamame and daikon radish. It's a true power meal that's elegant, incredibly light, and low calorie!

Bring a large pot half filled with lightly salted water to a boil. Add the edamame beans and boil for 5 minutes or until tender (or according to package directions).

Pour the boiling water through a fine-mesh sieve or colander (to catch and drain the beans) and into a large bowl. Add the rice threads to the bowl and soak to al dente in the boiled water according to the package directions (usually 5 to 7 minutes).

While the threads are soaking, whisk together the tamari, sake, and toasted sesame oil.

In a large bowl, toss together the edamame, rice threads, daikon, cilantro, and ginger. Dress to taste and divide among four plates. Top with equal portions of curly lettuce and garnish with the gomasio. Serve the sashimi on the side with the wasabi and tamari.

Yield: 4 servings

Per Serving: 574 Calories; 11g Fat (16.3% calories from fat); 50g Protein; 78g Carbohydrate; 7g Dietary Fiber; 43mg Cholesterol; 1105mg Sodium

*Prepared pickled ginger is a popular sushi condiment. You can find the conventional version in jars in large grocery stores. You can also find an unsweetened version (usually in bags) in the macrobiotics section of most natural food stores.

**Gomasio is a Japanese condiment made from sesame seeds and salt. Find it in the macrobiotics section of natural food stores. It's useful if you are cutting your salt consumption, as the nutty flavor of the sesame makes the small amount of salt strong enough to pop the flavors of vegetables, soups, and salads.

***To slice the tuna yourself, use a very sharp knife and, in one fluid motion, slice each piece very thinly (¼ inch or 0.5 cm) against the grain of the tuna.

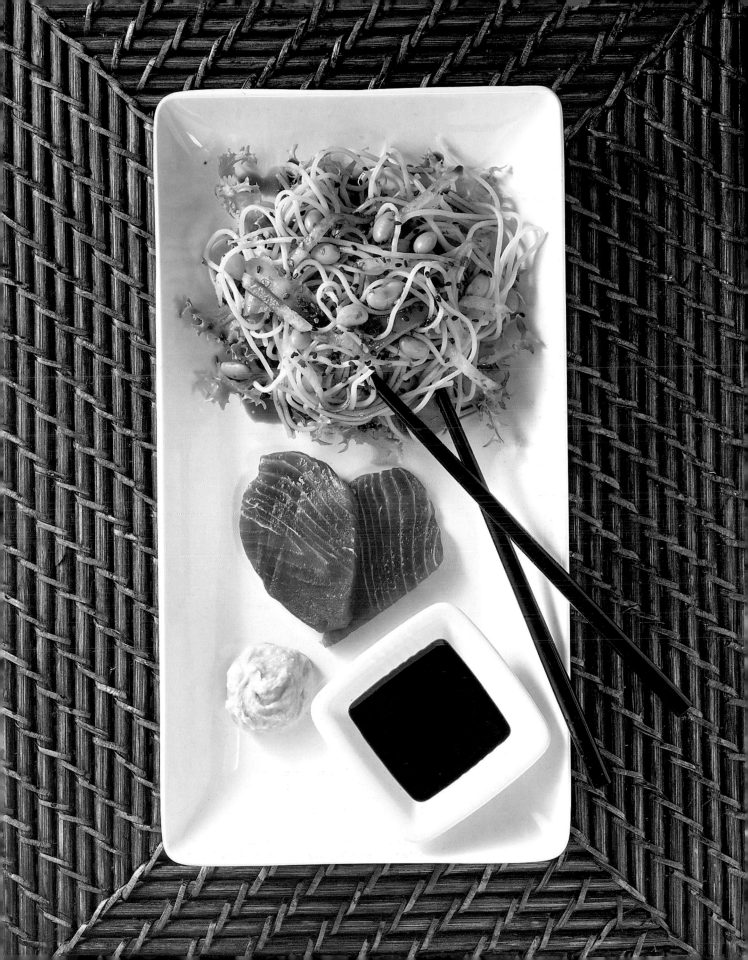

Ingredients

4 bluefish fillets (6 ounces or 170 g each)
$\frac{1}{2}$ teaspoon salt
$\frac{1}{2}$ teaspoon cracked black pepper
$\frac{1}{4}$ teaspoon chipotle pepper (or cayenne),
    or to taste
$\frac{1}{4}$ cup (85 g) maple syrup

From Chef Jeannette

To Complete the Meal: Serve with quick-cooking grits and tomatoes. Follow the directions on the package to make 2 cups grits, then stir in 1 cup (180 g) of chopped fresh tomatoes, $\frac{1}{2}$ teaspoon of dried thyme, and $\frac{1}{2}$ teaspoon of salt, and fresh ground pepper to taste.

If You Have an Extra Hour: Brine the fillets to remove some of the intense fishy flavor of bluefish. I live in Newport, Rhode Island, and it's common for a friend or neighbor to bring over a bluefish from time to time when the fishing is good. Blue is a rich, oily fish, and even when it's superfresh, the flavor is strong and distinctive. To mellow that somewhat (and tenderize the flesh), stir $\frac{2}{3}$ cup (200 g) of kosher salt into 1 quart (946 ml) of cold water. Place the fillets in the water and store in glass in the fridge for an hour. Rinse well and pat dry before grilling.

Super-Selenium Bluefish in a Snap

From Dr. Jonny: A little bluefish trivia, if you ever find yourself on *Jeopardy!*: This aggressive little fish clicks its teeth as it attacks other fish, so the small ones are called "snappers" and the adults are called "choppers." Regardless, they taste delicious, are plentiful along the Atlantic coast, and probably kept a lot of hungry Americans alive during the Great Depression of the 1930s, when they were a dietary staple. These fish are really good for you, too. One 4-ounce (115 g) fillet has a whopping 30 grams of high-quality protein, much more potassium than a banana, and is an excellent source of selenium, niacin, and vitamin B_{12}. The distinctive taste of the blue in this recipe is offset by the sweetness of the syrup and the kick of the peppers. My recommendation: Use 100 percent pure grade B maple syrup (not grade A)—it has more minerals!

Preheat the grill to medium heat (or heat a broiler).

Rinse the fillets well and pat very dry. In a cup, mix together the salt and peppers. Add the syrup to a pie plate and run the fillets through it, flipping and/or brushing them with the syrup to coat well. Spray the grill lightly with olive oil. Sprinkle the salt and pepper mix evenly over the fillets and grill (or broil) for 2 to 4 minutes per side, basting with the syrup at least once, until the fish flakes easily with a fork.

Yield: 4 servings
Per Serving: 267 Calories; 7g Fat (25.2% calories from fat); 34g Protein; 14g Carbohydrate; trace Dietary Fiber; 100mg Cholesterol; 371mg Sodium

Ingredients

¼ cup (10 g) fresh basil leaves

4 fresh flounder fillets (4 to 6 ounces [115 to 170 g] each)

Salt and fresh ground black pepper

2 tablespoons (28 g) butter

2 tablespoons (28 ml) fresh-squeezed lemon juice

¼ cup (28 g) slivered almonds

From Chef Jeannette

To Complete the Meal: Serve with chopped Swiss chard and yellow onion with a teaspoon of lemon zest and a few pinches of salt, steam-sautéed until tender in olive oil.

Variation Tip: For an unusual, folate-rich option, try substituting 3 tablespoons of fresh-squeezed orange juice (45 ml) for the lemon.

Light and Lemony 10-Minute Flounder

From Dr. Jonny: Flounder without butter is like a day without sunshine. Okay, maybe I exaggerate. But I'm kind of sick of hearing butter trashed as a "cooking oil." It's a perfectly good food, especially when it comes from grass-fed cows and is organic. It's also a perfectly healthy fat, and cooking with it may even have some advantages over vegetable oil. (I say "may" because I'm being polite and cautious; in my opinion, it has a *ton* of advantages over vegetable oil, but explaining why would take more pages than you're likely to want to read in a recipe introduction!) Anyway. Add the rich taste of butter to the light, incredibly low-calorie white fish, season with almonds and lemon, and you've got the core of a perfect light, high-protein meal that works in any season. Tip from Jonny: Chef Jeannette takes no responsibility for the cooking opinions expressed by the resident nutritionist in this duo (me) but for what it's worth, I think this dish works equally well when cooked in high-quality organic coconut oil (such as Barlean's brand), or even with a mix of half butter, half coconut oil. And as long as I'm putting my two cents in, why not try sprinkling a few coconut flakes on top of it as well? I'm just saying.

Stack the basil leaves on top of each other and roll them up together like a cigar. Slice or snip widthwise into thin strips. Set aside.

Lightly season the fillets all over with salt and pepper, to taste. Heat the butter in a Dutch oven or large skillet over medium heat. Once melted, stir in the lemon juice and add the fish and almonds. Cook the fish for 2 to 3 minutes per side or until just cooked through (flakes with a fork). Sprinkle the basil over all to serve.

Yield: 4 servings

Per Serving: 248 Calories; 11g Fat (41.8% calories from fat); 34g Protein; 2g Carbohydrate; 1g Dietary Fiber; 97mg Cholesterol; 196mg Sodium

Choosing the Healthiest Salmon—Farmed Fish versus Wild

I have some bad news: There's a world of difference between farmed and wild salmon.

Now before I tell you why, let me give you a spoiler alert: If you can't get wild salmon, you should probably still eat the farmed kind, because some salmon is better than none. But if you have a choice, and most people do, choose and insist on wild salmon. Is it more expensive? Yes. Is it worth it? You be the judge.

At salmon farms, thousands of fish are crowded into small, roped-off areas known as "net pens," the fish equivalent of factory farms for cows. They're packed tightly and disease spreads rapidly (much like on farms), so antibiotics are the order of the day, both in feed and through injections. That's just for starters.

Salmon are natural carnivores and prefer to dine on mackerel, sardines, krill, and other crustaceans. In fact, the natural, bright red-pink color they have comes from a powerful (and red-colored) antioxidant known as astaxanthin, which is found in krill, a main staple of the salmon diet. But salmon raised in pens don't swim around hunting for krill. Instead, they exist on grain, a food that is completely unnatural for them, which results in their fat being much higher in inflammatory omega-6 fats than the fat of their wild brethren.

But wait, there's more. (Sorry, I warned you.)

Seven of ten farmed salmon purchased at grocery stores were contaminated with PCBs, according to independent laboratory tests by the wonderful consumer advocate agency Environmental Working Group. On average, farmed salmon have a whopping 16 times (that's 1,600 percent) higher content of PCBs than that found in wild salmon, and about 3½ times the amount found in other seafood.

That said, if you can't get any other kind of salmon, it's still worth it to eat this fish, but farmed is the poor cousin of the real deal, which is wild salmon.

And may I put in a plug for my friends at Vital Choice, a company in which I have absolutely no financial interest, but believe to be one of the most responsible and environmentally conscious food companies in America. This company, headed by third-generation Alaskan fishermen, strives to provide fish that have been caught by line, from pristine waters, are tested every which way and back for toxic metals, and are environmentally sustainable. I get all my fish sent to me from them, and once you've tasted it, you'll never go back to supermarket fish. You can find a link to Vital Choice directly on my website, www.jonnybowden.com, under Online Store/ Healthy Foods.

Ingredients

¼ cup (60 g) plain Greek yogurt

1 tablespoon (15 g) prepared horseradish sauce, or more to taste

2 teaspoons Dijon mustard

1 tablespoon (15 ml) lemon juice

¼ teaspoon cracked black pepper

4 roasted red peppers, drained (prepared) and diced

2 cold-smoked trout fillets (7 ounces or 195 g each), flaked

4 large whole-grain wraps (or serve open face on toasted slices of hearty bread, such as Mestemacher Sunflower Seed or Rye Bread)

4 cups (220 g) watercress or baby spring greens

⅓ English cucumber, peeled and grated, optional

From Chef Jeannette

To Complete the Meal: Serve these wraps with modest portions (¾ ounce or 21 g) of prepared roasted vegetable chips, such as Terra Exotic Vegetable chips and/ or fresh, ripe Anjou pears.

Fast and Fiery Smoked Trout Wraps

From Dr. Jonny: Trout, found in rushing streams of cold clear water, are probably one of the most sought-after sport fish. If you're lucky enough to eat one of these guys fresh from the stream, you'll understand why fishermen stand for hours in the water wearing big, high, uncomfortable rubber boots trying to outsmart them. They're simply delicious. (The fish, not the boots!) They're interesting, too; some species actually spend part of their lives in fresh water and part in saltwater. (Unfortunately, most of the trout in the United States is farm raised, and the taste varies considerably depending on the food that it's fed and the conditions under which it's raised.) But enough trout trivia. Trout is a protein powerhouse (about 20 grams in a mere 3 ounces [85 g]), low in calories (144 calories for 3 ounces [85 g] cooked fish), and an excellent source of both niacin and vitamin B_{12}. I'm particularly fond of the yogurt-based sauce in this recipe. The snap of the horseradish and the tang of the lemon nicely mellow the salty smokiness of the trout in this elegant and delicious wrap. Enjoy!

In a large bowl, whisk together the yogurt, horseradish, mustard, lemon juice, and black pepper. Add the diced red peppers and flaked trout and mix gently to combine. Lay out the wraps and place 1 cup (55 g) of greens in the middle of each one.

Divide the cucumber, if using, equally among the wraps and add to the greens.

Spoon one quarter of the dressed trout mixture over the greens and cucumber, roll the wraps closed, slice in half, and serve them, edges down, on the plate.

Yield: 4 servings
Per Serving: 273 Calories; 9g Fat (30.2% calories from fat); 26g Protein; 21g Carbohydrate; 5g Dietary Fiber; 61mg Cholesterol; 336mg Sodium

Meatless

Neither of us thinks meat is something you need to avoid at all costs, but we realize there are many situations that call for meatless dishes, and even carnivores like a break from the "hard stuff" once in a while. Hence this section. There are all kinds of scrumptious choices featuring beans (high-fiber and protein), soy foods (preferably fermented), and other delicious options. Feel free to enjoy and experiment. These dishes offer lots of variety with no sacrifice in the nutrition or taste department.

Potassium Powerhouse: Quickest Artichoke Pasta

Ingredients

12 ounces (340 g) whole-grain spaghetti or linguine (e.g., Barilla Plus)

4 packed (80 g) cups baby arugula, baby spinach, or combo (6-ounce [170 g] bag)

1 can (14.5 ounces or 413 g) cannellini beans, drained and rinsed

1 jar (10 ounces or 280 g) high-quality artichoke hearts in oil, drained and roughly chopped

1/3 cup (37 g) sun-dried tomato strips in oil, drained (optional)

1/3 cup (33 g) chopped black olives, optional

Olive oil, to taste

Salt and fresh ground black pepper

Crumbled feta or fresh grated Parmesan cheese

From Dr. Jonny: Being something of a low-carb guy, pasta isn't something I eat every day, but I do confess that I love the stuff. Here's a fast way to get your pasta fix in a healthy way. Artichokes are high in potassium, folate, and the eye-healthy nutrients lutein and zeaxanthin. The cheese adds protein (and rich flavor!), the olives add monounsaturated fat and a bunch of compounds known as phenols that have all kinds of health benefits (anti-inflammatory, immune boosting), and the beans add a ton of fiber. The result is a superfast, supereasy, heart-healthy Mediterranean meal that won't send your blood sugar skyrocketing.

Cook the pasta al dente as directed on the package. As soon as it is drained, pour it back into the empty pasta pot. Stir the greens into the hot pasta and allow them to wilt for a minute or two. Gently stir in the beans, artichoke hearts, tomatoes, and olives, if using.

Warm over low heat for a couple of minutes, if desired, adding a drizzle of olive oil to moisten. Season to taste with salt, pepper, and cheese.

Yield: 4 servings

Per Serving: 708 Calories; 4g Fat (5.3% calories from fat); 40g Protein; 137g Carbohydrate; 28g Dietary Fiber; 0mg Cholesterol; 202mg Sodium

From Chef Jeannette

Superspeed Tip: The fastest way to do a Mediterranean pasta is to simply dump the whole jar of artichokes with about half the oil into the cooked pasta after wilting the greens. Stir in some olives and feta for protein and great fats, and you have a hot, healthy, satisfying meal in just a few minutes.

To Complete the Meal: Serve with a side of Greek salad and a glass of wine. Try Duuton Estate Kylie's Cuvée Sauvignon Blanc or Santa Carolina Sauvignon Blanc.

Ingredients

8 ounces (225 g) whole grain penne (e.g., Barilla Plus)

1 tablespoon (15 ml) olive oil

1 cup (160 g) prepared diced onions (or 1 yellow onion, diced)

1 small zucchini, unpeeled, grated (food processor is fastest for this)

3 teaspoons prepared garlic (or 3 large cloves, minced)

2 prepared roasted red peppers, drained and quartered

1 teaspoon dried thyme (or 1 tablespoon [2.4 g] minced fresh)

½ teaspoon salt

¼ teaspoon black pepper

1 can (14.5 ounces or 413 g) diced fire-roasted tomatoes, undrained

1 tablespoon (15 ml) red wine vinegar

2 tablespoons (32 g) sun-dried tomato paste, or regular

1 can (15 ounces or 435 g) cannellini beans, drained and rinsed

Grated Parmigiano-Reggiano cheese, optional, to taste

Not Your Average Penne

From Dr. Jonny: I'm generally an advocate of lower carb consumption. But that doesn't mean I don't enjoy pasta. When I do eat it, I try to go for a dish that is balanced in protein and fat, not necessarily a carb orgy like your typical pasta dish. Well, this isn't your typical pasta dish. The cheese is high in calcium, and the beans—well, let's just say that eating beans on a regular basis is one of the greatest predictors for long life. This dish has a taste of Italy with its light, immune-boosting sauce, high-protein pasta, and rich, lacy cheese wafers!

Cook the pasta until tender according to the package directions. Heat the oil in a Dutch oven. Add the onions, zucchini, and garlic, and sauté them for 4 minutes. Stir in the peppers, thyme, salt, and pepper, and sauté for 2 minutes. Add the diced tomatoes, red wine vinegar, and tomato paste, and simmer for 3 minutes. Puree the sauce with an immersion blender—or in batches in a regular blender—adding a few tablespoons of water (or vegetable broth) if it's too thick. Add the beans, correct the seasonings, and simmer for 1 minute to heat through.*

Toss four equal servings of the pasta with sauce, to taste, topping with cheese, if using.

Yield: 4 servings

Per Serving: 673 Calories; 7g Fat (8.9% calories from fat); 35g Protein; 127g Carbohydrate; 21g Dietary Fiber; 0mg Cholesterol; 300mg Sodium

*If you have finicky eaters who won't be excited about beans in their pasta sauce, puree them. Tender white beans will "disappear," leaving you with a thick, flavorful sauce.

From Chef Jeannette

To Complete the Meal: Make up a batch of superquick and tasty Parmigiano-Asiago Wafers. While the vegetables are sautéing, in a small bowl, mix ¼ cup (25 g) of grated Asiago cheese, ¼ cup (25 g) of grated Parmigiano-Reggiano cheese, 1 ½ teaspoons of whole wheat pastry flour, and ⅛ teaspoon cayenne pepper—the mixture will be dry and crumbly. Using a large teaspoon, spoon eight small mounds of the mixture onto a nonstick baking sheet (or use a Silpat). Gather any stray pieces into the mounds and flatten them slightly with the back of the spoon. Bake for 4 to 5 minutes until melted and bubbly with lightly browned edges. Cool for at least 5 minutes before serving.

If You Have 30 More Minutes: Roast fresh peppers yourself for higher nutrient and flavor concentrations. Preheat the oven to broil, stem 2 fresh red bell peppers, slice them in half, and clap their open sides together over a disposal or trash can to remove the seeds. Lay the cut peppers face down on a broiling sheet and broil for about 10 to 15 minutes until charred. Remove from the oven and place in a bowl, covering tightly with plastic wrap for about 10 minutes until they are cool enough to handle. Slip the skins off with your hands.

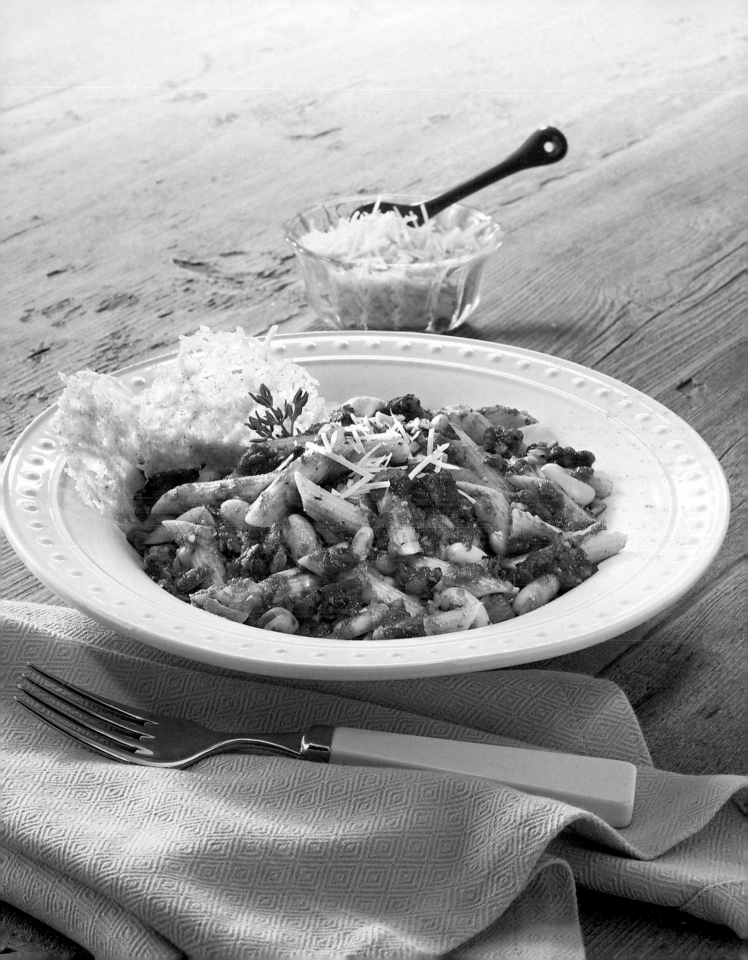

Ingredients

4 large whole-grain tortillas

1½ cups (240 g) ripe, fresh cantaloupe or
    honeydew melon chunks (or frozen,
    thawed)

½ fresh jalapeño, seeded, chopped, or to
    taste, optional

1 tablespoon (15 ml) lemon juice (preferably
    fresh squeezed)

1 teaspoon honey

1 teaspoon lemon zest, optional

Pinch salt

4 ounces (115 g) Camembert cheese, sliced
    thinly

1 ripe Anjou pear, cored and thinly sliced

From Chef Jeannette

To Complete the Meal: Serve with a
salad of 4 cups (80 g) of baby arugula
and 2 cups (290 g) of sliced seasonal fruit
dressed lightly with 2 tablespoons (28 ml)
of fresh-squeezed lime or lemon juice,
1 tablespoon (20 g) of raw honey, and
1 tablespoon (15 ml) of almond oil. Garnish
with toasted, sliced almonds or chopped
hazelnuts.

Variation Tip: Vary the fruit in this
dish with the seasons. Try sliced fresh
strawberries or peaches (not too juicy!)
in place of the pears, or substitute mango
for the melon in the salsa.

Quick, Whole-Grain Camembert Quesadillas

From Dr. Jonny: One reason I managed to stay out of Mexican restaurants for years was that the gummy, starchy, tasteless white tortillas
filled with boring old Jack cheese just didn't do it for me. But as the
saying goes, these ain't your parents' quesadillas! Chef Jeannette's
come up with some bold new flavor pairings coupled with whole-grain
wraps for a new experience in fast food. This quesadilla is accompanied
by melon salsa (the other version features chicken chutney—see page
46). Melon is the ultimate "high-volume" food, meaning it packs a lot
of nutrients into very few calories—being mostly water, it helps fill you
up without filling you "out." The melon salsa takes a few extra minutes
to make but hey, it's worth it—it'll be oh-so-fresh and you'll love the
way the creamy richness of cheese blends beautifully with the snappy
freshness of the melon salsa. Pears are very low on the glycemic load
scale, and high in the fiber department, delivering 6 full grams per fruit.

Preheat the broiler. Lay the tortillas out in a single layer on a large broiling
or baking sheet. When the broiler is almost at full heat, slide the sheet under the broiler for about 1 minute to quickly toast the tortillas and set aside.

While the broiler is preheating, place the melon, jalapeño, if using, lemon juice, honey, zest, if using, and salt in a blender and process until well
combined but still a little chunky. Set aside.

Heat a large, dry griddle over medium heat and lay out two of the tortillas. Place one quarter of the Camembert slices over half of each tortilla.
Place half the sliced pear over the same half and spread a layer of salsa
over the other half, to taste. Fold the quesadilla closed and grill until hot.
You can flip it once, if desired, to toast more evenly.

Repeat with the remaining two tortillas. Cut each tortilla into two
pieces and serve.

Yield: 4 servings

Per Serving: 277 Calories; 11g Fat (33.7% calories from fat); 12g Protein;
35g Carbohydrate; 6g Dietary Fiber; 20mg Cholesterol; 382mg Sodium

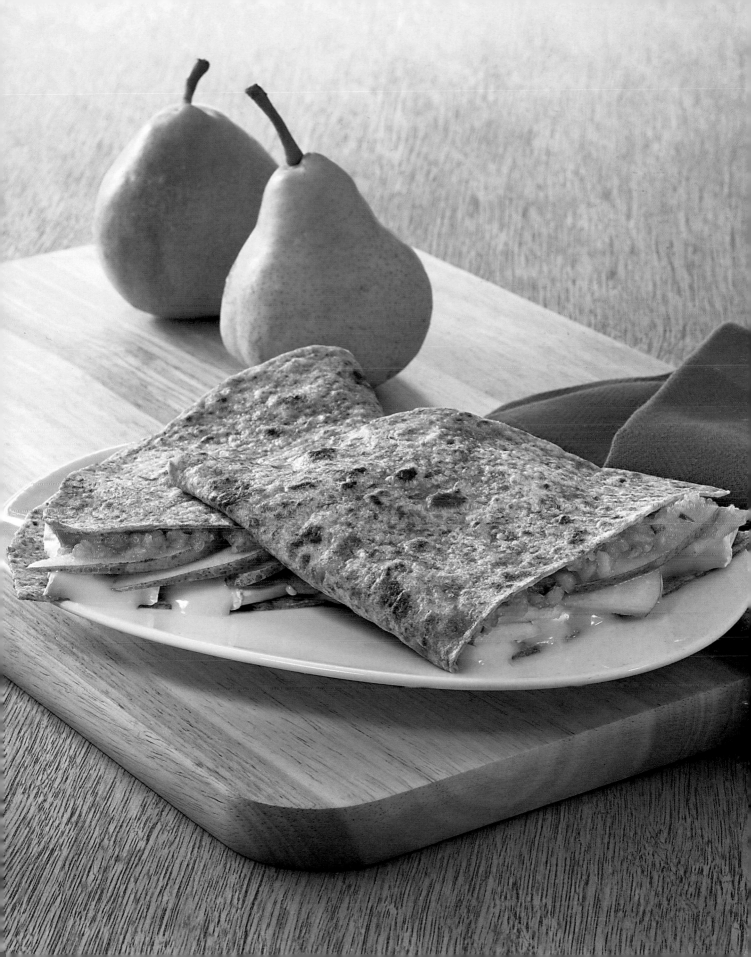

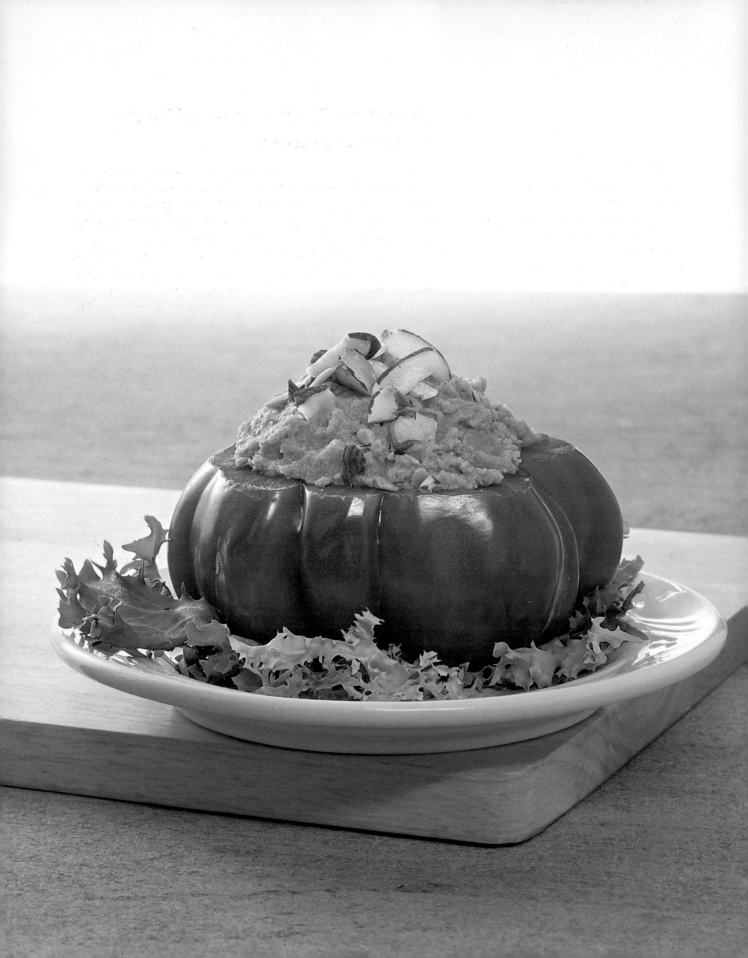

Nutritious Hummus-in-a-Hurry-Stuffed Tomatoes

Ingredients

1 can (15 ounces or 425 g) chickpeas, drained and rinsed

3 tablespoons (45 g) roasted tahini (or raw)

1 teaspoon minced prepared garlic (or 2 cloves, minced)

½ cup (120 ml) orange juice (fresh-squeezed, if possible)

1 tablespoon (15 ml) apple cider vinegar

2 teaspoons orange zest, optional

¼ teaspoon ground fennel

¼ teaspoon ground ginger (or ½ teaspoon prepared ginger juice)

Pinch ground cardamom

½ teaspoon salt

4 large heirloom tomatoes

¼ cup (28 g) toasted sliced almonds or pine nuts, optional

From Chef Jeannette

To Complete the Meal: Nestle the tomatoes in a bed of tender lettuce, mild sprouts (such as clover or alfalfa), and sliced red onion. Drizzle olive oil over all, if desired.

From Dr. Jonny: One of the big misconceptions about hummus is that it's fattening. Yes, a cup of conventional prepared hummus is high in calories (435), but who eats a cup? More important, it's rich in protein, healthy fat, and fiber (from those wonderful chickpeas), plus it has a decent amount of calcium, iron, phosphorus, and potassium. In this dish, Chef Jeannette uses a hint of orange to lighten up the classic hummus in this nontraditional salad. The recipe makes a terrific light, cooling meal, perfect for a summer afternoon or evening. Brimming with antioxidants from the heirloom tomatoes and the red onion, this dish is refreshing and satisfying without being heavy.

In a food processor, combine the chickpeas, tahini, garlic, orange juice, vinegar, zest, fennel, ginger, cardamom, and salt, and process until smooth, scraping down the sides, as necessary. Set aside.

Slice off the tops of each tomato and, using a spoon, remove and discard (or eat!) the seeds, hollowing out the centers.

Spoon each tomato full of hummus and garnish with nuts, if using.

Any extra hummus can be added to the suggested salad greens or refrigerated for later.

Yield: 4 servings

Per Serving: 538 Calories; 17g Fat (26.6% calories from fat); 25g Protein; 78g Carbohydrate; 22g Dietary Fiber; 0mg Cholesterol; 317mg Sodium

Ingredients

3 large, ripe heirloom tomatoes, halved

2½ tablespoons (40 ml) rosemary olive oil

¾ teaspoon prepared minced garlic (or 1 clove, minced)

½ teaspoon salt

½ teaspoon cracked black pepper

Pinch Sucanat

1½ tablespoons (25 ml) red wine vinegar

½ teaspoon anchovy paste, optional

1 can (15 ounces or 425 g) Great Northern beans, drained and rinsed

⅓ cup (33 g) fresh grated Parmesan cheese

6 cups (120 g) baby greens mix (spring mix, arugula, spinach, etc.)

From Chef Jeannette

To Complete the Meal: Serve this warm, tasty salad with bowls of hot, high-quality, low-sodium canned soup. Minestrone and lentil are great choices. We like Muir Glen or Health Valley. For an additional nutrient boost, grate some fresh vegetables into the soup while it is warming. Try zucchini, yellow squash, or colored bell peppers.

If You Have 10 More Minutes: Make your own rosemary garlic oil. Heat 3 tablespoons (45 ml) of olive oil with 4 crushed garlic cloves and a 4-inch (10 cm) sprig of fresh rosemary in a small sauté pan over medium heat for 1 to 2 minutes until the rosemary starts to bubble. Reduce the heat to low and continue cooking for 5 minutes or until the rosemary starts to brown. Remove from the heat, remove and discard the solids, and use the oil as directed.

Effortless Antioxidant Tomato Salad

From Dr. Jonny: The first time I tasted an heirloom tomato I couldn't believe it was a tomato. If you're used to the commercial, pink, crunchy, and tasteless tomatoes that populate the supermarket aisles, you'll be astounded to learn what a real tomato can taste like. Tomatoes are loaded with a powerful antioxidant known as lycopene. (A Harvard Medical School study that examined the dietary habits and health of more than 47,000 men found that four foods were associated with a lower risk of prostate cancer—tomato sauce, pizza (with tomato sauce!), strawberries, and…tomatoes! In this study, men who ate ten or more servings of foods containing tomatoes each week were 45 percent less likely to develop prostate cancer, and even those who ate four to seven weekly servings were 20 percent less likely to develop the disease.) While association is not necessarily cause, it does make you think! The lycopene in tomatoes is better absorbed with fat (hence the olive oil), and the white beans add not only a perfect taste complement, but a ton of fiber and nutrients as well. With its deceptively rich flavor from the touch of salty anchovy paste and the "quick" garlic rosemary oil, you'll love this easy-to-put-together dish.

Preheat the broiler. Place the tomatoes cut side up on an ungreased broiler pan and cook for 10 minutes or until soft.

While the tomatoes are broiling, in a medium saucepan over medium heat, whisk together the oil, garlic, salt, pepper, Sucanat, vinegar, and anchovy paste, if using, until lightly emulsified. Stir in the beans to coat well and cook for 3 to 4 minutes or until warm. Remove from the heat. Taste and adjust the seasonings to your liking, if necessary.

When the tomatoes are soft, remove from the oven and sprinkle with the Parmesan. Pour the warm bean mixture over a bed of greens and nestle the tomato halves in the mixture.

Serve immediately.

Yield: 4 servings

Per Serving: 509 Calories; 13g Fat (22.9% calories from fat); 29g Protein; 73g Carbohydrate; 23g Dietary Fiber; 6mg Cholesterol; 467mg Sodium

Prepared Meat Substitutes

There is a lot of controversy about whether or not to use the vegan "meatless meat" products out there. Though they are a processed food, we chose to include them in this book because of their generally high protein content and convenience of delivery. We love the fact that many are frozen and thus you can always have a ready protein at hand without needing to thaw it overnight (as with meats). Also, their cook time is only a few minutes, so they are among the fastest "pantry to plate" proteins in town. In addition, when incorporated into a recipe, they have a comparable look, mouth feel, and taste to many types of meats. This is particularly helpful if your family is used to eating conventional, factory farmed meats and you are trying to wean off of them. They are also very low in saturated fat, generally low in calories, and relatively inexpensive. We prefer the soy-free Quorn products over any that are made primarily from TVP (textured vegetable protein). We recommend keeping your consumption of these products to a minimum, but think they are a good choice for taste, familiarity, and variety in speedy dinner prep. When you have the time, go for grass-fed and wild caught meat and fish, but in a pinch, using the meat substitutes can get a good, nutrient-filled dinner on the table in a hurry.

Keen on Quinoa

Quinoa—pronounced *keen-wah*—is a seed that looks like a grain, cooks like a grain, and tastes like a grain. It originated in the Andean region of South America and has been an important food for more than 6,000 years. High in protein, it can be served in place of a starch or as a substitute for morning cereal.

So what's with the "heirloom" quinoa mentioned occasionally in this book? Well, in 1998, a group of families in Los Angeles agreed to cultivate quinoa in the traditional, organic way for a group called the Heirloom Quinoa Project. It is grown without chemical fertilizers, pesticides, or herbicides. It has a nice red shade, tastes delicious, and is as healthy as the day is long.

Quick and Hearty Vegetable-Bean Quinoa

Ingredients

1 cup (170 g) quinoa
2 cups (475 ml) vegetable broth
1 can (15 ounces or 425 g) black beans, drained and rinsed
1 jar (15 ounces or 425 g) high-quality prepared salsa
¼ cup (12 g) chopped chives, optional
½ cup (8 g) chopped fresh cilantro
½ cup (70 g) toasted pepitas

From Dr. Jonny: If you're a vegetarian and have wondered whether you're getting enough high-quality protein, this dish is perfect for you. In fact, even if you're like me and not a vegetarian, this is a great way to get your protein fix. Unlike most protein dishes, this one also comes with a ton of fiber. Beans are high in fiber, with all the accompanying benefits such as blood sugar control, digestive health, and a lowered risk of many illnesses. It's probably no accident that in all the areas of the globe where people live the longest, beans of some kind are a staple in the diet. And quinoa is the highest in protein of any cereal-type food on the planet. Quick and hearty, this dish tastes just as good reheated the next day as it does when you first make it!

In a medium saucepan, toast the quinoa dry for 2 minutes over medium heat. Add the broth and bring to a quick boil. Reduce the heat, cover, and simmer for about 12 minutes or until the quinoa is tender and the tails have popped. When the quinoa is done, add the beans, salsa, chives, if using, and cilantro, stirring gently to combine well. Cover and cook for 1 minute or until the dish reaches desired temperature. Fold in the pepitas and serve.

Yield: 4 servings
Per Serving: 712 Calories; 10g Fat (11.8% calories from fat); 36g Protein; 125g Carbohydrate; 24g Dietary Fiber; 1mg Cholesterol; 1296mg Sodium

From Chef Jeannette

To Complete the Meal: Sauté two medium zucchini sliced into thin coins in a little olive oil with 1 cup (150 g) of diced tricolor peppers and a sprinkling of salt and pepper for 6 to 8 minutes until desired tenderness.

In-a-Flash Frittatas I: Heart-Healthy Mediterranean

From Dr. Jonny: In the olden days, quiche used to be one of my favorite dishes. Then, during the insane "low-fat" era of the '80s, I would avoid it because of the eggs! When I came to my senses and realized eggs (and fat) were not the problem in our diet, I still tended to avoid quiche, only this time it was because of the high-carb crust. Enter Chef Jeannette's "in-a-flash frittatas"—not only superfast but also crustless. You get the taste and texture of a quiche without the heavy crust calories, poor-quality fat, and processed carbs. Chef Jeannette has put together a frittata with Mediterranean ingredients such as olives, olive oil, and feta cheese—great for the heart and the brain, and not so bad for your waistline either!

Preheat the oven to broil.

In a large bowl, whisk together the eggs, milk, oregano, basil, salt, and pepper.

Heat the oil in a 10-inch (25.5 cm) cast-iron skillet over medium heat. Swirl the oil to coat the entire inner surface of the pan, including the sides (you may need to oil a paper towel and "wipe" the sides to oil completely). Add the garlic, if using, and sauté for 1 minute. Add the artichoke hearts and olives and stir gently to combine. Sprinkle the feta over the top and gently pour the prepared eggs evenly over the top of all. Evenly distribute the tomato slices and sprinkle the surface lightly with the oregano. Cook for about 5 minutes until the outer edges are cooked and the center is still wet. Place under the broiler and cook for 3 to 4 minutes until the center is set and the surface has begun to brown.

Yield: 4 servings
Per Serving: 247 Calories; 17g Fat (57.9% calories from fat); 9g Protein; 19g Carbohydrate; 6g Dietary Fiber; 28mg Cholesterol; 866mg Sodium

Ingredients

6 eggs
2/3 cup (160 ml) milk (cow's, unsweetened plain soy, or almond)
1 teaspoon dried oregano plus extra
3/4 teaspoon dried basil (or 1/4 cup fresh, chiffonade cut*)
1/2 teaspoon salt
1/4 teaspoon cracked black pepper
2 tablespoons (28 ml) olive oil
1 teaspoon prepared minced garlic, (or 2 cloves fresh, minced), optional
1 can (14 ounces or 400 g) artichoke hearts in water, drained and coarsely chopped
1/2 cup (50 g) sliced and pitted Kalamata olives
2/3 cup (100 g) crumbled feta cheese
2 plum tomatoes, thinly sliced across the middle (to make circles, not ovals)

*Roll the leaves together like a cigar and slice or snip with scissors into thin ribbons.

From Chef Jeannette

To Complete the Meal: Serve with a large Caesar salad. To reduce starchy carbs and add antioxidant punch, replace the traditional salad croutons with jarred, sliced, roasted red peppers.

Ingredients

6 eggs

½ cup (120 ml) milk (cow's, unsweetened plain soy, or almond)

¼ teaspoon salt

¼ teaspoon cracked black pepper

2 tablespoons (28 ml) olive oil

1½ cups (240 g) prepared diced onion (or 1 medium sweet onion, diced)

1 teaspoon prepared minced garlic (or 2 large cloves garlic, minced)

1 package (8 ounces or 225 g) thinly sliced mushrooms (button or shiitake work well)

1 teaspoon dried basil

1 teaspoon dried marjoram

2 teaspoons low-sodium tamari

2 cups (60 g) packed baby spinach

From Chef Jeannette

To Complete the Meal: Serve with lightly grilled or broiled tomatoes drizzled with olive oil and a sprinkle of salt and fresh ground pepper.

If You Have 5 More Minutes: Use broccoli, a nutrient powerhouse, in place of the spinach. Chop 2 cups' (142 g) worth of bite-size broccoli florets and add them when you add the mushrooms, cooking a couple of minutes longer to soften. Continue with the rest of the recipe as directed.

To boost your calcium and vitamin D, add ½ cup (58 g) of shredded cheese to the top of the eggs after pouring them over the mushroom mixture. Gruyère or ¼ cup (25 g) fresh grated Parmesan both work well.

In-a-Flash Frittatas II: Immune Vitality Mushroom and Spinach

From Dr. Jonny: This is the second recipe in what I call Chef Jeannette's "frittata madness" series, and it features two great foods for the immune system—mushrooms and spinach. A 2009 study said mushrooms appear to give the immune system a nice big hand in attacking foreign invaders, which fits nicely with traditional wisdom about the healing properties of mushrooms. What's more, the common white button mushroom had even stronger immune-boosting effects than more exotic (and expensive) varieties such as oyster and shiitake mushrooms. Spinach is loaded with antioxidants, and regular consumption of garlic and onions is associated with lower blood pressure and reduced rates of certain cancers. Can't get more immune boosting than that!

Preheat the oven to broil.

In a large bowl, whisk together the eggs, milk, salt, and pepper. Heat the oil in a 10-inch (25.5 cm) cast-iron skillet over medium heat. Swirl the oil to coat the entire inner surface of the pan, including the sides (use a paper towel and "wipe" the sides to oil completely). Add the onion, garlic, and mushrooms, and cook for 4 to 5 minutes, stirring occasionally. Add the basil, marjoram, tamari, and spinach, stirring well to combine, and sauté for 1 to 2 minutes, stirring frequently, until the spinach is wilted and the mushrooms have softened. Drain any excess liquids from the pan, return to the heat, and gently pour the prepared eggs evenly over the top of all. Cover and cook for about 5 minutes until the outer edges are cooked, the frittata is mostly solid, but the center is still a little wet. Place under the broiler and cook for 1 minute or until the center is set and the surface is firm.

Yield: 4 servings

Per Serving: 229 Calories; 15g Fat (57.9% calories from fat); 14g Protein; 11g Carbohydrate; 2g Dietary Fiber; 322mg Cholesterol; 371mg Sodium

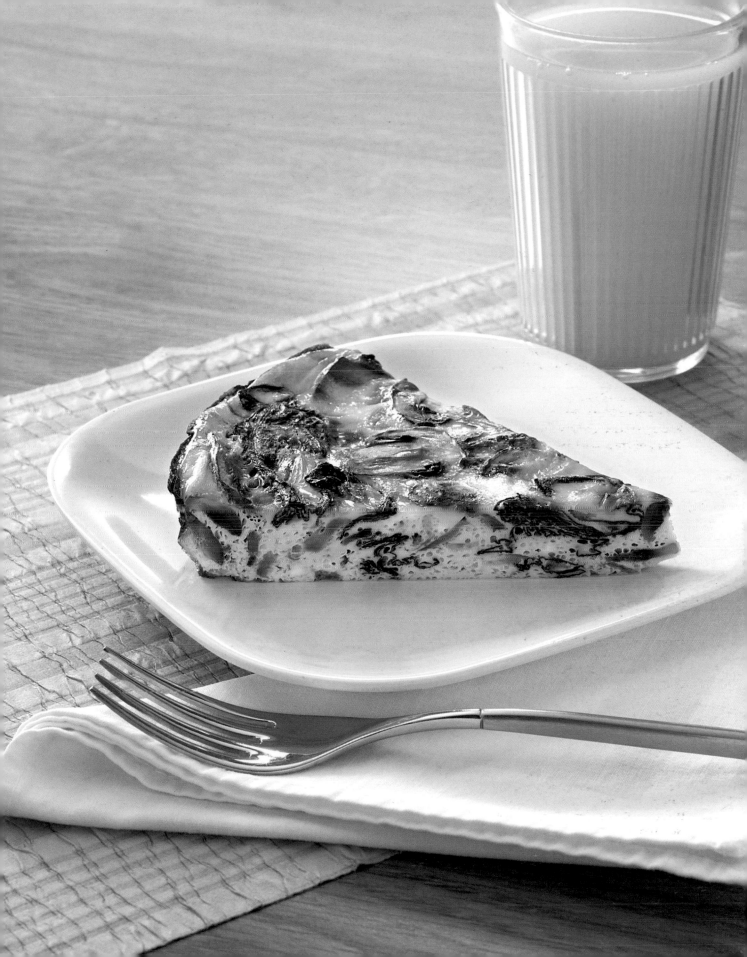

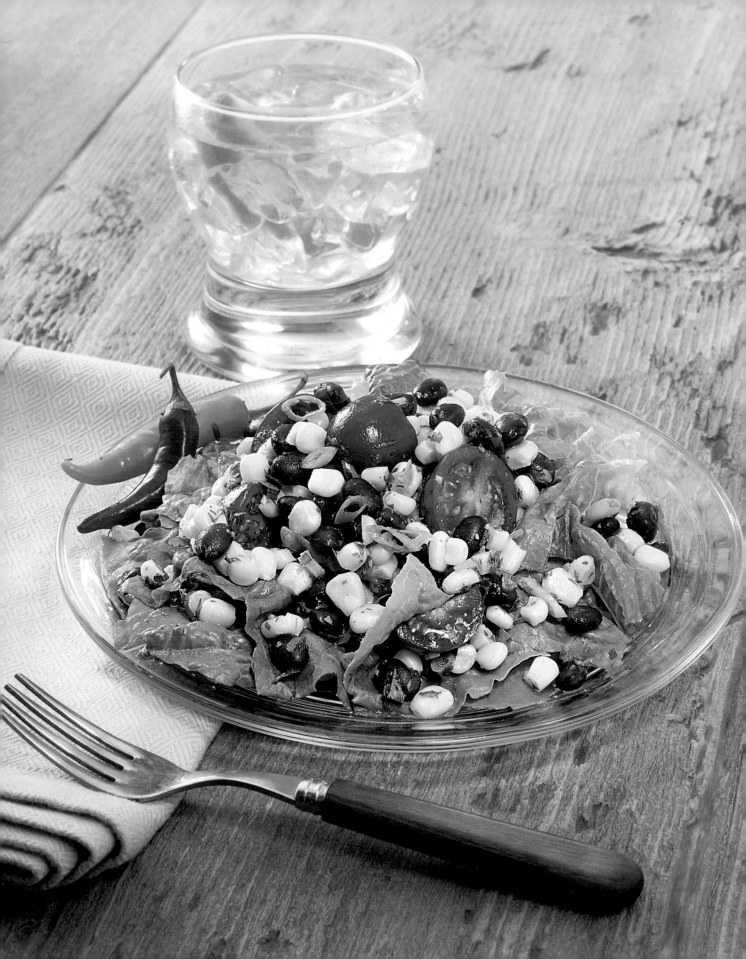

Fast and Fiberful Black Bean Salad

From Dr. Jonny: Black beans are my favorite variety of beans, even though nutritionally all beans are powerhouses. They taste great and are especially "friendly" to spices, which can make them taste anything from mild to wild. This salad is a perfect example. The jalapeño peppers give the salad a little bit of fire, the raw honey and spices balance the spicy taste with a touch of sweetness, and the limes give it a citrusy, summery—almost Caribbean—feel. I can easily imagine eating it at my favorite beach bar on Orient Bay in St. Martin!

Ingredients

Dressing

½ to 1 small jalapeño pepper, stemmed, to taste*

2 garlic cloves, crushed

Juice of 2 limes

2 teaspoons raw honey

2 teaspoons Dijon mustard

½ teaspoon ground cumin

¼ teaspoon ground coriander

½ teaspoon salt

⅓ cup (80 ml) olive oil

Salad

1 can (15 ounces or 425 g) black beans, drained and rinsed

2 cups (260 g) frozen corn, thawed

1 pint (300 g) heirloom mini tomatoes (yellow, teardrop, cherry, etc.)

1 bunch fresh cilantro, chopped

½ cup (80 g) sliced scallions, optional

1 bag (6 ounces or 170 g) chopped romaine lettuce (or 1 head, torn or chopped into bite-size pieces)

In a blender or food processor, pulse the jalapeño and garlic a few times until minced. Add the lime juice, honey, Dijon, cumin, coriander, and salt and pulse once or twice to briefly mix. Drizzle in the olive oil while processing until emulsified, scraping down the sides, if necessary.

In a large bowl, gently combine the beans, corn, tomatoes, cilantro, and scallions, if using.

Make a bed of romaine in a large salad bowl. Dress the bean mixture to taste and pour over the greens bed.

Yield: 4 servings

Per Serving: 598 Calories, 21g Fat (29.7% calories from fat); 26g Protein; 84g Carbohydrate; 19g Dietary Fiber; 0mg Cholesterol; 321mg Sodium

*The white membranes of the chile peppers store most of the pungent capsaicin, so for a milder "bite," remove both the membranes and seeds and use just the outer pepper. For a spicier bite with more metabolic power, dice and use the entire stemmed pepper. To protect your skin from burning, always use rubber gloves when handling raw or dried chile peppers and never touch your eyes!

From Chef Jeannette

If You Have 15 More Minutes: For the freshest, healthiest version, shuck three or four ears of summer corn and cook them in a pan of boiling water for 5 to 8 minutes or right on a hot grill for 10 to 12 minutes, or until cooked through. Using a sharp knife, slice the kernels off down the length of the cob on four sides and use in place of frozen corn as instructed.

To Complete the Meal: This salad can stand alone, or serve it with grilled bell peppers and zucchini, or grilled fish or chicken. See page 102 for veggie shish kebabs or page 73 for simple instructions for grilling fish.

Capsaicin: Hot Stuff

You'll love this story. It's 2008, and the presidential campaign is in full swing. I get a call from Tara Parker Pope, the terrific health writer for the *New York Times*. She asks me whether I'd care to comment on a statement by Hillary Clinton. I'm a bit taken aback because I usually don't get requests for political commentary. Turns out that Clinton had been quoted as saying that she attributed her indefatigable energy to eating hot peppers.

Well, I don't know whether you can get Clintonian energy from hot peppers, but there's more than a bit of truth embedded here. Peppers contain a chemical called *capsaicin*, which is actually what makes them hot. (The hottest peppers have the most capsaicin; green peppers have none because of a genetic weirdness, but I digress.) It's capsaicin that puts the nasty sting in pepper spray. And it's that very same capsaicin that was probably partly responsible for Hillary's energy. Why? Because in addition to burning the heck out of your tongue, capsaicin also stimulates circulation (maybe giving you a bit of a buzz?) and triggers pain receptors to release pain-killing endorphins.

No wonder she can put in eighteen-hour days!

Low-Cal Sloppy Joe-matoes in Minutes

From Dr. Jonny: The first time I ever tasted a sloppy Joe was at sleepaway camp, and I remember loving it. (Ah, to be young and completely clueless about health and nutrition!) The thing of it is, you can enjoy these childhood favorites and not feel guilty—it just takes a little bit of tweaking to turn a nutritional nightmare into something healthy. In this case, these bunless "Joe-matoes" are several cuts above the average sloppy Joe for health quality. They're low in fat yet still have that "mouth taste" I remember so well from childhood. And by the way, they are meant to be eaten sloppy! Chop up that tomato and spoon it into your mouth with the hot, faux-beef mix and pickle. Go on, enjoy—that's what napkins are for! The whole thing tastes great and will definitely satisfy the kid in you!

In a large skillet over medium heat, combine the tomato sauce, mustard, Worcestershire sauce, syrup, chili powder, salt, pepper, crumbles, and beans, stirring gently to mix well. Cook for 6 to 8 minutes or until hot throughout.

While the mix is cooking, slice the tops off the tomatoes, scoop out the seeds with a spoon, and discard (or eat them while you're waiting for dinner to be ready!). Spoon the Joe mix into the tomatoes to fill them up and spill over.

Yield: 4 servings
Per Serving: 490 Calories; 3g Fat (5.5% calories from fat); 35g Protein; 88g Carbohydrate; 33g Dietary Fiber; 0mg Cholesterol; 1218mg Sodium

Ingredients

1 can (14 ounces or 400 g) tomato sauce
2 tablespoons (30 g) Dijon mustard
2 tablespoons (28 ml) Worcestershire sauce (choose organic to avoid high fructose corn syrup, e.g., Annie's Worcestershire Sauce)
1 tablespoon (20 g) maple syrup
1 tablespoon (7.5 g) chili powder
1/2 teaspoon salt
1/2 teaspoon cracked black pepper
1 bag (12 ounces or 340 g) vegan "beef" crumbles (e.g., Quorn Meatless Soy-Free Grounds)
1 can (15 ounces or 425 g) kidney beans, drained and rinsed
4 large heirloom tomatoes

From Chef Jeannette

To Complete the Meal: Place the tomatoes over several large leaves of green lettuce before filling and garnish with chopped dill pickles.

Variation Tip: If you'd prefer "tidy Joes," use eight tomatoes instead of four. Or you can stuff the filling into baked potatoes, or roll it up in warm corn tortillas with a sprinkle of grated Cheddar.

Quick and Comforting Black Bean Chili

Ingredients

2 cans (14.5 ounces or 413 g each) fire-roasted diced tomatoes, undrained

2 cans (15 ounces or 425 g each) black beans, drained and rinsed

1 package (12 ounces or 340 g) frozen vegan "beef" crumbles (e.g., Quorn Meatless and Soy-Free Grounds)

1 cup (235 ml) chicken broth or water

¼ cup (60 ml) red wine

2 tablespoons (15 g) chili powder, or to taste

1 teaspoon ground cumin

¾ teaspoon dried basil

¼ teaspoon chipotle pepper (or cayenne), or to taste, optional

½ teaspoon salt

⅓ cup (37 g) sun-dried tomato strips in oil, drained

2 tablespoons (28 ml) balsamic vinegar

From Dr. Jonny: Once, many hundreds of years ago, I was a traveling theater musician on the road with *Joseph and the Amazing Technicolor Dreamcoat*, and one night the cast and crew had a chili-making contest. My group cheated: We found a fabulous little lady who owned a local restaurant and got her to whip up some homemade chili that we then brought to the contest. Okay, I'm confessing now—don't hate me—but the reason I tell you this is because this chili reminds me of that night. There are few dishes as rich and pleasantly filling as well-made chili, and if you're looking for something hot and satisfying on a cold night—something that you can whip up in 15 minutes—you won't do much better than this. In this meatless version (and in the one we cheated with), black beans are the featured ingredient (read about the health benefits of beans opposite). The sun-dried tomatoes add a touch of brightness to the classic flavors. Highly recommended should you get invited to participate in a chili-making contest!

Place the tomatoes, beans, crumbles, broth, wine, chili powder, cumin, basil, chipotle pepper, if using, and salt in a large sauté pan or Dutch oven over high heat and bring to a quick boil. Reduce the heat to medium, cover, and simmer for 7 minutes. Stir in the tomato strips and simmer for 3 minutes. Stir in the balsamic vinegar and serve.

Yield: about 10 cups

Per Serving: 347 Calories; 3g Fat (7.1% calories from fat); 23g Protein; 61g Carbohydrate; 16g Dietary Fiber; 0mg Cholesterol; 259mg Sodium

From Chef Jeannette

If You Have 5 More Minutes: Deepen the flavor and boost the nutrient content of the dish by sautéing 1 cup (160 g) of prepared diced onions (or dice 1 small yellow onion) in a tablespoon (15 ml) of olive oil over medium-high heat for 2 minutes. Add 2 teaspoons of prepared minced garlic (or 2 to 3 cloves, minced) and sauté for 1 more minute before adding the rest of the ingredients and increasing the heat to high. Superspeed option: Add 1 teaspoon of onion powder and ½ teaspoon of granulated garlic.

To Complete the Meal: Serve the chili with grilled zucchini or eggplant. Slice two large unpeeled zucchini lengthwise (about ¼ inch or 0.5 cm thick) or two unpeeled young (or Japanese) eggplants widthwise (about ⅓ inch or 0.7 cm thick); toss with olive oil, salt, and pepper; and grill until tender, about 3 minutes per side.

For an ultrafast option that will get those green-veggie minerals in, chop or tear kale into bite-size pieces (about 2 cups [110 g]) and add it when you add the liquid ingredients. You may need another few minutes of simmer time for it to get completely tender.

The Benefits of Beans

You can't really talk about beans without discussing fiber. Fiber, basically a nondigestible kind of starch, is associated with lower risks of diabetes, obesity, heart disease, and even some cancers. By no one's estimation do Americans get enough. The National Cancer Institute recommends at least 25 grams a day, the American Gastroenterological Association suggest 30 to 35 grams, and the Institute of Medicine recommends between 25 and 38 grams. Americans get a paltry amount anywhere from 4 to 18 grams (at best). Fiber normalizes bowel movements, helps maintain digestive and bowel health, lowers blood cholesterol levels, helps control blood sugar levels, and aids in weight loss.

Enter beans. If beans aren't the highest-fiber food on the planet, they're pretty close. A single cup of cooked beans provides anywhere from 11 grams (kidney beans) to an astonishing 17 grams (adzuki beans).

But even though fiber is an excellent reason to eat beans, it's not the only thing beans offer. A number of studies investigating health properties of foods have put beans among the top ten in antioxidant power. In the Nurses' Health Study II (a long-running study of thousands of people and their dietary habits), women who consumed beans as few times as twice a week had a 24 percent reduced risk of breast cancer, possibly because of the many phytochemicals found in beans such as diosgenin (which tends to lower the rate at which cancer cells multiply).

In 2005, the U.S. Food and Drug Administration approved a health claim stating "diets including beans may reduce your risk of heart disease and certain cancers." Apparently, even cultures that have never heard of the FDA seem to understand this intuitively. For what it's worth—and I think it's worth a lot—beans were one of the few foods found in the diet of every long-lived society investigated by reporter Dan Buettner for *The Blue Zones*, his book on healthy centenarians.

Ingredients

1 ½ cups (355 ml) chicken broth (or vegetable)

¾ cup (126 g) kasha*

2 tablespoons (28 ml) low-sodium tamari

1 teaspoon onion powder, optional

Fresh ground black pepper, to taste

2 tablespoons (28 ml) olive oil (or 1 tablespoon [15 ml] olive oil and 1 tablespoon [14 g] butter)

2 shallots, diced

8 ounces (225 g) sliced fresh shiitake mushrooms (prepared)

1 teaspoon dried thyme (or 1 tablespoon [2.4 g] fresh), optional

¼ cup (60 ml) unseasoned rice wine or white wine

1 can (15 ounces or 425 g) adzuki beans, drained and rinsed

From Chef Jeannette

To Complete the Meal: Prepare a 12-ounce (340 g) bag of frozen Chinese stir-fry veggies as directed, and toss with a dressing of 1 tablespoon (15 ml) of fresh-squeezed lemon juice, 2 teaspoons of low-sodium tamari, 1 teaspoon of toasted sesame oil, and a good sprinkling of sesame seeds.

Fiber Fest: Shiitake Adzuki Kasha

From Dr. Jonny: Buckwheat isn't really wheat at all. It's the fruit seed of a plant originally from Asia. The hulled grains of buckwheat, known as the buckwheat groats, are awfully nutritious, but they're pretty hard to chew. To make them edible they're usually soaked and cooked. When they're roasted they're known as kasha (or kashi). And they're terrific. Shiitake mushrooms are one of the trifecta of healing mushrooms (shiitake, reiki, and maitake) and have been used as medicinal foods for centuries. And adzuki beans have the distinction of being the highest in fiber of any bean in the U.S. Department of Agriculture's database! This dish is a nutritional wonder. Even more amazing is the fact that you can whip it up in no time.

Bring the broth to a boil in a medium saucepan over high heat. When the broth is boiling, reduce the heat to medium low and stir in the kasha, tamari, onion powder, and pepper. Cover and cook for about 12 minutes or until tender and all liquid has been absorbed.

While the broth is coming to a boil, heat the olive oil in a sauté pan over medium. Add the shallots, mushrooms, and thyme, if using, and sauté until tender, about 5 minutes. Add the wine, increase the heat to medium high, and sauté an additional 2 minutes until most of it is absorbed or evaporated.

When the kasha is tender, gently stir in the mushrooms and adzukis and adjust the seasonings to taste.

Yield: 4 servings

Per Serving: 552 Calories; 8g Fat (12.8% calories from fat); 37g Protein; 91g Carbohydrate; 20g Dietary Fiber; 0mg Cholesterol; 635mg Sodium

*Kasha is toasted buckwheat groats. As Dr. Jonny points out, although it has the word *wheat* in it, it is actually gluten free. Buckwheat, like quinoa, is a seed, and when toasted to make kasha, has an earthy, nutty flavor that combines well with mushrooms. It's a good grain to get to know for quick, healthy cooking as it is high in fiber and magnesium and cooks up in a short time. The consistency is somewhat mushy, so pair it with a crisp salad or green veggies for texture contrast. Look for it packaged or in bulk bins in natural food stores.

Ingredients

2 cups (475 ml) vegetable broth (or water)

1 cup (140 g) bulgur wheat (fine grind)

12 to 14 good-size collard leaves

1 can (15 ounces or 425 g) cannellini beans, drained and rinsed

3 tablespoons (48 g) sun-dried tomato paste

4 teaspoons prepared garlic (or 5 cloves, minced)

2 tablespoons (8 g) chopped fresh parsley, optional

½ teaspoon salt

½ teaspoon red pepper flakes, or to taste

Juice of 1 lemon (or 3 tablespoons [45 ml] prepared)

2 tablespoons (28 ml) olive oil

3 prepared roasted red peppers, sliced into strips, optional

From Chef Jeannette

To Complete the Meal: Serve with a tangy tomato salad. Slice four heirloom tomatoes thickly and combine with half of a sliced red onion. Dress with equal parts lemon juice and olive oil, and add sprinkles of salt and fresh ground black pepper.

Superspeed Tip: If you want to trim some time off this preparation, skip the stuffing step and simply tear or chop the collards into bite-size pieces before boiling. Serve the bulgur beans "open-faced" over a bed of the cooked collards and garnish with red pepper strips.

Low-Cal Stuffed Collards

From Dr. Jonny: Some of you know that I often speak of my childhood as a young black child, which of course, technically I was not, but *believed* myself to be, largely because of my love of gospel music, jazz, and what was then lovingly called soul food. And when you talk about soul food, you're talking about collard greens. This green hardly ever gets the respect it deserves, even though it's loaded with calcium, potassium, folate, and iron, has almost no calories, and is high in fiber. Stuff it with one of the healthiest foods on the planet—beans—and mix with bulgur wheat and you've got a dish for the ages! Okay, we admit, with the stuffing this recipe tips the timer at a little more than 15 minutes, but the cooking time is so minimal and it's so tasty that it's worth it. (And if you absolutely must cut the prep time, see Chef Jeannette's superspeed tip!)

Bring a large pot halffull of salted water to a boil, and in a small saucepan, bring the broth to a boil. Once the broth is boiling, pour it over the bulgur in a medium bowl. Soak for 7 minutes (it takes 15 for medium grind) and drain any excess liquid (or follow the package directions).

Lay the collards down and slice away the stems with a sharp knife from 3 to 4 inches (7.5 to 10 cm) into the bottom of the leaves (you can do this in three stacks of four leaves). You should be left with oval leaves with narrow Vs cut out where the stems came out.

Place the leaves gently into the boiling salted water and cook for 5 minutes. Without tearing the leaves, drain them carefully into a colander, letting them cool a bit while you prepare the stuffing.

In a food processor, pulse together the beans, tomato paste, garlic, parsley, if using, salt, red pepper flakes, lemon juice, and olive oil until well combined but still chunky. Turn out into a bowl and mix in the bulgur until well combined. Adjust the seasonings, if necessary.

To stuff the collards, lay a collard leaf in front of you—the V will be at the top of the leaf. Spoon a few tablespoons of the bulgur mixture onto the bottom of the leaf and roll the bottom edge up to cover it. Roll the sides in over the bottom fold and roll it, gently but tightly, away from you, from the bottom up.

Lay it on your serving platter, seam side down, and lay the red pepper strips over the tops of the rolls to garnish, if using.

Yield: 4 servings

Per Serving: 449 Calories; 7g Fat (13.2% calories from fat); 24g Protein; 78g Carbohydrate; 20g Dietary Fiber; 1mg Cholesterol; 816mg Sodium

Low-Glycemic Caesar Salad Pizza in a Snap

From Dr. Jonny: Being a pizza lover and not wanting to OD on carbs presents a bit of a problem, so I'm always looking for nutritious solutions to my pizza cravings that won't break my carb budget. This recipe fits the bill and then some—it just might be the lightest pizza ever. And no pizza I've ever seen is particularly high in fiber—but this one is, lowering the glycemic impact even further. Chef Jeannette nicknamed it "vegetarian salad pizza," but don't let the healthy-sounding nickname put you off. This is a delicious pie, loaded with colorful vegetables and high-fiber beans. You can make this meal rock by pairing it with a good red wine (see suggestions in To Complete the Meal!). Remember, there's a reason red wine is one of the seven "magical" foods that constitute the polymeal (the concept on which we built our book *The Healthiest Meals on Earth*). That reason is spelled *resveratrol*, the most promising anti-aging substance on the planet (see Nutritional Note on resveratrol on page 245).

Ingredients

1 teaspoon olive oil

1 whole-grain, premade, thin pizza crust (10 ounces or 280 g, about 12 inches (30 cm); we like Rustic Pizza organics)

3 cups (115 g) prepared chopped romaine lettuce

²/₃ cup (73 g) prepared grated carrots

4 Campari tomatoes, quartered (or use 2 large plum tomatoes, sliced)

3 small lemon cucumbers, unpeeled, quartered (or use ½ peeled regular cucumber, chopped)

2 prepared roasted red peppers, drained and chopped

1 can (15 ounces or 425 g) navy beans, drained and rinsed

³/₄ cup (53 g) prepared sliced mushrooms, optional

4 ounces (115 g) crumbled feta cheese (or use 2 ounces [55 g] fresh-grated Parmesan)

3 to 4 tablespoons (45 to 60 ml) high-quality prepared Caesar dressing, or to taste (we like Annie's Natural Organic Caesar Dressing)

Preheat the oven to 450°F (230°C, gas mark 8).

Lightly oil a baking sheet (or you can use a pizza stone) and place the crust in the center. Brush lightly with olive oil. Reduce the oven temperature to 425°F (220°C, gas mark 7) and cook the crust for 8 to 9 minutes or until lightly browned.

While the crust is toasting, in a large bowl, combine romaine, carrots, tomatoes, cucumbers, red peppers, beans, mushrooms, if using, feta, and dressing and toss gently to combine. Slice the pizza crust into quarters and serve as "scoops" under the salad.

Yield: 4 servings

Per Serving: 743 Calories; 17g Fat (20.1% calories from fat); 38g Protein; 117g Carbohydrate; 37g Dietary Fiber; 26mg Cholesterol; 717mg Sodium

From Chef Jeannette

To Complete the Meal: Enjoy it with a glass of Castello Delle Regine Sangiovese or Banfi Chianti Classico.

If You Have 10 More Minutes: Make your own Caesar dressing from scratch:

1 ½ tablespoons (23 g) anchovy paste
2 cloves garlic, crushed
2 tablespoons (28 ml) fresh-squeezed lemon juice
1 raw or lightly poached organic egg (or can use equivalent pasteurized)
1 teaspoon Dijon mustard
1 dash Worcestershire sauce, to taste (choose organic to avoid high-fructose corn syrup; we like Annie's)
⅓ cup (80 ml) extra-virgin olive oil
¼ cup (25 g) freshly grated Parmesan cheese

In a blender or food processor, combine the anchovy paste, garlic, lemon juice, egg, mustard, Worcestershire, olive oil, and Parmesan cheese, and process until blended.

If You Have 30 More Minutes: Roast fresh peppers yourself for higher nutrient and flavor concentrations. Preheat the oven to broil, stem two fresh red bell peppers, slice them in half, and clap their open sides together over a disposal or trash can to quickly remove the seeds. Lay the cut peppers face down on a broiling sheet and broil for about 10 to 15 minutes until they are charred all over. Remove them from the oven and place in a bowl, covering tightly with plastic wrap for about 10 minutes until they are cool enough to handle. Slip the skins off with your hands and use in the recipe as directed. Make some extra for sandwiches, salads, or for Not Your Average Penne (page 116)!

Ingredients

1 cup (170 g) quinoa, rinsed

2 cups (475 ml) vegetable broth

1 tablespoon (15 ml) olive oil

2 teaspoons prepared minced garlic (or 4 cloves, crushed and chopped)

1 pound (455 g) escarole, stemmed and chopped

½ teaspoon salt

1 cup (150 g) grape tomatoes (or halved cherry tomatoes)

3 tablespoons (45 ml) vegetable broth, white wine, or water

1 can (15 ounces or 425 g) chickpeas, drained and rinsed

⅓ cup (45 g) toasted pine nuts or chopped hazelnuts

4 to 5 dashes hot sauce, or to taste

¼ cup (20 g) shredded Parmesan cheese, optional

From Chef Jeannette

If You Have 5 More Minutes: Substitute kale for the escarole for a hardier, cooler-weather dish. Just add 5 minutes (and a tablespoon or two of extra liquid if the greens are tough) to the cooking time when you add the broth and chickpeas.

Easy, "All-Star" Escarole Quinoa

From Dr. Jonny: If meals were baseball teams, this terrific one-pot would be considered an all-star. It has all the biggies: foods that have been consistently found to be staples in the diets of the longest-lived people on earth. I'm talking about high-fiber beans (associated with lower rates of digestive issues, diabetes, and obesity), nuts (linked to lower rates of heart disease), and greens and tomatoes, which are filled with antioxidants. These are all mixed with quinoa, a grainlike seed that was once blended with fat into what the Incans called "war balls" for their ability to sustain marching armies for days on end. (In fact the Incas held the crop to be sacred and referred to quinoa as *chisaya mama* or "mother of all grains.") Quinoa is also the highest-protein "cereal" on the planet. Did I mention that this dish tastes great, too?

In a medium saucepan, add the quinoa and broth and bring to a quick boil over high heat. Reduce the heat slightly, cover, and simmer for about 12 minutes or until the quinoa is tender and tails have popped.

While the quinoa is cooking, in a 4- to 6-quart (3.8 to 5.7 L) sauté pan, heat the oil over medium.

Add the garlic and escarole, turning gently to combine. Cover for 1 minute, remove lid, stir, add the salt and tomatoes, and cook for 1 minute. Add the broth and chickpeas and cook for about 2 minutes until the beans are hot, the tomatoes are soft, and the escarole is tender.

When the quinoa is done, gently fold in the escarole mixure and nuts. Add the hot pepper sauce to taste, and correct the seasonings, if necessary. Garnish with the Parmesan, if using.

Yield: 4 servings

Per Serving: 793 Calories; 23g Fat (25.5% calories from fat); 36g Protein; 117g Carbohydrate; 27g Dietary Fiber; 5mg Cholesterol; 1329mg Sodium

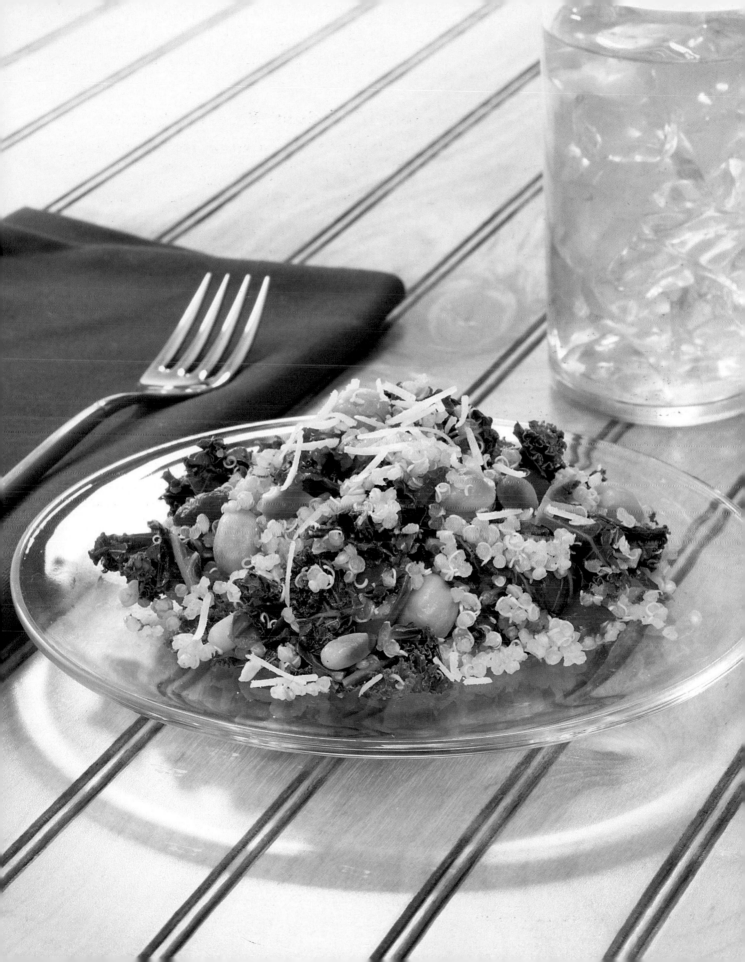

Ingredients

4 cups (950 ml) vegetable broth

2 cans (14.5 ounces or 413 g each) diced tomatoes with basil, garlic, and oregano, undrained

2 tablespoons (28 ml) red wine

1 teaspoon dried basil

3/4 teaspoon dried oregano

1/2 teaspoon salt

1/2 teaspoon fresh ground black pepper, or to taste

1/3 cup (53 g) whole wheat orzo (we like Rice Select)

1 can (15 ounces or 425 g) chickpeas, drained and rinsed

1 can (15 ounces or 425 g) kidney beans, drained and rinsed

3 cups (210 g) frozen or fresh, prepared vegetables of your choice (e.g., corn, broccoli florets, cauliflower florets, red bell pepper strips, sliced carrots, cut green beans, etc.)

1 1/2 cups (45 g) prepared chopped or baby spinach

1/4 cup (25 g) grated Parmesan cheese, for garnish, optional

The Healthiest Minestrone Stew

From Dr. Jonny: This stew is a perfect example of what I spoke about in my introductory chapter: nutrient density. The minestrone-like stew is simply brimming with vitamins, minerals, and phytochemicals, not to mention fiber from the double helping of beans. Best of all, you don't have to sacrifice a thing in the taste department. There's a small amount of whole wheat orzo for your toothy carb fix, a huge improvement over a bucket of white noodles! You also get some fat from the Parmesan cheese, which won't hurt you but will help make you feel full and add some sparkle to the mix. The canned tomatoes are filled with antioxidants such as lycopene. As a bonus, the whole shebang is low in calories—and high on flavor! Enjoy!

In a large soup pot, combine the broth and tomatoes and bring to a boil over high heat. Stir in the red wine, basil, oregano, salt, pepper, orzo, chickpeas, beans, and frozen or fresh-cut veggies. Reduce the heat and simmer for about 6 minutes. Stir in the spinach and simmer for 2 to 3 more minutes or until all the veggies are tender. Garnish with the Parmesan and serve.

Yield: 4 to 6 servings

Per Serving: 687 Calories; 9g Fat (11.9% calories from fat); 39g Protein; 116g Carbohydrate; 35g Dietary Fiber; 5mg Cholesterol; 1399mg Sodium

From Chef Jeannette

If You Have 10 More Minutes: Drop in a 10-ounce (280 g) "block" of chopped frozen spinach when you add the other veggies (in place of the fresh spinach). The longer cooking time will melt it down and fix you with a concentrated dose of "green" in this nutritionally souped-up soup.

Fresh and Fast Whole Wheat Pasta with Ricotta and Sun-Dried Tomatoes

Ingredients

1 package (10 ounces or 280 g) chopped frozen spinach, thawed and drained

¾ cup (188 g) fresh ricotta cheese

1 teaspoon dried basil

⅔ cup (74 g) sun-dried tomato strips in oil, drained

¼ cup (12 g) finely chopped chives or scallions (greens only)

½ teaspoon salt

¼ teaspoon black pepper

9 ounces (255 g) fresh, whole wheat pasta

1 tablespoon (15 ml) olive oil, or to taste

¼ cup (25 g) grated Parmesan cheese

From Dr. Jonny: Well-done, wet-noodle type pasta not only tastes like cardboard, it also affects your blood sugar in a much more negative way than cooking pasta al dente, which is actually the proper way to make pasta anyway. Why? Because overcooking destroys fiber and turns a perfectly good food into a mush that doesn't have to be broken down by the body. When this food is high in carbs—as pasta is—the result is a much higher glycemic impact on your blood sugar than you get from a food that is more chewy and fibrous. This tender fresh pasta cooks up in seconds—all it really needs is a hot bath—and the carb load is offset by the protein and healthy fat in the fresh ricotta. Bonus nutrition points for the calcium and vitamin D in the cheese, the antioxidant lycopene in the tomatoes, and the iron, calcium, magnesium, potassium, and fiber in the spinach!

Put a large pot half full of salted water on to boil over high heat. In a medium bowl, mix the spinach, ricotta, basil, sun-dried tomatoes, chives, salt, and pepper together well (a mixer will do this in seconds). When the water is boiling, add the pasta and cook according to the package directions (usually only for a minute to two), and drain. Combine the hot pasta and ricotta mixture, drizzle the oil over all to moisten, and garnish with the Parmesan to serve.

Yield: 4 servings

Per Serving: 428 Calories; 13g Fat (25.8% calories from fat); 22g Protein; 63g Carbohydrate; 10g Dietary Fiber; 29mg Cholesterol; 871mg Sodium

From Chef Jeannette

If You Have 10 More Minutes: With a few substitutions, you can turn this dish into a veritable fresh fest! The spinach is frozen, cooked, but if you have an extra few minutes, chop up a couple of packed cups of fresh baby spinach and use that instead. Sun-dried tomato strips are packed with flavor, but to lighten up on calories, substitute three fresh ripe heirloom tomatoes, chopped. You can even substitute the dried basil for ¼ cup fresh chopped!

Fresh whole-grain pasta has a light, delicious feel. Fresh ricotta cheese doesn't even taste like the same animal as supermarket ricotta—airier, with a melt-in-your mouth quality. Look for it at a local dairy, cheese shop, or natural food store. Many whole foods and high-end grocers also carry it.

To Complete the Meal: Serve it with a salad made with 6 ounces (170 g) of chopped romaine lettuce; one can of artichoke hearts, drained and halved; one small red onion, sliced; two sliced fresh tomatoes; and a prepared red wine vinaigrette (if you're making the pasta with fresh tomatoes, use jarred roasted red pepper strips instead). Garnish with a little Parmesan, if desired.

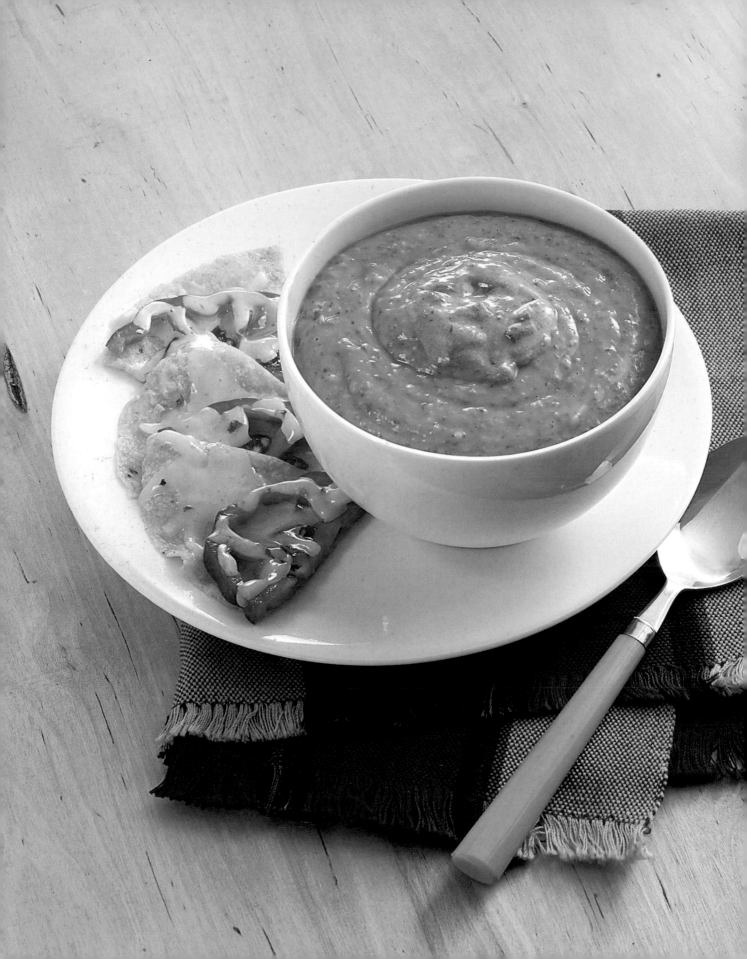

Avocado Soup with Cheesy Tortillas in No Time

Ingredients

Avocado Soup

2 ripe Hass avocados, peeled, pitted, and coarsely chopped
2 cups (60 g) baby spinach
2 cups (475 ml) low-sodium vegetable broth
Juice of 1 lime
¼ teaspoon salt
¼ teaspoon black pepper
Few dashes hot sauce, optional, to taste
⅓ cup (77 g) plain Greek yogurt
⅓ cup (87 g) jarred salsa

Cheesy Tortillas

4 sprouted corn tortillas (6 inches or 15 cm)
Drizzle olive oil
2 medium heirloom tomatoes, sliced thick
⅔ cup (75 g) shredded jalapeño Jack cheese

From Dr. Jonny: Here's a little-known fun fact about avocados that I'll bet you didn't know: They have fiber. Lots of it. A whopping 13.5 grams per avocado, which puts them right smack in the middle of the category of food with the most fiber on the planet, beans. Sure, avocados have a reputation as being "fattening," but that's only because they're moderately high in calories, not because there's anything inherently "fattening" about them. Fact is, they're loaded with some of the healthiest fat on the planet (the same monounsaturated fat found in olive oil). They have twice the potassium of a banana, a decent amount of folate (163 mcg), and provide about 4 grams of protein. What a superstar food! And what a rich, satisfying soup you can make from them, which is exactly what Chef Jeannette has whipped up in this creamy soup recipe, which you can put together in literally minutes with zero cooking. Wait till you try it!

Preheat the broiler.

Place the avocados, spinach, and broth in a strong blender or food processor, blending until smooth. Season with the lime juice, salt, pepper, and hot sauce, if using, to taste and pulse briefly to incorporate.

In a small bowl, combine the yogurt and salsa and mix well.

Lay the sprouted corn tortillas on a broiler pan and drizzle or brush lightly with olive oil. Lay two slices of tomato on each tortilla and sprinkle with the cheese, dividing evenly. Broil the tortillas for about a minute or until the cheese is melted and the tomatoes are hot, watching carefully to prevent burning.

Divide the soup among four bowls and garnish with the yogurt salsa, to taste. Serve the soup with the tortillas.

Yield: 4 servings
Per Serving: 369 Calories; 20g Fat (46.8% calories from fat); 12g Protein; 40g Carbohydrate; 10g Dietary Fiber; 2mg Cholesterol; 433mg Sodium

Ingredients

4 medium baking potatoes (choose Idaho, russet, or Yukon Gold)

1 package (12 ounces or 340 g) fresh or package (10 ounces or 280 g) frozen broccoli florets

2 medium heirloom tomatoes, quartered

⅔ cup (100 g) prepared, diced, colored bell peppers

⅔ cup (74 g) sun-dried tomato strips in oil, lightly drained

1 tablespoon (15 ml) olive oil

¾ teaspoon garlic powder

1 teaspoon dried basil, plus extra

1 teaspoon dried oregano, plus extra

Pinches salt and fresh ground black pepper, to taste

½ cup (60 g) shredded mozzarella cheese (or feta), or to taste

From Chef Jeannette

To Complete the Meal: Add a prepared protein, such as a free-range rotisserie chicken. You can also add additional cooked proteins to the potato with the broccoli, such as cooked chicken, diced organic ham, or drained and rinsed canned navy or black beans. If you don't want the extra protein, finish the meal with a large dark green salad with the remainder of the prepared diced peppers and a drizzle of Caesar or balsamic dressing.

Nourishing Potatoes Series I: Better Broccoli Pizza Potato

From Dr. Jonny: I admit it: One of my guilty pleasures is pizza, though I rarely eat it. One reason is the dough, which offers little more than empty calories and a lot of starch and carbs. Enter Chef Jeannette's clever turn on the old favorite. Potatoes, while not the most nutritious vegetable on the planet, are nonetheless a lot better than the white dough used for conventional pizzas, and recent research ranked russet potatoes fifth among 100 different foods tested for antioxidant activity! One medium potato with the nutritious skin (very important to keep that in there!) has way more potassium than two medium bananas, not to mention about 4 grams of fiber. Stuff that baby with nutrient-rich vegetables such as broccoli, tomatoes, and peppers, and you've got a real winner. This dish is filling, satisfying, and cheesy, nicely complemented by the fresh-tasting sauce.

Preheat the broiler.

Scrub the potatoes well and pierce with a fork. Place potatoes in the microwave with 3 tablespoons (45 ml) of water in a small bowl or cup. Microwave on high for 8 to 10 minutes or until tender, turning the potatoes once at 4 minutes for even cooking.

While the potatoes are cooking, bring water to boil in a large pot with a steamer basket. When the water is boiling, place the broccoli in the steamer and cook until tender-crisp (about 3 minutes for fresh, 4 to 5 for frozen). Set aside.

While the broccoli and potatoes are cooking, combine the tomatoes, peppers, sun-dried tomato strips, olive oil, garlic powder, basil, oregano, salt, and pepper in a food processor.

Process until mostly smooth (about 35 seconds), scraping down the sides as necessary. Adjust the seasonings if necessary.

When the potatoes are tender, remove from the microwave and place on a broiler sheet.

Working carefully so you don't burn your hands, slice each one lengthwise down the middle and gently pull the halves apart. Stuff each potato with one quarter of the broccoli, pizza sauce to taste, and one quarter of the mozzarella, sprinkling the basil and oregano over the cheese.

Broil for 2 to 3 minutes or until the cheese is melted and bubbly.

Yield: 4 servings
Per Serving: 300 Calories; 10g Fat (29.5% calories from fat); 10g Protein; 46g Carbohydrate; 7g Dietary Fiber; 13mg Cholesterol; 143mg Sodium

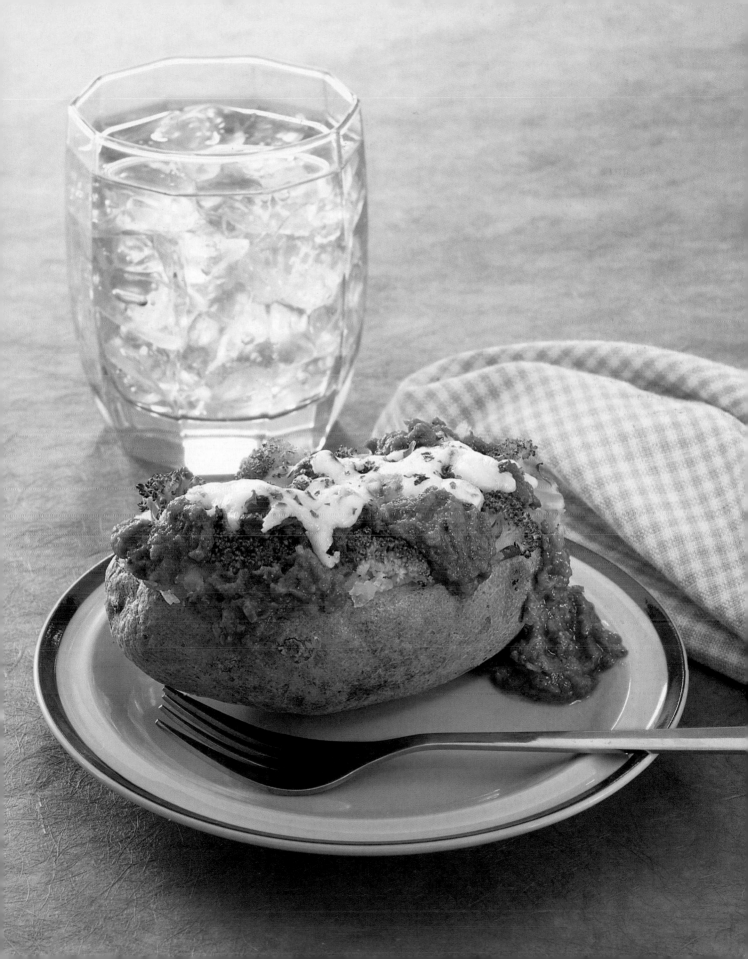

Nourishing Potatoes Series II: Beany Greenie Potato

From Dr. Jonny: Ask almost anyone for a list of healthy foods and you're sure to hear broccoli mentioned pretty quickly. But the thing of it is, broccoli has a couple of lesser-known relatives that are frequently overlooked, and both of them bring a lot to the table, no pun intended! Broccoli rabe is a fiber heavyweight—one bunch provides more than 12 grams of the stuff, putting it right up there with beans, also included in this recipe, on the list of fiber all-stars. It also has more potassium than almost any other food I've researched—one bunch provides an almost unbelievable 1,499 mg (a medium banana has 422 mg). And baby broccoli, or broccolini, is just delicious. It's less crunchy than the regular kind and has a nice, almost sweet, taste, more similar to asparagus without the sulfurlike smell! Both rabe and baby broc are members of the brassica family of vegetable royalty (which also includes Brussels sprouts and cabbage) and are loaded with plant compounds called *indoles*, which are known to have cancer-fighting activity. There's probably not a more guilt-free way to enjoy a potato than this one!

Ingredients

4 medium baking potatoes

1 tablespoon (15 ml) olive oil

3 cloves garlic, minced (or 1½ teaspoons prepared)

1 teaspoon chili powder, or to taste

1 teaspoon ground cumin

Pinch salt

Pinch cayenne pepper, optional

⅔ cup (73 g) shredded carrots

6 cups (180 g) baby spinach (or baby arugula or chopped escarole)

1 can (15 ounces or 425 g) kidney beans, drained and rinsed

1 jar (16 ounces or 455 g) salsa

½ cup (8 g) chopped fresh cilantro, optional

½ cup (58 g) shredded pepper Jack cheese (or regular Monterey Jack, mozzarella, or Cheddar)

Scrub the potatoes well and pierce with a fork. Place potatoes in the microwave with 3 tablespoons (45 ml) of water in a small bowl or cup. Microwave on high for 8 to 10 minutes or until tender, turning the potatoes once at 4 minutes for even cooking.

While the potatoes are cooking, heat the olive oil in a large skillet or Dutch oven over medium heat. Add the garlic, chili powder, cumin, salt, cayenne, if using, and carrots and sauté for 2 minutes, stirring frequently to combine. Stir in the spinach and cover for 2 minutes or until starting to wilt. Remove the cover and stir in the beans and salsa. Cook for 2 to 3 more minutes or until the mixture is hot and the vegetables have reached their desired tenderness. Stir in the cilantro, if using, and remove from the heat.

Working carefully so you don't burn your hands, slice each potato lengthwise down the middle and gently pull the halves apart. Stuff each potato with one quarter of the bean mixture and top with one quarter of the cheese.

Yield: 4 potatoes

Per Serving: 596 Calories; 10g Fat (13.9% calories from fat); 35g Protein; 98g Carbohydrate; 32g Dietary Fiber; 13mg Cholesterol; 657mg Sodium

From Chef Jeannette

To Complete the Meal: These potatoes need only a light accompaniment, such as a green leafy salad topped with sliced avocado, a sprinkling of pepitas, and a drizzle of olive oil with salt—or a glass of homemade sangria. Try it with a bottle of Spanish Rioja, 2 cups (450 ml) of seltzer, ⅔ cup (160 ml) of fruit juice (try pineapple or orange), 4 cups (640 g) of chopped fruit (try unpeeled orange, lemon, lime, pineapple, berries, or mango), and a tablespoon or two of honey to sweeten.

If You Have 5 More Minutes: To add a little variety, substitute 4 cups (280 g) of chopped broccoli rabe or chopped broccolini for the spinach. Add 3 to 5 minutes more for cooking to soften, adding a couple of tablespoons of water and covering for a minute or two.

Quick-Fix Stuffed Peppers with Chèvre

Ingredients

2 cups (475 ml) vegetable broth (add ¼ teaspoon salt if using low-sodium broth)

1 cup (184 g) quick-cooking barley

2 large green or colored bell peppers, stemmed, seeded, and halved

1 tablespoon (14 g) butter

4 ounces (115 g) presliced shiitake mushrooms

2 shallots, chopped

3 tablespoons (48 g) tomato paste

¾ teaspoon dried thyme

½ teaspoon dried oregano

⅓ cup (37 g) toasted pecan pieces

¼ cup (38 g) chèvre

From Dr. Jonny: Everyone digs stuffed peppers, but they usually take a heck of a long time to make. Not these babies. Our vegetarian quick-fix version is high in the flavor department but low on prep time—a winning combination if you're in a time crunch. Barley is high in fiber, the peppers are loaded with cell-protecting antioxidants, and the shiitake mushrooms are one of the most immune-boosting foods on the planet. And oregano doesn't just make food taste great, it also contains two important plant compounds, carvacrol and thymol, which have been shown to inhibit the growth of all kinds of microbes. (That's one reason oregano oil is considered such a good "purifier" for the system and one of the first things I turn to when I feel like I'm getting a stomach bug.) The pecans nicely balance the texture of the peppers and grain with a sweet crunchiness, all the more satisfying because it comes from one of the healthiest nuts on earth.

Bring the broth to a boil in a large saucepan over high heat. Add the barley, reduce the heat, and simmer for about 10 minutes or until tender.

Place the pepper halves face down in a sealed glass, microwave-safe container and microwave on high for 6 to 7 minutes or until tender-crisp.

While the barley and peppers are cooking, heat the butter in a large skillet over medium. Add the mushrooms and shallots and cook for 4 to 5 minutes or until the mushrooms are tender. In a medium bowl, gently mix together the hot, cooked barley, mushroom mixture, tomato paste, thyme, oregano, and pecans until combined. Stuff each pepper half with one quarter of the barley mixture and top with 1 tablespoon (9 g) of chèvre to serve.

Yield: 4 servings

Per Serving: 385 Calories; 14g Fat (30.5% calories from fat); 12g Protein; 59g Carbohydrate; 9g Dietary Fiber; 13mg Cholesterol; 978mg Sodium

From Chef Jeannette

To Complete the Meal: Serve with grilled (prepared) strips of smoky tempeh "bacon" (e.g., Lightlife Organic Smoky Tempeh Strips).

If You Have 5 Extra Minutes: Broil the peppers for 2 minutes to melt the goat cheese just before serving.

Variation Tip: Make this dish with cooked brown rice or a wild rice blend, both of which would be excellent with green peppers. You could also "beef" it up with a cup of vegan "beef" crumbles, or rinsed, canned adzuki beans. Try switching the goat cheese for blue cheese for a zippy alternative.

Ingredients

8 ounces (225 g) whole-grain or sprouted spaghetti (we like Barilla Plus)

¾ cup (195 g) prepared high-quality pesto

2 tablespoons (30 g) whole-grain Dijon mustard

½ cup (120 ml) vegetable or chicken broth

½ cup (24 g) snipped chives

2 cups (512 g) skinned fava beans, frozen or canned, drained and rinsed*

1 cup (100 g) cooked peas

½ cup (60 g) crushed walnuts

From Chef Jeannette

To Complete the Meal: Steam-sauté 1 pound (455 g) of chopped greens in 1½ tablespoons (25 ml) of olive oil with 2 teaspoons of garlic, salt, and fresh ground black pepper until tender. Try escarole or mature spinach, which are faster cooking, or kale or collards (which are slower cooking and need a few tablespoons of liquid).

If You Have 10 More Minutes: Make your own pesto. See page 95 for lemon pesto or page 154 for arugula pesto.

Lightning-Fast Legume-Pesto Spaghetti

From Dr. Jonny: All the areas around the globe where people routinely live the longest, known as the Blue Zones, have one dietary staple in common: beans. They're one of the few foods that just about every healthy, long-lived society eats. And in the Nurses' Health Study, one of the longest-running studies of dietary habits and health, women who ate four or more servings of legumes a week decreased their risk of heart disease by 22 percent and their risk of colorectal adenomas by 33 percent. Not bad for a few servings of these fiber-rich beauties! Adding fava beans to peas, pesto, and spaghetti is a fabulous and tasty way to get beans into your diet. The crushed walnuts add some plant-based omega-3 fats to boot!

Prepare the spaghetti according to the package directions.

While the spaghetti is cooking, place the pesto, mustard, and broth in a large skillet over medium heat and whisk to combine. Sir in the chives, fava beans, and peas, and cook for about 2 minutes or until hot throughout. Stir in the walnuts.

Spoon the pesto mixture into the hot pasta and toss well to combine. Season with salt and pepper to taste, if necessary.

Yield: 4 servings

Per Serving: 688 Calories; 35g Fat (43.5% calories from fat); 30g Protein; 72g Carbohydrate; 13g Dietary Fiber; 15mg Cholesterol; 1299mg Sodium

*It can be a little tricky to find prepared fava beans (or broad beans). If you are lucky enough to have a Middle Eastern market nearby, you will likely find both the canned and frozen variety. Most Whole Foods stores sell frozen favas. Fresh is far better for flavor, but they are labor and time intensive and generally only available in the spring and part of summer. If you have no luck, substitute canned white kidney beans or Great Northern beans.

Ingredients

2 sprouted corn tortillas (6 inches or 15 cm; we like Food for Life Organic Sprouted Corn Tortillas)

½ cup (119 g) no-fat, vegetarian refried beans

½ peeled and pitted avocado, sliced

¼ cup (65 g) prepared, high-quality salsa

4 thin heirloom tomato slices

1 cup (50 g) broccoli sprouts

1 tablespoon (9 g) toasted pepitas, optional

A Healthier Sandwich: Open-Faced Veggie-Mex

From Dr. Jonny: Okay, I'll be the first to admit I'm not a huge fan of the sandwich as a go-to meal. Why? Because your basic deli sandwich uses junky, low-quality, high-carb bread and meats that are filled with nitrate and sodium, not to mention sauces loaded with sugar. But there's no doubt that a sandwich can make an excellent quick (and healthy!) meal, providing you build it with the right materials.

We use sprouted-grain wraps and pockets, but you can also use whole-grain options. Sprouted grains retain their natural plant enzymes, which are beneficial for digestion and are also nutrient rich. Some argue that the nutrients in sprouted-grain breads are easier to absorb, but others claim that the effect is minor. No matter. Sprouted, and whole-grain, wraps are preferable to the bulky rolls made with refined white flour that come with the average deli sandwich. Whole grains are fine, but make sure the first ingredient is whole wheat or whole oats, and look for at least 2 grams of fiber per slice, preferably 3. As a vegetarian protein source it's hard to beat beans. Sprouts add enzymes and nutrients, and the avocado is not only creamy and smooth, it's also a wonderful source of heart-healthy fat, and—surprisingly—fiber!

Toast the tortillas briefly in a toaster oven to warm and soften them. Spread each tortilla with half the refried beans and top with half the avocado slices. Spoon half the salsa on each and top with tomato slices. Top with the sprouts and a sprinkling of pepitas, if using.

Yield: 4 servings

Per Serving: 481 Calories; 23g Fat (40.6% calories from fat); 16g Protein; 60g Carbohydrate; 16g Dietary Fiber; 0mg Cholesterol; 808mg Sodium

Ingredients

1 tablespoon (15 ml) olive oil

1 1/2 cups (240 g) prepared diced onion (or 1 yellow onion, chopped)

2 cups (475 ml) vegetable or chicken broth

1 can (28 ounces or 795 g) crushed tomatoes

1 tablespoon (15 ml) balsamic vinegar

1 teaspoon Sucanat, or to taste

1/2 teaspoon salt

1/2 teaspoon cracked black pepper

1 can (15 ounces or 425 g) small white beans (e.g., cannellini, navy, etc.)

From Chef Jeannette

To Complete the Meal: Serve it with the Italian or Caesar salad on pages 175 or 136. For a little calcium blast, add the Parmigiano-Asiago wafers on page 116

If You Have 5 More Minutes: To add nutrient-rich greens, stir in 2 cups (40 g) of watercress or chopped baby arugula after pureeing. Heat for 1 to 2 minutes or until just wilted and serve.

For more protein, add a cup of cooked meat after pureeing. Try ground beef, or shredded or diced chicken or turkey.

To beef up the "good carbs" and make it more filling, stir in 3/4 cup cooked brown rice or quinoa after pureeing.

If You Have 15 More Minutes: To capture the flavor and vital nutrients of fresh tomatoes, substitute 5 to 6 ripe, chopped, fresh heirloom tomatoes for the canned tomatoes, and simmer for 10 minutes longer. Choose a blend of tomatoes for flavor variations: zebras, oranges, and yellows are milder and less acidic than reds. (Blanch and skin them first for the smoothest consistency.)

Easy, Protein-Rich Tangy Tomato Soup

From Dr. Jonny: I'm always amused by "absolute truths" in the food world, like the belief that it's always better to eat raw foods. Tomatoes are a perfect case in point. They're actually better for you lightly cooked, as the cooking breaks down their cell walls and releases the valuable antioxidant lycopene, which is far more available to you in the cooked version than in raw form. (Not that raw tomatoes are bad, mind you!) Tomatoes are always a go-to vegetable where soups are concerned, and this tomato soup has the added benefit of being high in fiber and protein, largely because of the wonderful white beans that feature both important constituents of a healthy meal. This is a great low-calorie meal with all the familiar comforting flavor of Mom's tomato soup. And it passes the "Jonny" test for being really easy to make. Enjoy.

Heat the oil in a large soup pot over medium heat. Add the onion and sauté for 4 minutes. Add the broth, tomatoes, vinegar, Sucanat, salt, and pepper, increase the heat, and bring to a low boil for 5 minutes.

Using an immersion blender, puree the soup until smooth (or process in batches using a regular blender). Add the beans and leave intact for a thinner soup, or puree them partially or fully into the soup for a thicker consistency—cook's choice. Adjust the seasonings, if necessary, to serve.

Yield: 4 servings

Per Serving: 551 Calories; 7g Fat (10.8% calories from fat); 32g Protein; 97g Carbohydrate; 23g Dietary Fiber; 1mg Cholesterol; 1364mg Sodium

Ingredients

4 cups (50 ml) vegetable or chicken broth

1/3 cup (37 g) shredded carrots

1 can (14.5 ounces or 413 g) fire-roasted diced tomatoes, undrained

3 cans (15 ounces or 425 g each) black beans, drained and rinsed

1/4 cup (60 ml) sherry

2 teaspoons prepared garlic (or 2 large cloves, minced)

3/4 teaspoon salt, or to taste

1/2 teaspoon cracked black pepper

1 teaspoon cumin

1 teaspoon onion powder

1 cup (130 g) frozen corn (roasted, if possible–try Trader Joe's)

1/3 cup (5 g) chopped fresh cilantro, optional

From Chef Jeannette

To Complete the Meal: Prepare sun-dried tomato grits. While the soup is cooking, follow package directions for four servings of quick-cooking grits (usually about 2 cups [475 ml] of boiling water or broth to 1/2 cup grits). For the last 2 minutes of cook time, stir in 1 cup (130 g) of frozen corn, 1/3 cup (37 g) of drained sun-dried tomato strips in oil, 1/2 teaspoon of salt, and fresh ground pepper, to taste.

If You Have 10 More Minutes: Sauté 2 to 3 chopped shallots with the carrots in a tablespoon of olive oil over medium heat for 3 to 4 minutes before adding the broth. This will both enrich the flavor and provide you with a liver-supportive dose of sulfur from the shallots. You may also add 1/4 teaspoon of red pepper flakes for a little heat and/or squeeze a half a lime into the cooked soup when you add the cilantro for a fresh burst of vitamin C.

Black Bean Slenderizer Soup

From Dr. Jonny: I'll be honest: I'd make soup a lot more often if it didn't take so darn long to make. Why? First, soup is one of the great secrets of weight control—something about eating our nutrients in a liquid base fills us up more and signals "full" to the appetite centers in the brain in ways that aren't fully understood but make it a lot easier to resist overeating. Second, soup can be incredibly nutritious, especially when made with beans or vegetables as a base. But there's that pesky issue of time. Now Chef Jeannette has conquered the problem and come up with a fabulous soup that takes—get this—only 15 minutes of prep time. If you make the (recommended) grits as well, you'll wind up with a corn-and-beans combo reminiscent of a core staple dish for many indigenous peoples around the globe. Whip it up and enjoy over and over again—it reheats really well!

In a soup pot over high heat, combine all ingredients from the broth through the onion powder and bring to a boil. Reduce the heat slightly, cover, and simmer for about 8 minutes.

Using an immersion blender (or regular blender), puree the soup to a chunky-smooth consistency. Always have caution working with hot liquids. Stir in the corn and cilantro, if using. Adjust the seasonings, if necessary. Let the soup rest for 1 minute (to heat the corn) before serving.

Yield: 4 to 6 servings

Per Serving: 290 Calories; 2g Fat (4.9% calories from fat); 17g Protein; 52g Carbohydrate, 12g Dietary Fiber; trace Cholesterol; 339mg Sodium

Ingredients

Salad

2 cups (475 ml) vegetable broth

1 cup (170 g) red heirloom quinoa, rinsed (we like Ancient Harvest Organic Inca Red)

¼ cup (38 g) dried currants

⅓ cup (45 g) toasted cashews or almond slices

2 tablespoons (16 g) toasted sesame seeds

1½ cups (187 g) chopped apple (or presliced apples, such as green or crisp red)

1½ cups (210 g) precooked protein (e.g., canned beans, diced chicken, cubed firm tofu, etc.), optional

½ cup (80 g) sliced scallions, optional

Dressing

Superspeed Option

⅓ cup prepared fruity dressing, or to taste (e.g., Annie's Naturals Organic Pomegranate Vinaigrette, or Cuisine Perel Cranberry Orange Vinaigrette—just swap the currants for dried cranberries!)

Make-Your-Own Option

¼ cup (60 ml) orange juice*

2 tablespoons (28 ml) olive oil

1 tablespoon (15 ml) low-sodium tamari

1 tablespoon (15 ml) mirin (or sherry)

½ teaspoon powdered ginger

*For the best flavor, use fresh-squeezed juice plus 1 teaspoon orange zest

One Main, Two Meals I

From Dr. Jonny: These recipes are in Chef Jeannette's "one main, two meals" series. Heirloom Quinoa Salad was actually inspired by a little side dish I found in a gourmet airport delicatessen. I bought it on a whim 'cause it looked healthy but was pleasantly surprised to find that it was one of the tastiest and most satisfying salads I ever enjoyed! This recipe combines quinoa, currants, and nuts, dolled up with Chef Jeannette's special touches, and I'll bet you love it as much as I do. The second recipe, Red Quinoa Burgers, is deliciously easy and there's not a "moo" to be heard anywhere—"no animals were harmed in the making of this burger!" And quinoa and beans make a great, high-fiber protein!

Fast Fruit 'n' Fiber Quinoa Salad

In a medium saucepan bring the broth to a boil over high heat. Add the quinoa, stir, reduce the heat slightly (keep a strong simmer), and cook until tender and the tails have popped, about 12 minutes.

While the quinoa is cooking, prepare the dressing, if using make-your-own option. In a small bowl, whisk together (or use an immersion blender) juice, olive oil, tamari, mirin, and ginger.

In a large bowl, mix together the currants, nuts, sesame seeds, apple, protein, and scallions, if using. Set aside 1 cup (185 g) of the quinoa to refrigerate or freeze for the Red Quinoa Burgers (following) or something else. Add the remaining quinoa to the bowl and mix gently to combine. Pour in the dressing to taste and mix gently to thoroughly coat.

Yield: 4 to 6 servings

Per Serving: 341 Calories; 12g Fat (31.1% calories from fat); 12g Protein; 49g Carbohydrate; 7g Dietary Fiber; 1mg Cholesterol; 794mg Sodium

(Superspeed Option)

Per Serving: 326 Calories; 11g Fat (29.8% calories from fat); 10g Protein; 49g Carbohydrate; 7g Dietary Fiber; 1mg Cholesterol; 788mg Sodium

From Chef Jeannette

To Complete the Meal: Add 1 pound (455 g) of fresh green beans. Microwave for 3½ minutes on high in a microwave-safe glass container with a slightly vented lid. Toss with ⅓ cup (50 g) of feta cheese or chèvre, ½ teaspoon of salt, and ¼ teaspoon of fresh ground pepper. Add a teaspoon of orange zest if you like.

Ingredients

Burgers

1 can (15 ounces or 425 g) kidney beans, drained and rinsed

¼ cup (20 g) quick-cooking rolled oats

2 ounces (55 g) grated or crumbled cheese (or ¼ cup [32 g] nutritional yeast for a vegan option)

½ teaspoon salt

1 cup (185 g) cooked heirloom quinoa

2 tablespoons (28 ml) olive oil

Dressing

½ cup (130 g) prepared salsa

2 tablespoons (30 g) plain low-fat yogurt

1 tablespoon (15 ml) lime juice

1 teaspoon maple syrup or agave nectar

1 teaspoon ground cumin

½ teaspoon chili powder

From Chef Jeannette

To Complete the Meal: Serve the burgers over a big salad or on a whole grain wrap or sprouted corn tortilla. Use plenty of shredded lettuce, sliced heirloom tomatoes, and sliced avocado.

Superspeed Tip: Flavor up the patties a bit more with 1 teaspoon each of onion powder and garlic granules, skip making the dressing altogether, and serve them up with a generous helping of prepared salsa.

Quick Quinoa Burgers

Place the beans, oats, cheese, and salt in a food processor in that order and pulse until combined and holding together but still chunky, about ten quick pulses. Turn the bean mixture out into a medium bowl, add the quinoa, and mix with your hands just until it holds together well.

Heat the oil in a large, nonstick skillet over medium heat (or just below medium in a regular skillet to prevent sticking), and form the quinoa mixture into four patties.

Place the burgers in the pan and cook for 3 to 4 minutes per side or until heated through. Patties will be soft, so handle gently.

While the burgers are cooking, place the salsa, yogurt, lime juice, syrup, cumin, and chili powder into a blender (or a small bowl and use an immersion blender), and blend until smooth. Serve the burgers with a generous helping of the dressing.

Yield: 4 servings

Per Serving: 565 Calories; 12g Fat (18.8% calories from fat); 35g Protein; 84g Carbohydrate; 31g Dietary Fiber; 12mg Cholesterol; 602mg Sodium

Calcium-Rich Caprese Salad in Seconds

Ingredients

¼ cup (35 g) pine nuts, plus extra for garnish

1 packed (20 g) cup chopped baby arugula

⅓ cup (13 g) fresh basil

2 tablespoons (10 g) Parmesan cheese (grated or shaved)

¼ teaspoon salt

¼ teaspoon cracked black pepper

2 tablespoons (28 ml) balsamic vinegar, plus extra to drizzle

¼ cup (60 ml) olive oil

1 pint (300 g) cherry or grape tomatoes

½ English cucumber, peeled and sliced

6 cups spring or mesclun mix

1 large or 2 medium balls fresh mozzarella cheese, thinly sliced or diced (6 ounces or 170 g)

From Dr. Jonny: Though you would hardly know it from listening to commercials from the dairy industry, milk is not the only way to get calcium in your diet. (According to some folks, including me, it's not even the best. But I digress.) Mozzarella cheese, for example, is an excellent source of calcium, ounce for ounce even better than milk! But this caprese salad has more to recommend it than just calcium, important as that nutrient is. Pine nuts, in addition to adding a wonderful taste and texture to the salad, are rich in minerals and fiber, and olive oil is loaded with healthy monounsaturated fat plus plant compounds known as phenols, which have multiple health benefits. Together with the greens, they make a rich, fresh-tasting pesto you could eat by the spoonful! Complement this salad with a great source of light protein such as fish and you have a flavorful, nutritious meal that comes together in minutes.

Place the pine nuts, arugula, basil, Parmesan, salt, pepper, and vinegar in a food processor and pulse five times or so to break down the greens. Process until well combined and at desired consistency, scraping down the sides as necessary. Pulse or process briefly as you add the olive oil in a thin stream to incorporate.

On a large platter or in a salad bowl, arrange the tomatoes and cucumber over a bed of the greens. Lay the mozzarella slices on top and spoon the pesto to taste over all.

Finish with an extra drizzle of balsamic and/or a sprinkle of pine nuts, if desired.

Serve at room temperature.

Yield: 4 servings

Per Serving: 343 Calories; 29g Fat (73.0% calories from fat); 14g Protein; 10g Carbohydrate; 3g Dietary Fiber; 40mg Cholesterol; 372mg Sodium

From Chef Jeannette

To Complete the Meal: Add an extra lean protein for more heartiness, or just serve as is for light summer fare. Try four 4- to 6-ounce (115 to 170 g) fillets of fresh grilled fish or a high-quality rotisserie-style chicken from the grocer. To grill fish, lightly oil with macadamia nut or avocado oil and salt and pepper to taste. Grill over medium-high heat for 2 to 3 minutes per side, depending on the thickness of your fillets, until they are opaque and flake easily, turning carefully so they don't fall apart. Squeeze fresh lemon juice over the cooked fillets and serve.

Ingredients

1 cup (160 g) prepared diced onion
3/4 cup (109 g) raw almonds
1/4 cup (32 g) toasted sesame seeds
1 cup (165 g) cooked brown rice
3/4 teaspoon powdered ginger
1 egg
1½ tablespoons (24 g) sweet white or
    mellow miso
1/4 cup (4 g) chopped fresh cilantro, optional
1 tablespoon (15 ml) low-sodium tamari
2 tablespoons (28 ml) sesame oil

Optional Wasabi Sauce (or just use a drizzle of prepared ginger dressing, such as Organicville's Miso Ginger Vinaigrette, to taste)

2 tablespoons (30 g) plain Greek yogurt
2 tablespoons (28 g) high-quality mayonnaise (we like vegan: Nayonaise or Vegenaise)
1½ teaspoons wasabi powder or paste, or
    more to taste
1 tablespoon (1 g) minced fresh cilantro,
    optional

From Chef Jeannette

To Complete the Meal: Serve over dressed greens. Dress watercress (2 large bunches) or baby arugula (4 cups) with 2 tablespoons (30 ml) of olive oil, 1 tablespoon (15 ml) of red wine vinegar, a teaspoon (4 g) of mustard, and pinches of salt and fresh ground pepper, to taste.

Nuts about Croquettes: Nutritional Powerhouses in 15 Minutes

From Dr. Jonny: I don't have anything against a good hamburger, especially when it's made from grass-fed, hormone-free meat. But how about a great nut burger, just for variety? What's that, you say? Simply put, it consists of nuts and a whole grain held together with a little egg. (Some might call it a "veggie burger," but a true nut croquette isn't made primarily with veggies, though they make the perfect accompaniment, either as a cooked side dish or in a nice colorful salad.) You'll find two outstanding variations on the nut croquette concept right here. The Asian Nutty features almonds, sesame seeds, and brown rice, and a (highly recommended) optional sauce with probiotic-rich miso and wasabi; the Middle Eastern Nutty is made from quinoa, the high-protein "food of the Incan gods," cashews, and raisins. It's slightly reminiscent of falafel, only, with its sweet nuttiness, even better. See the Nutritional Note on page 158 on the additional benefits of nuts and seeds.

Easy, Appetizing Asian Croquettes

Place the onion in a food processor and process until minced. Add the almonds and sesame seeds, and pulse a few times to chop. Add the rice and pulse a few times until a coarse mixture is formed. Avoid creating a fine texture by overprocessing. Add the ginger, egg, miso, and cilantro, if using, and process for a few seconds to combine, scraping down the sides to evenly mix. Add the tamari (if needed for moisture) a little at a time just until a moist mixture forms; it should not be too wet, but should hold together well.

Heat the oil over medium heat in a large nonstick skillet, and form 4½-inch (11 cm)-thick patties.

Cook the patties for 3 to 4 minutes on one side and 2 to 3 minutes on the other until lightly browned and hot throughout. Reduce the heat to medium low if the patties are browning too quickly.

While the croquettes are cooking, whisk together the yogurt, mayo, wasabi, and cilantro, if using. Serve the croquettes with a dollop of the wasabi sauce, if using.

Yield: 4 servings
Per Serving: 373 Calories; 27g Fat (61.0% calories from fat); 14g Protein; 25g Carbohydrate; 6g Dietary Fiber; 56mg Cholesterol; 442mg Sodium

Ingredients

²/₃ cup (110 g) coarsely chopped scallions
    (including white bulbs)

¼ cup (35 g) raisins

1 cup (145 g) raw cashews

1 egg

2 tablespoons (30 g) tahini

2 tablespoons (32 g) sun-dried tomato
    paste

¾ teaspoon prepared garlic (or 1 clove,
    minced)

¾ teaspoon salt

½ teaspoon cumin

1 cup (185 g) cooked quinoa*

1 tablespoon (15 ml) lemon juice, optional

2 tablespoons (28 ml) olive oil

Optional Tangy Sauce (or just use a
    drizzle of tahini, to taste)

¼ cup (60 g) plain Greek yogurt

1 tablespoon (15 ml) lemon juice

½ teaspoon prepared minced garlic
    (or 1 clove garlic, minced)

1 tablespoon (4 g) minced fresh parsley,
    optional

Pinch salt

Fresh ground black pepper to taste

*If you don't have cooked quinoa on hand, use cooked brown rice or uncooked whole, rolled oats.

Mouth-Watering Middle Eastern Croquettes

Place the onions and raisins in a food processor and process until minced. Add the cashews and pulse a few times until a coarse mixture is formed. Avoid making too fine a mixture by overprocessing. (If using oats instead of quinoa, add them now.) Add the egg, tahini, tomato paste, garlic, salt, and cumin, and process for a few seconds to combine well, scraping down the sides to evenly mix. Turn the mixture out into a bowl and add the quinoa and lemon juice, if using, mixing well. The mixture will be very moist.

Heat the oil over medium heat in a large nonstick skillet. Form 4½-inch (11 cm)-thick patties and cook for 3 to 4 minutes on one side and 2 to 3 minutes on the other until lightly browned and hot throughout. Reduce the heat to medium low if the patties are browning too quickly.

While the croquettes are cooking, whisk together the yogurt, lemon juice, garlic, parsley, if using, salt, and pepper, and set aside for the flavors to develop.

Serve the croquettes with a dollop of the sauce, if using.

Yield: 4 servings

Per Serving: 435 Calories; 30g Fat (59.4% calories from fat); 13g Protein; 33g Carbohydrate; 5g Dietary Fiber; 55mg Cholesterol; 543mg Sodium

From Chef Jeannette

To Complete the Meals: Serve them in whole-grain or sprouted wraps or over a salad. Either way, use lots of crisp green lettuce and raw or steamed veggies with a dollop of the sauce. With the Asian Croquettes try baby bok choy, shredded Napa cabbage, mung bean sprouts, snow peas, stir-fried veggies, sesame seeds, and so on. With the Middle Eastern Croquettes try chopped tomatoes, sliced celery, banana rings, shredded carrots, sliced dill pickles, drained and rinsed canned chickpeas, and so on.

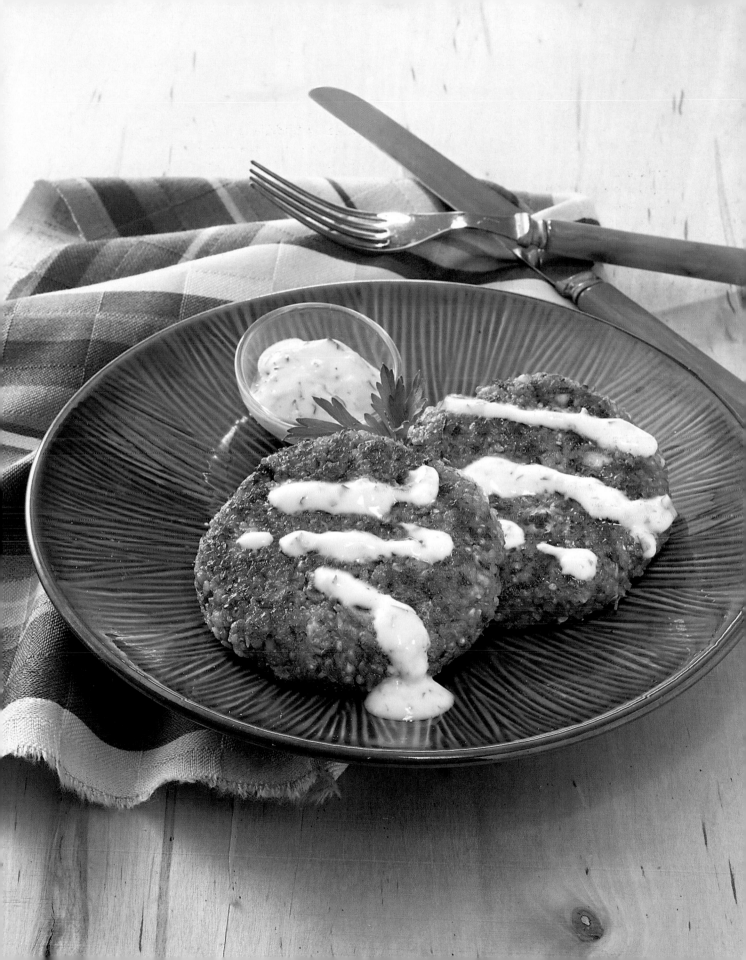

Snack on Heart-Healthy Nuts and Seeds

What if I told you there was a pill you could take that would reduce your risk of heart disease by 35 percent? Oh, and the pill had exactly zero side effects.

Would you take it?

Of course you would.

Well, I don't know of any pill like that, drug company advertising to the contrary. But I do know of a class of food that will do the same thing: nuts and seeds.

Eating nuts on a regular basis lowers the risk of heart disease by anywhere from 30 to 50 percent, according to a ton of research. In the Nurses' Health Study from Harvard University—one of the longest ongoing studies of dietary habits and disease ever done—people who ate more than 5 ounces (140 g) a week of nuts had a 35 percent lower risk of heart disease than people who didn't. Those numbers have been essentially duplicated in other studies, such as the Iowa Women's Health Study and the Adventist Study.

It gets better. Research from Loma Linda University examined the lifestyle habits of 34,000 Seventh-Day Adventists (who are already known for living pretty long lives to begin with) and found that those who ate about five servings of nuts a week lived an extra 2.9 years! How great is that?

Nuts and seeds contain an awful lot of protective compounds, including magnesium, vitamin E, fiber, and potassium. According to Harvard Health Publications, Harvard Medical School:

- Nuts may help lower cholesterol, partly by replacing less healthy foods in the diet.
- Nuts contain mono- and polyunsaturated fats, known to benefit the heart.
- The omega-3 fats found in walnuts may protect against irregular heart rhythms.
- Nuts are rich in arginine, a substance that may improve blood vessel function.
- Other nutrients in nuts, such as fiber and vitamin E, may also help lower cardiovascular risk.

Seeds are a pretty close cousin of nuts and have many of the same benefits. In addition, some seeds have special "extras." Pumpkin seeds, for example, contain beta-sitosterol, a plant chemical that has some benefit in treating benign prostate hyperplasia, that annoying condition that makes men over forty have to go to the bathroom several times a night! Beta-sitosterol also lowers cholesterol.

So the bottom line is this: Eat your nuts. Regularly. At least 5 ounces (140 g) a week.

The only caution is this: They're high in calories. So don't buy a 3-pound (1¼ kg) bag of almonds and eat them mindlessly all day long, at least not if you're not also cutting back on calories from other sources.

Other than the calorie warning, there's no reason to stay away from nuts.

In fact, there's every reason not to.

Feel-Great Feta-Fig Tabbouleh

From Dr. Jonny: This is another of my favorite Chef Jeannette concoctions because it exemplifies her signature ability to combine unexpected flavors, textures, and foods into dishes that sing off the tongue. Just picture figs with feta cheese, seasoned with mint and sprinkled with walnuts. Add some finely ground bulgur wheat, make a sweet and sour dressing with a base of orange juice and vinegar, and you've got the perfect "one-pot" meal for a summer's evening. And as far as health goes, remember that lentils and nuts are two of the dietary staples in most of the areas of the globe where people routinely live the longest, healthiest lives. Lentils (and beans) are both enormously high in fiber and loaded with antioxidants. Put them together with the bulgur, figs, and cheese and you've got a fruity twist on a Middle Eastern favorite. Best of all, the amount of cooking involved is...let's see...that would be...zero.

Ingredients

Tabbouleh

1½ cups (355 ml) vegetable broth (or water)

¾ cup (105 g) bulgur wheat (fine grind)

1 can (15 ounces or 425 g) lentils, drained and rinsed

3 ounces (85 g) crumbled feta

8 to 10 dried figs, chopped (pulse briefly in the food processor to save time)

½ cup (60 g) toasted walnuts, roughly chopped

2 tablespoons chopped fresh mint, or to taste

½ head of Bibb or other tender lettuce

Dressing

⅓ cup (80 ml) orange juice (fresh squeezed is best)

2 tablespoons (28 ml) fig vinegar (or 1½ tablespoons [25 ml] apple cider vinegar, but the fig is worth getting—its unique, sweet tang is utterly delicious and works well on meats and veggie sides, too!)

3 tablespoons (45 ml) walnut oil

2 teaspoons orange zest, optional

Bring the broth to a boil and pour over the bulgur. Soak for 7 minutes (it takes 15 for medium grind—faster if you simmer it, but add a little water so it doesn't get too dry) and drain any excess liquid (or follow the package directions for cooking), pressing it against a double-mesh sieve to squeeze out any excess moisture. While the bulgur is soaking, in a small bowl, whisk together the juice, vinegar, walnut oil, and zest, if using. When the bulgur is tender and drained, gently fold together the bulgur, lentils, feta, figs, walnuts, and mint. Dress to taste and mix gently to combine well. Line a salad bowl with lettuce leaves and spoon the tabbouleh into the center.

Yield: 4 servings

Per Serving: 860 Calories; 27g Fat (26.7% calories from fat); 43g Protein; 121g Carbohydrate; 44g Dietary Fiber; 20mg Cholesterol; 869mg Sodium

Ingredients

2 eggs
1 tablespoon (15 ml) water
Pinch salt
Pinch fresh ground black pepper
1 teaspoon coconut oil or butter

From Chef Jeannette

Variation Tip: For additional calcium and vitamin D, add a tablespoon or two of grated or crumbled cheese to your omelet just before you fold it over. Try feta, Parmesan, or sliced string cheese.

To Complete the Meal: You can add any number of high-fiber, low-sugar carbohydrates. Try sliced apples and pears with a squeeze of fresh lemon juice; a bowl of plain instant oatmeal with cinnamon and a sprinkling of xylitol; or chopped spinach and diced tomatoes steam-sautéed in a spray of olive oil with sprinkles of salt and pepper.

Perfect Protein: Two-Minute Omelet

From Dr. Jonny: There's one trick I know about making omelets, and I learned it from an old girlfriend who learned it from her mother and it was this: Make the pan really hot and cook the eggs quickly. And use really high-quality fat. So when I got this recipe from Chef Jeannette, with whom I've never actually discussed my omelet-making prowess, I smiled to myself when I read the cooking instructions. Ah, I thought to myself, my ex-girlfriend's mother must have taught her the same thing! Just kidding. Fact is, the quick, high-heat cooking in a small amount of healthy, delicious fat is the key to the simple richness of this egg dish. The omelets are fluffy and tender and a cinch to whip up on a moment's notice. They work equally well as a quick light lunch or dinner as well as making a terrific breakfast. Worth knowing: Studies show that eating eggs for breakfast helps with weight loss, probably because the protein makes you feel fuller for longer.

Lightly whisk the eggs, water, salt, and pepper together in a small bowl and set aside.

Heat the coconut oil in a small sauté or omelet pan over high heat, swirling to coat the pan for about 1 minute or until fully melted and distributed evenly across the bottom and side surfaces of the pan. When the pan is well coated and hot, pour the eggs into the pan and do not disturb for about 30 seconds. When eggs are bubbling and the bottom surface has solidified, gently lift one half of the omelet and fold it over the other side (about 30 seconds). Let it cook for another 20 seconds or until desired doneness and slide out onto your plate. If you prefer your eggs to be well cooked, you may flip the omelet over and cook for another 10 to 20 seconds before plating.

Yield: 1 omelet
Per Serving: 250 Calories; 21g Fat (78.1% calories from fat); 13g Protein; 1g Carbohydrate; 0g Dietary Fiber; 455mg Cholesterol; 257mg Sodium

Eggs, Eggs, Who's Got the Eggs?

Eggs are one of the most perfect foods on the planet.

And, wait for it not, that includes the yolk.

Yup, the yolk, that poor misunderstood but essential component of the egg that too often gets thrown out in a misguided attempt to avoid cholesterol and fat. So let's clear a few things up about eggs, cholesterol, fat, and health.

Number one: The cholesterol in eggs has virtually no effect on the cholesterol in your blood.

Number two: The fat in the egg yolk is mostly monounsaturated fat, the same kind found in olive oil! Yes, you heard that right. Of the approximately 5 grams of total fat in one large egg, only 1.6 grams are saturated (2 grams are monounsaturated, and the rest is polyunsaturated).

Number three: Many of the nutrients that make eggs so incredibly healthy are found in the yolk. Examples: lutein and zeaxanthin, two members of the carotenoid family that are essential for eye health. The yolk also contains choline—important for brain health—and vitamin D.

The idea that eating eggs is bad for your heart is a myth. No study has linked egg eating to greater risk of heart disease. In fact, quite the opposite. "The only large study to look at the impact of egg consumption on heart disease...found no connection between the two," according to *Harvard Health*, a publication of Harvard Medical School, in 2000.

Research has also shown that eggs eaten at the start of the day can reduce your daily calorie intake, prevent snacking between meals, and keep you satisfied.

Worth noting: Stay away from scrambled eggs at open buffets. Although the cholesterol in eggs poses no real harm to you, when that cholesterol is "scrambled" and then exposed to oxygen for a long time, it becomes damaged by a process known as oxidation, similar to what happens when you leave metal outside in the rain and it rusts. When cholesterol is oxidized, it accelerates the development of heart disease. Bottom line: Oxidized cholesterol is not something you really want in your body. Better to poach, soft-, or hard-boil. If you do scramble eggs, eat them quickly and don't let them sit around for a long time!

CHOOSE WISELY

When it comes to eggs, and any animal food, for that matter, quality matters a great deal. Free range eggs supposedly come from chickens that roam free and are able to peck at insects and seeds rather than being confined to feedlots and fattened on grain. The fat (and the eggs) of such chickens is a lot healthier, as are the chickens themselves. (Some eggs of free-range chickens are even a decent source of omega-3 fats!).

Problem is, the term *free-range* has been watered down to the point where it's almost meaningless. In some cases, *free-range* simply means that the chicken has access to the outdoors via a little "doggy gate," even if it rarely actually takes advantage of it. Even so, we strongly recommend that you buy free-range eggs, as those are the only ones that come from chickens that have a fighting chance of seeing the outdoors and eating a diet more suited to their metabolism.

Ingredients

2 tablespoons (28 ml) coconut oil

½ cup (62 g) whole wheat pastry flour or oat flour

½ cup (120 ml) any milk (cow's, unsweetened soy, or almond)

2 tablespoons (13 g) ground flaxseed

2 eggs

1 teaspoon ground cinnamon

1 to 1½ cups (220 g) berries (bite-size), diced peaches (unpeeled), diced mango (peeled), or diced ripe pears (unpeeled), fresh or frozen, partly thawed (leave them on the countertop while pan cake is cooking)

2 tablespoons (24 g) Sucanat, xylitol, or erythritol

½ large lemon

From Chef Jeannette

Cooking many rounds of traditional pancakes can be time consuming. For the speediest pan-cake breakfast, use this recipe to get four servings on the table in just over 15 minutes!

Anytime Fast Fruity Skillet Cake

From Dr. Jonny: This quickie cake in a pan is so darn easy to make, even your kids can do it. And it works in all seasons—all you have to do is choose any soft fruit growing out of the ground right now. The combinations are endless. And let's talk about coconut oil for a minute: Forget everything you've heard; this is a superfood. (We highly recommend Barlean's Organic Coconut Oil, available everywhere.) Coconut oil has important fatty acids that are antiviral and antimicrobial, such as lauric acid. And the flax adds cancer-fighting lignans, fiber, and a bit of omega-3s. This dish satisfies just like a baked product—better, actually, because it has only a small amount of flour and sweetener and not a hint of syrup in sight. It does triple duty—great for breakfast, brunch, or a mini-meal snack!

Preheat the oven to 425°F (220°C, gas mark 7). Place the coconut oil in a cast-iron skillet and place the skillet in the oven while preparing the batter.

In a medium bowl, combine the flour, milk, flax, eggs, and cinnamon. Mix with a fork until just combined, leaving some lumps. Remove the pan from the oven and pour the batter into the melted oil. Return the pan to the oven and cook for 12 minutes.

Remove the pan, spoon the fruit evenly over the pan cake (it may have puffed way up in places), sprinkle the sweetener over the fruit, and squeeze lemon over all. Return the pan to the oven and cook for another 5 minutes, or until the edges are lightly browned. Remove, cut into quarters, cool slightly, and serve.

Yield: 4 servings

Per Serving: 201 Calories; 11g Fat (48.6% calories from fat); 7g Protein; 20g Carbohydrate; 4g Dietary Fiber; 110mg Cholesterol; 52mg Sodium

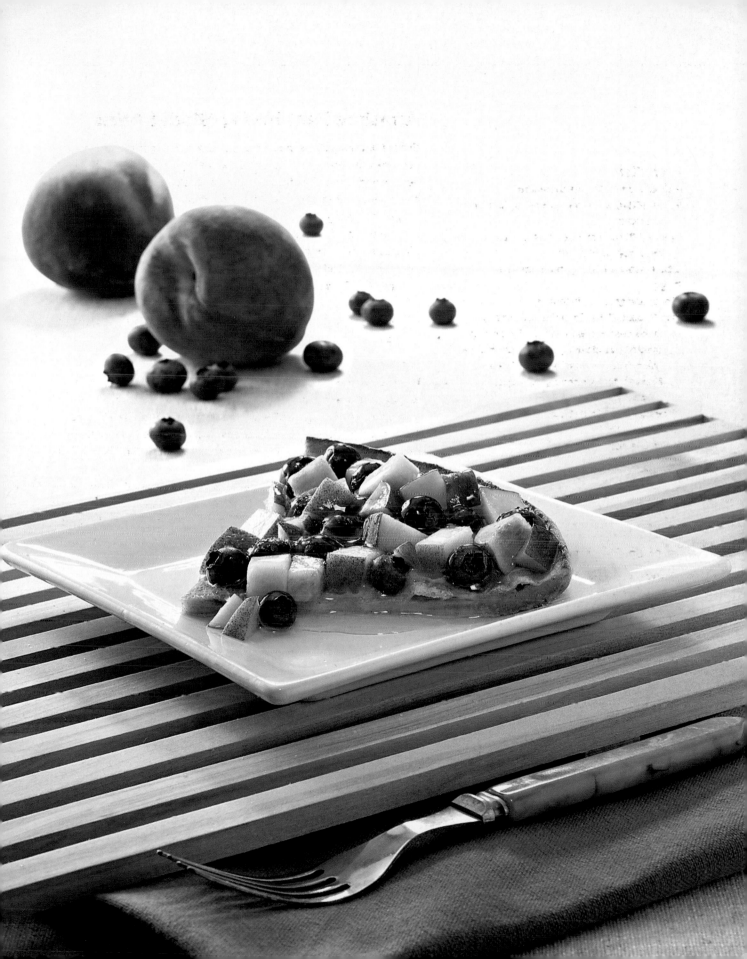

Apple Power Breakfast to Keep You on the Go

Ingredients

²/₃ cup (160 ml) water

4 small crisp apples (Gala or Pink Lady work well), cored and diced, unpeeled

1 cup (164 g) cooked chickpeas (drained and rinsed, if canned)

1 cup (120 g) grated Cheddar cheese

1 cup (145 g) toasted tamari sunflower seeds

From Dr. Jonny: My friends make fun of me when I suggest having beans for breakfast, but when they try this dish they see what I'm talking about! To me, the secret of managing weight (and eating less food in general) is to keep your blood sugar from going on a roller-coaster ride. (When blood sugar shoots up, as it does when you eat high-carb foods, it also crashes back down, leaving you ravenously hungry.) The best way to keep your blood sugar even (and keep cravings at bay) is to eat high-fiber foods. They enter the bloodstream slowly and keep you full and satisfied longer. And no food accomplishes this better than beans! Mix with cheese, seeds, and apples, and you have a hearty breakfast that will keep you going all morning. P.S. This also makes a quick but satisfying snack with great staying power!

Bring the water to a simmer over medium heat in a large cast-iron (or regular) skillet. Add the apples and cook, uncovered, until the water has evaporated, 5 to 7 minutes. Add the chickpeas and toss gently to warm them. Sprinkle the cheese over all and cook for 1 minute or until the cheese is melted.

Top with the sunnies and serve immediately.

Yield: 4 servings

Per Serving: 458 Calories; 29g Fat (53.9% calories from fat); 18g Protein; 37g Carbohydrate; 9g Dietary Fiber; 31mg Cholesterol; 310mg Sodium

Cinnamon: A Superspice for Super Health

Cinnamon has gotten an impressive reputation of late, largely because of studies showing that it helps lower blood sugar. Research by C. Leigh Broadhurst and others at the U.S. Department of Agriculture tested the effects of 49 different herbs, spices, and medicinal plants on blood sugar and found cinnamon was the star of the show. Its active ingredient—MHCP (methylhydroxychalcone polymer, if anyone ever asks)—actually mimics the function of insulin, increasing the ability of cells to take up sugar.

But this isn't all cinnamon has to recommend it. It's a spice that contains *anthocyanins*, which improve the function of your capillaries. It's also great for digestion, and, believe it or not, for relieving gas and nausea.

I find cinnamon to be a great spice to use in high-carb dishes. It also seems to lower triglycerides (which can go up on high-carb diets), and according to some research, also lowers "bad" cholesterol in people with type 2 diabetes. One animal study even showed that dietary cinnamon reduced blood pressure. Best of all, the health benefits are available in the cheapest kind of store-bought cinnamon. You don't need the fancy stuff at all!

Instant Fruit-and-Nut, Hot-and-Healthy Cereal

Ingredients

¾ cup (175 ml) water, plus more if needed

1 to 2 tablespoons (7.5 to 15 g) dried berries (try cherries, cranberries, or blueberries)

⅓ cup (80 g) instant whole-grain hot cereal (plain, no additives, such as cream of wheat, quinoa cream, or buckwheat cream)

¼ teaspoon vanilla extract

1 tablespoon (8 g) unsweetened vanilla whey protein powder

½ teaspoon ground cinnamon

1 tablespoon (20 g) sweetener, or to taste (try blackstrap molasses, honey, xylitol, or a packet of stevia powder/a few drops of liquid stevia)

1 teaspoon ground flaxseed

2 tablespoons (18 g) toasted chopped nuts (try slivered almonds, walnuts, pecans, or sunflower seeds)

¼ to ⅓ cup (60 to 80 ml) milk (use cow's, or unsweetened vanilla almond, soy, or rice milk), optional

½ cup (75 g) bite-size fresh seasonal fruit, optional (berries, sliced banana, peaches, or pears work well)

From Dr. Jonny: So if you've read anything I've written about food, you probably know I'm not a fan of prepared instant oatmeal. And that's putting it mildly. It tends to have a ton of sugar, little fiber, a bunch of artificial flavors and colors, and is way more processed than the "real" kind of oatmeal. Try our version for a superfast, satisfying, and nutrient-loaded start to your day. Just be sure to use a whole-grain version of the instant cereal as Chef Jeannette indicates. (If you have just a bit more time, use the regular kind—it doesn't take that much longer to make!) Our version offers real fruit (berries and cherries are nutritional powerhouses). This dish is actually a variation on a favorite of bodybuilders everywhere—oatmeal mixed with high-quality whey protein powder. (I do this all the time—they mix well and taste terrific.) Regarding nuts: Let's remember that research shows clearly that eating nuts on a regular basis significantly lowers the risk of cardiovascular disease—and does not contribute to obesity (especially if you keep the portions small). This dish is a super way to start your day and tastes pretty good even when you save it in the fridge and eat it cold the next day. The flavors and sweetness meld together perfectly!

In a small saucepan, bring the water to a quick boil over high heat. Stir in the berries and cereal and remove from the heat or lower the heat and cook for 30 seconds to 2 minutes (read the package directions or judge by consistency). If the cereal gets too thick, add a few more tablespoons of water to thin. Stir in the vanilla, whey protein powder, cinnamon, sweetener, flaxseed, and nuts until well incorporated. If using, stir in the milk and/or fruit and serve immediately.

Yield: 1 servings

Per Serving: 578 Calories; 14g Fat (21.9% calories from fat); 19g Protein; 95g Carbohydrate; 9g Dietary Fiber; 16mg Cholesterol; 63mg Sodium

From Chef Jeannette

If You Have 15 More Minutes: Grind your own grains fresh. Many companies sell instant whole-grain cereals; some even have healthy nutrient boosters such as added whey protein or flaxseed. But if you don't have any on hand, make your own out of almost any dried grain that will cook up in minutes. This makes about the healthiest and cheapest quick cereal you can imagine!

To make your own, grind about ½ cup (250 g) of dried grains in your blender for 30 seconds to 2 minutes (depending on the strength of your blender) until it reaches a fine sand consistency. You may need to scrape down the sides occasionally, and let it settle before removing the lid. To cook it, add the grains and 2 cups (475 ml) of water to a medium saucepan. Whisk the mixture well to combine and bring it to a boil over high heat. Once boiling, switch it to another burner set to low and cook for about 5 minutes or until a smooth consistency is reached, whisking often. You may need to add a little more water if the mixture gets too thick. Smaller grains tend to need more water than larger grains. Try it with brown rice, millet, or quinoa.

This method also works with beans, and the proportions are about the same: ¼ cup (125 g) of dried whole grain or bean to 1 cup (235 ml) of water. Incorporating ground beans into your cereals is a great way to increase fiber and vegan protein (but prepare them as a savory dish—the taste isn't great with fruit). These fresh-ground grains and beans make terrific baby foods, too, by the way!

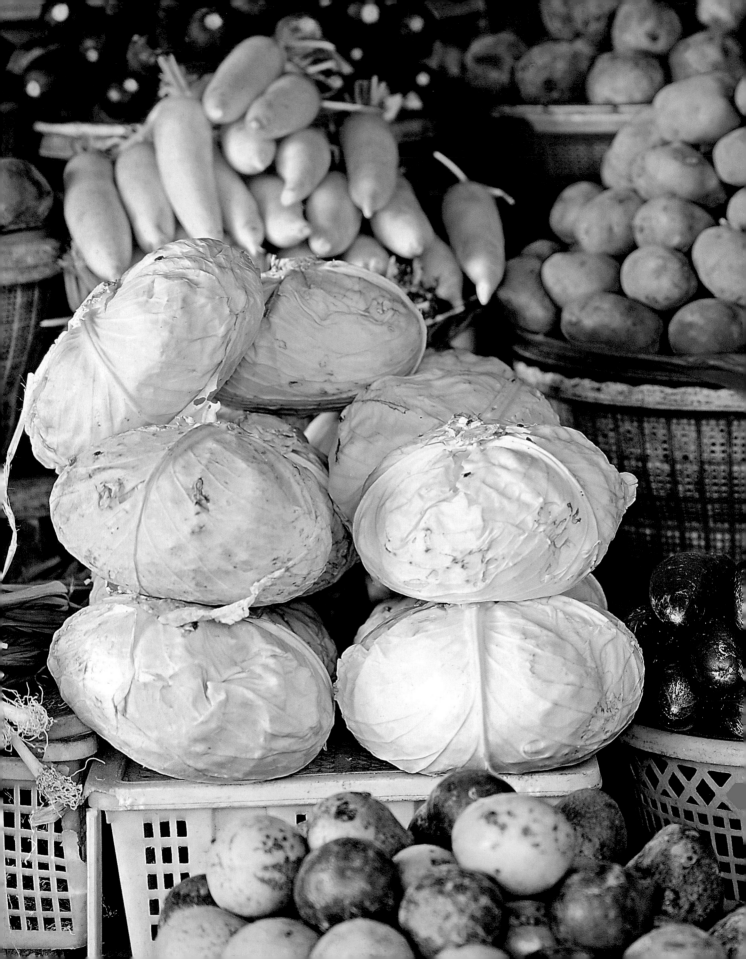

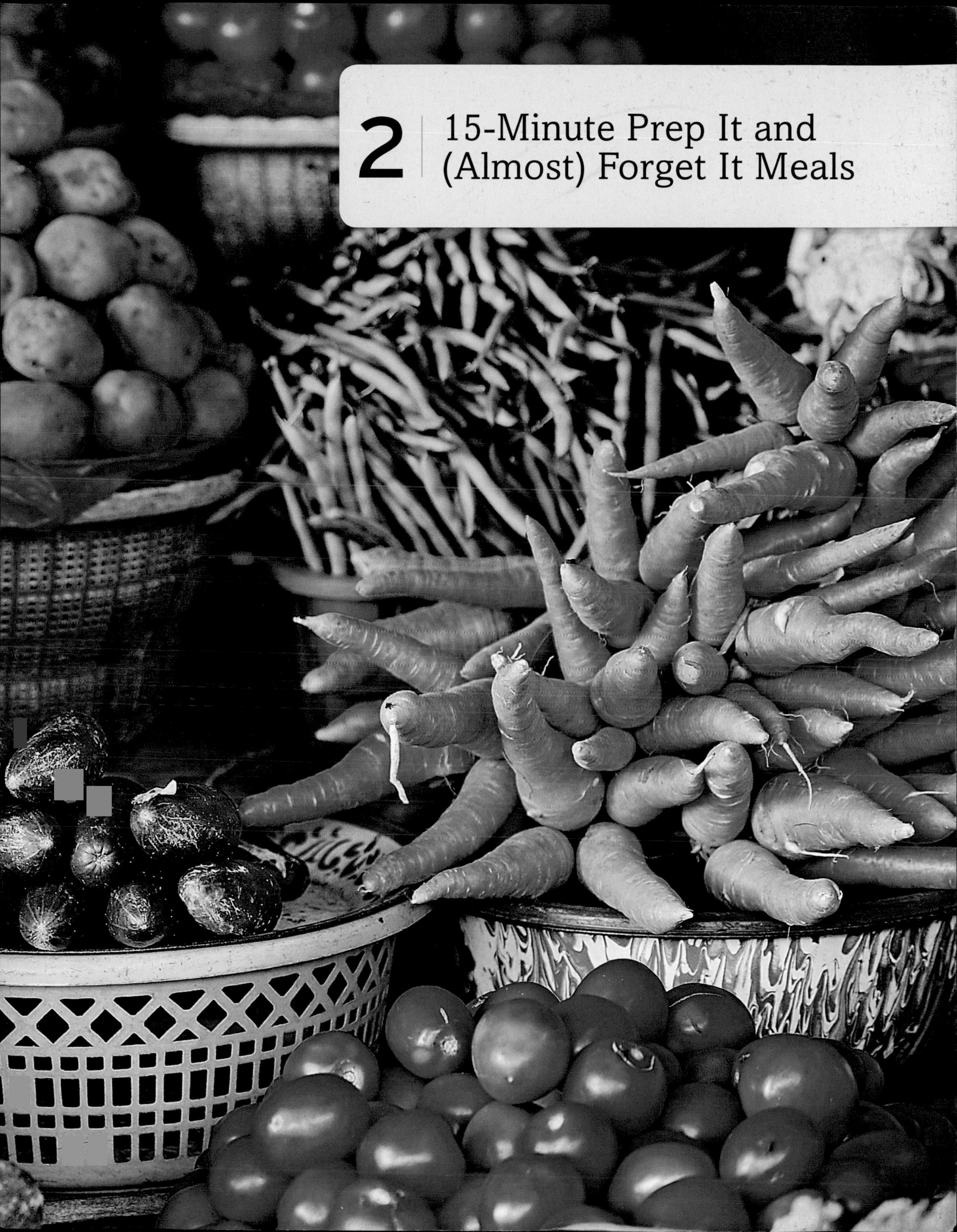

2 | 15-Minute Prep It and (Almost) Forget It Meals

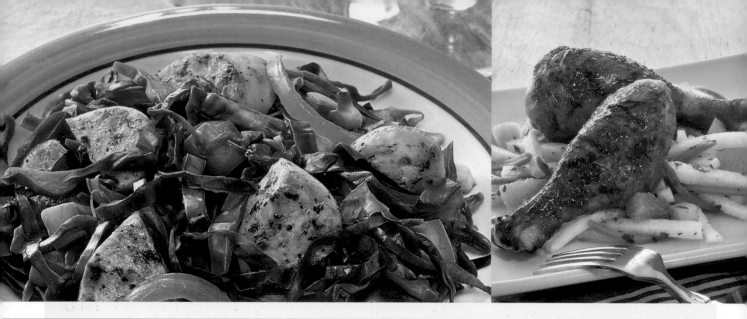

Poultry

As a lean source of protein, poultry is hard to beat for its versatility, as shown in these flavorful recipes. Just be sure to purchase poultry without the hormones, steroids, and other unhealthy additives. These dishes require a bit more cook time, but are both easy and delicious to make. Bonus: They incorporate superspices such as turmeric and antioxidant-rich additions like cranberries and cabbage.

One-Pot 5-Spice Chicken and Shrimp
  Soup

Honey Drumsticks with Calorie-Burning
  Cayenne

Light and Quick Caribbean Chicken Thighs

Quick-Dash Baked Hash

Healthy-in-a-Hurry Chicken Apple
  Sausage and Red Cabbage

A Healthier Meatloaf with Chutney

One Main, Two Meals II

  Easy Roasted Turkey Tenderloin
with Cranberry Salsa

  Low-Cal Turkey Barley Soup

One-Pot 5-Spice Chicken and Shrimp Soup

Ingredients

3 cups (684 ml) chicken broth

2 tablespoons (12 g) five-spice powder

1 tablespoon (15 ml) low-sodium tamari

1 tablespoon (15 ml) honey

1 sweet potato, peeled and chopped (or 2 cups [220 g] prepared diced Yukon Gold potato)

1 can (13.5 ounces or 385 g) light coconut milk (or 1½ cups [455 ml] plain unsweetened almond milk)

4 heads baby bok choy, roughly chopped (or 1 small head of mature bok choy, chopped)

1 bunch scallions, sliced into 1-inch (2.5 cm) pieces

1½ cups (210 g) cooked chicken breast, cubed*

¾ pound (340 kg) precooked fresh or frozen peeled and deveined medium shrimp

From Chef Jeannette

Variation Tip: For a pescatarian version (and to reduce saturated fat), use 1 cup (460 g) of prepared baked tofu, cubed, in place of the chicken. In the fall, substitute diced winter squash for the sweet potato for a fresh, seasonal alternative.

From Dr. Jonny: Typically, Chinese five-spice powder is made with star anise, fennel, Szechuan peppercorns, cloves, and cinnamon, but there are different variations. The formula is based on the Chinese philosophy of balancing yin and yang in food, and the five-spice powder is designed to encompasses all five flavors used in Chinese cuisine: sweet, sour, bitter, spicy hot, and salty. Here Chef Jeannette has given us a lovely one-pot meal with the subtle soft sweetness of the five spices. Worth mentioning is that bok choy—also known as Chinese cabbage—is an amazing nutritional bonanza. One of the lowest-calorie vegetables on earth (9 calories for 1 cup because it's mostly water), it nevertheless contains 74 mg of calcium, 25 mcg of bone-building vitamin K, 176 mg of potassium, and a whopping 3,128 IU of vitamin A and 1,877 mcg of beta-carotene. And even this isn't the whole story, as bok choy, a member of the cabbage group, also contains cancer-fighting plant chemicals called glucosinates. The mix of sweet potatoes and coconut milk is an especially pleasant and satisfying treat for your taste buds.

In a large soup pot, combine the chicken broth, five-spice powder, tamari, honey, and sweet potato, and bring to a boil. Reduce the heat, cover, and simmer for about 15 minutes or until the potato is tender (but not falling apart). Stir in the coconut milk, bok choy, and scallions, and cook until the bok choy is almost tender, about 3 minutes. Add the chicken and shrimp and cook for 1 to 2 minutes or until both are just heated through.

Yield: 4 servings

Per Serving: 321 Calories; 11g Fat (29.6% calories from fat); 38g Protein; 20g Carbohydrate; 2g Dietary Fiber; 165mg Cholesterol; 846mg Sodium

*If you don't have precooked chicken, add one boneless, skinless chicken breast, sliced into 1-inch (2.5 cm) pieces, in last the 15 minutes of cook time. For raw shrimp, allow 2 to 3 minutes of cook time until they turn pink. Do not overcook.

Honey Drumsticks with Calorie-Burning Cayenne

Ingredients

8 chicken drumsticks
  (about 2½ pounds or 1 kg)
1 teaspoon garlic granules
1 teaspoon onion powder
1 teaspoon paprika
¾ teaspoon chili powder
¾ teaspoon cayenne pepper
1 teaspoon ground cumin
¾ teaspoon turmeric
½ teaspoon salt
2 tablespoons (28 ml) lemon or lime juice
  (preferably fresh-squeezed)
¼ cup (85 g) honey

From Dr. Jonny: Chef Jeannette sent me this question a while ago: "Can chicken drumsticks be healthy?" The answer is yes. Just add a bunch of terrific spices such as metabolism-boosting cayenne pepper and the anti-inflammatory, anticancer superspice turmeric, accompany with the highly recommended fabulous salad featuring the underappreciated crunchy vegetable jicama, and you're in business! Jicama, a root vegetable that's sold as a street food in South America and is a staple of Mexican cuisine, is low in calories and remarkably high in fiber (6 grams per cup!). It's also got calcium, magnesium, potassium, vitamin C, vitamin A, and beta-carotene. The citrus tang and cool crunch of the salad offset the gentle spicy bite of the hot chicken. Note: Chef Jeannette offers a tip for skinning the drumsticks—which reduces the calories even more.

Preheat the grill to medium (or preheat the broiler). Make two deep diagonal cuts across the meaty part of each drumstick. In a gallon-size zip-closure bag, mix together the garlic powder, onion powder, paprika, chili powder, cayenne, cumin, turmeric, and salt.

Add the drumsticks to the bag and move them around until evenly coated, pressing the spices into the cut grooves. Place the drumsticks on a lightly oiled grill or broiler pan and cook for 15 to 20 minutes (depending on plumpness) or until nearly done.

While the chicken is cooking, in a small bowl, whisk together the lemon and honey. Divide the mixture and use half to baste the chicken for the last minute of cook time. When the chicken is off the heat, baste with the remaining citrus honey before serving.

Yield: 4 servings
Per Serving: 466 Calories; 29g Fat (55.3% calories from fat); 32g Protein; 20g Carbohydrate; 1g Dietary Fiber; 164mg Cholesterol; 400mg Sodium

From Chef Jeannette

To Complete the Meal: Whip up this delicious Citrus Jicama Salad while the chicken is cooking:

2 small navel oranges, peeled
1 large jicama, peeled and julienned
1 cup (110 g) prepared grated carrots or
  prepared diced tricolor peppers
1½ cups (205 g) diced or grated peeled
  English cucumber
⅓ cup (5 g) chopped fresh cilantro,
  optional
¼ cup (60 ml) fresh lime juice
2 teaspoons honey
1 tablespoon (15 ml) almond or
  macadamia nut oil

When the chicken first goes on the grill, make 4 cuts through the oranges "across the equator," and separate the segments on each of the ten slices (five per orange). In a medium bowl, combine the orange segments, jicama, carrots, cucumber, and cilantro, and mix gently. In a small bowl whisk the lime juice, honey, and oil together and pour over the salad. Toss gently to coat and allow to rest at room temperature. Toss again just before serving.

If You Have 15 Extra Minutes: To reduce the calories and saturated fat in this dish, skin the chicken legs before scoring them. Grab the skin at the top of the meatiest part of the leg and pull it downward toward the thinner section. It will peel downward easily to the bone at the bottom. Because this is slippery work, use a knife to pin the skin to a cutting board and then pull the chicken leg away from it to separate.

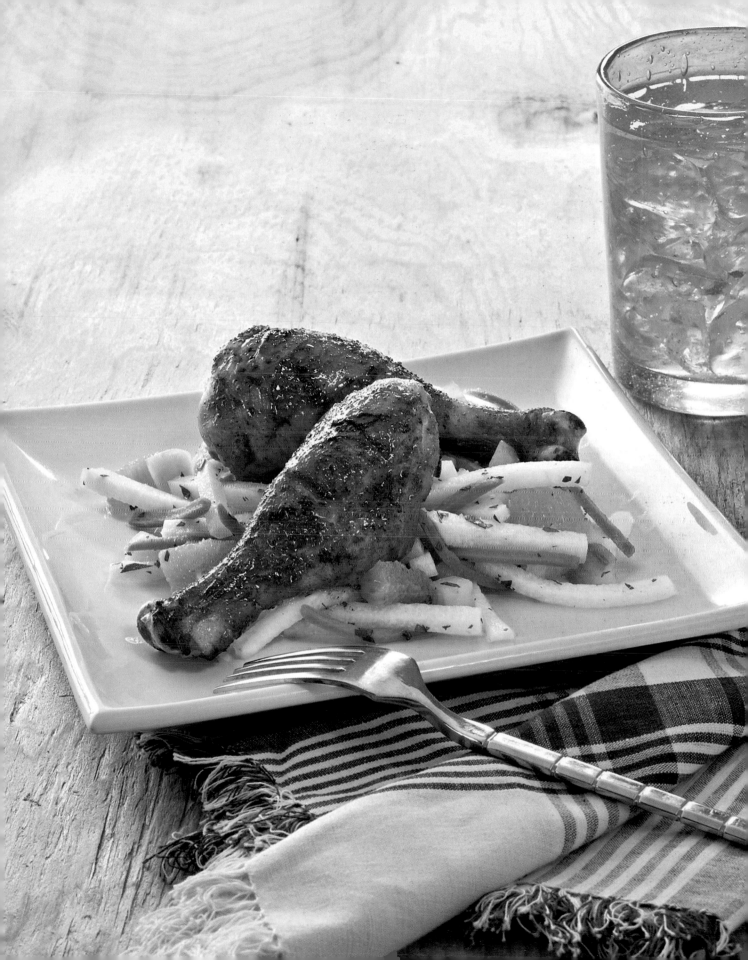

Ingredients

½ cup (120 ml) pineapple juice

¼ cup (60 ml) low sodium tamari

1 tablespoon (15 ml) dark rum

1 tablespoon (6 g) prepared minced ginger (or grated fresh)

1 teaspoon (10 g) prepared minced garlic (or 2 cloves minced)

1/8 teaspoon red pepper flakes

8 boneless, skinless chicken thighs (about 2 pounds [910 g])

From Chef Jeannette

To Complete the Meal: Serve with hot peas and rice. Prepare 1 cup (130 g) of frozen peas and 1½ cups (248 g) frozen cooked brown rice (or use leftovers or parboiled quick-cooking) according to package directions, combine and toss with 2 teaspoons (10 ml) low-sodium tamari and ¼ cup (28 g) toasted sliced almonds.

If You Have an Extra 30 Minutes:
Let the chicken soak in the marinade before cooking for a stronger flavor, up to overnight if you can prepare it the day before.

Light and Quick Caribbean Chicken Thighs

From Dr. Jonny: Almost every "health conscious" person has been indoctrinated with the idea that it's always best to choose white meat chicken, but I disagree. Dark meat—which we admittedly don't use all that often in these recipes—is a perfectly fine choice. Sure it's a bit higher in calories, but still not very caloric (178 calories per 100 grams), and the meat itself has iron, potassium, phosphorus, zinc, and selenium, not to mention a whopping 23 grams per cup of high-quality protein. The majority of the fat in dark meat chicken is actually monounsaturated (the same kind found in avocados and olive oil) and the few grams of saturated fat aren't a problem at all, "conventional" wisdom to the contrary. Skinless thighs provide a rich, quick-cooking protein the whole family will love. Just pair it with light fair, such as the classic Caribbean rice and peas dish recommended here!

Preheat oven to 425°F (220°C, gas mark 7).

Place the juice, tamari, rum, ginger, garlic, and red pepper flakes in a medium shallow roasting pan and mix to combine.

Add the thighs to the pan in a single layer and turn to coat.

Bake for 10 minutes, turn the thighs over to re-coat or baste, then cook for 10 to 15 more minutes or until chicken is cooked through but still very moist.

Yield: 4 servings

Per serving: 253 Calories; 10.8g Fat (38% calories from fat); 28.2g Protein; 4.9g Carbohydrate; Trace Dietary Fiber; 99mg Cholesterol; 436mg Sodium

Ingredients

2 teaspoons olive oil

4 organic chicken sausages, Italian-style

2 cups (220 g) prepared diced potatoes
    (½-inch [1 cm] "hash brown" potatoes)

1 cup (150 g) prepared diced tricolor pep-
    pers (or dice 1 large red or green bell
    pepper)

1 large zucchini, grated or diced

1 pint (300 g) cherry tomatoes, halved

1 teaspoon dried oregano

1 teaspoon dried basil

1 teaspoon garlic granules

Salt and fresh-ground pepper

From Chef Jeannette

To Complete the Meal: Serve with lightly
scrambled eggs for more protein, or a
large Italian salad for more antioxidants;
use plenty of romaine lettuce, diced
red onions, grated carrots, diced red
bell peppers, sliced mushrooms, and a
prepared balsamic or Italian vinaigrette.

Quick-Dash Baked Hash

From Dr. Jonny: For me, "hash" connotates low-quality fatty meat and a bunch of white potatoes highly salted and mixed into an unappetizing goo. (It also reminds me of my less-than-wonderful experiences at sleepaway camp, but that's a whole different story. Don't get me started.) Anyway, this version uses sausages—not just any sausage, mind you, but a nitrate-free (and lower-fat) version that is not only tasty but has fewer calories than regular sausage (not to mention it's not made of "mystery meat"). This baked hash will put you in mind of the Italian provinces—it's also a great way to use up any leftover vegetables. Bonus benefit: It will erase any pesky remnant memories of sleepaway camp. Or maybe that's just me.

Preheat the oven to 375°F (190°C, gas mark 5).

Spread the olive oil evenly over the bottom of a Dutch oven. Slit the sausages and spread their contents out in the bottom of the pan. Sprinkle the potatoes evenly over the sausages. Mix in the peppers and zucchini. Top with the tomatoes and sprinkle the oregano, basil, and garlic evenly over all. Season to taste with salt and ground pepper. If the sausage is low fat, drizzle a small amount of olive oil over the vegetables.

Top with a sprinkling of red pepper flakes, if using. Bake for 20 to 25 minutes or until all the vegetables are tender.

Yield: 4 servings
Per Serving: 286 Calories; 13g Fat (40.0% calories from fat); 25g Protein; 18g Carbohydrate; 4g Dietary Fiber; 75mg Cholesterol; 792mg Sodium

Ingredients

1 tablespoon (15 ml) coconut oil

4 links (3 ounces or 85 g each) high-quality chicken apple sausage (e.g., Applegate Farms Organic Chicken and Apple Sausage)

1 small red onion, sliced

1 pound (455 g) prepared shredded red cabbage (about 4 cups [280 g])*

2 cups (220 g) presliced green apples, unpeeled and roughly chopped

½ cup (120 ml) apple cider

1 tablespoon (15 ml) apple cider vinegar

1 tablespoon (12 g) Sucanat

2 tablespoons (28 ml) red wine

¼ teaspoon salt

½ teaspoon fresh ground black pepper

From Chef Jeannette

To Complete the Meal: Serve with 12 ounces (340 g) of prepared baked or roasted sweet or white potatoes (e.g., Cascadian Farms Organic Wedge Cut Oven Fries) for a hearty winter meal, or microwave four small garnet yams and serve with a sprinkling of ume plum vinegar for a calorie-free condiment (or use tiny pats of butter). (See page 181 for directions to microwave sweet potatoes). For a superspeed side with fewer carbs, prepare 10 ounces (280 g) of frozen cooked summer squash with a little coconut oil and a sprinkle of salt stirred in.

Healthy-in-a-Hurry Chicken Apple Sausage and Red Cabbage

From Dr. Jonny: I can't take credit for this recipe, but I am delighted that Chef Jeannette came to the same conclusion I came to years ago—protein foods taste great with apples! (I've cooked eggs and apples together, chicken and apples, just about anything and apples.) Here Chef Jeannette pairs a lean chicken sausage with my favorite cooking fruit. As usual, the sweetness from the apple balances the rich, warm, and satisfying meat, resulting in a taste delight. This particular dish has overtones of a heavier German dish but is light on calories, especially compared to, say, bratwurst and sauerkraut! The red cabbage and onions add a healthy dose of antioxidants and cancer-fighting plant chemicals, not to mention a hearty taste. (Note: You'll be surprised at how good this dish tastes stir-fried in my favorite cooking oil, Barlean's Organic Coconut Oil.)

Heat the coconut oil in a Dutch oven or large sauté pan over medium-high heat. Slit open the casings from the sausage and remove them from the meat (or slice thickly to save time). Break the skinless sausage up and add to the pan. Add the onion and cook for 4 minutes or until the sausage is lightly browned, stirring frequently. Add the cabbage, apples, cider, vinegar, Sucanat, red wine, salt, and pepper, stirring gently to combine. Reduce the heat, cover, and cook for 15 to 20 minutes or until the cabbage is tender, stirring occasionally.

Yield: 4 servings

Per Serving: 169 Calories; 5g Fat (27.4% calories from fat); 10g Protein; 22g Carbohydrate; 4g Dietary Fiber; 32mg Cholesterol; 389mg Sodium

*If you can't find prepared sliced red cabbage, quarter and core a 1½-pound (710 g) head and feed it through a food processor using the slicer attachment, or slice thinly (widthwise) by hand (do this after chopping the apple and before you heat the oil).

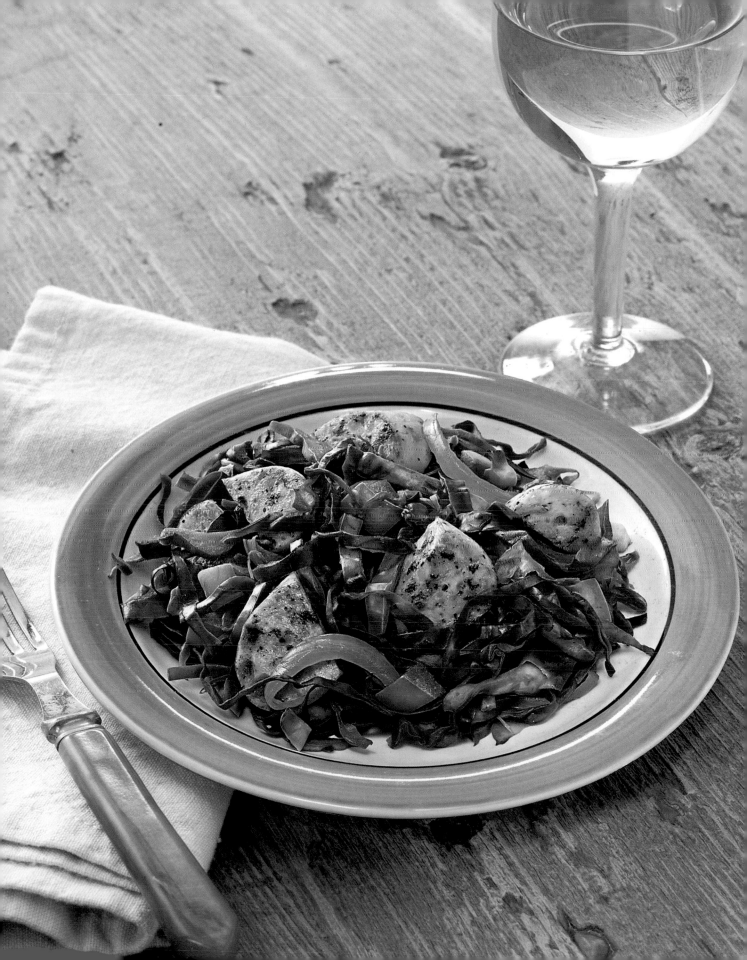

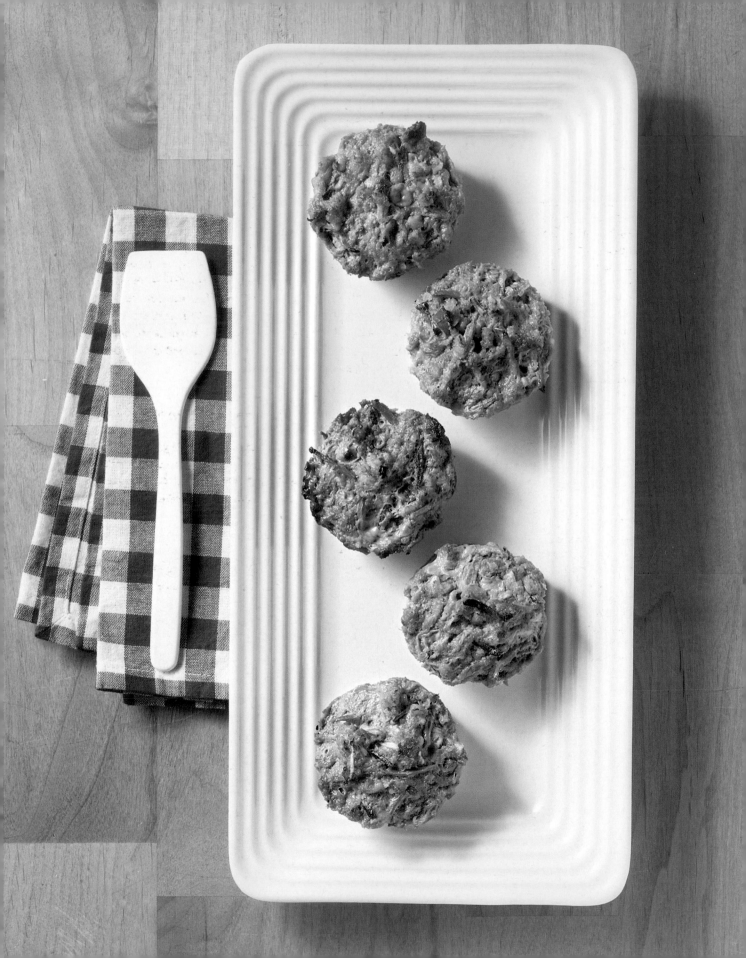

Ingredients

1 egg

½ cup (125 g) prepared chutney, or to taste for heat and sweet (e.g., Trader Joe's Mango Ginger Chutney or Native Forest Organic Pineapple Chutney)

1 to 1½ pounds (455 to 710 g) leanest ground turkey

⅓ cup (27 g) whole rolled oats

1 cup (110 g) prepared shredded carrots

1 cup (120 g) grated zucchini or summer squash, optional

1 teaspoon mustard powder

1 teaspoon onion powder

½ teaspoon salt

½ teaspoon cracked black pepper

From Chef Jeannette

To Complete the Meal: Steam 6 cups of fresh or 10 ounces (280 g) of frozen green beans, toss with 1½ tablespoons (25 ml) of Italian or balsamic salad dressing (or make your own with 1 tablespoon (15 ml) of lemon juice, 1 teaspoon of Dijon mustard, ½ teaspoon of garlic powder, and a pinch of salt), and top with ⅓ cup (37 g) of toasted sliced or slivered almonds.

A Healthier Meatloaf with Chutney

From Dr. Jonny: My mother, bless her heart, was not exactly a great cook. (True story: Until I was a teenager, I actually thought spaghetti and meatballs came out of a can.) But she knew how to make meat-loaf, which she actually did rather well. So meatloaf occupies a warm fuzzy spot in my culinary memory bank, just like it does for so many other people. Problem is, the conventional version is high in fat and calories, stuffed with bread crumbs (unnecessary carbs and calories), and most often made with meat that contains hormones, steroids, and antibiotics. This crowd-pleasing low-cal version makes some clever substitutions that won't lose you an iota of flavor or comfort, but will gain you a heck of a lot of healthy nutrition. Lean turkey instead of feedlot-farmed mystery meat, rolled oats instead of bread crumbs, and vegetables fill it out. The chutney lends a sweet and exotic spiciness. My mother would have loved it!

Preheat the oven to 375°F (190°C, gas mark 5). Lightly spray a twelve-cup muffin tin with cooking oil.

In a large bowl, whisk together the egg and chutney. Add the turkey, oats, carrots, zucchini, if using, mustard powder, onion powder, salt, and pepper, and mix with your hands until well combined. Gently spoon the meat evenly into twelve muffin cups (do not pack). Bake for about 30 minutes or until cooked through.

Yield: 12 mini loaves

Per Serving: 95 Calories; 3g Fat (29.5% calories from fat); 7g Protein; 9g Carbohydrate; 1g Dietary Fiber; 38mg Cholesterol; 120mg Sodium

Choose the Right Protein

Protein comes from the Greek, meaning "of prime importance." You need protein—or more accurately, the building blocks of protein known as amino acids—to construct just about everything your body needs to run effeciently. Muscle proteins known as actin and myosin enable every muscular movement under the sun, from flexing your biceps to blinking your eyes. A protein called hemoglobin carries oxygen throughout the bloodstream. Proteins make up bones and muscles, hormones and neurotransmitters. Without protein (and without fat) you would simply die. (The same can't be said of carbohydrates, interestingly enough, but that's a whole other discussion.)

You get protein from either animal foods (fish, chicken, turkey, meat, milk, eggs) or plant sources such as tofu and beans. Controversy ranges about protein quality, and several ranking systems have been developed to measure how well the body absorbs and uses protein from a given food source. (These systems include biological value, net protein utilization, protein efficiency ratio—you get the idea.) On most of these scales milk and eggs score very high, closely followed by beef and soybeans; protein from vegetables or grains, such as corn, scores much lower.

The fact that a protein food scores very high in one of the ranking systems isn't the whole story, however. Beef always scores pretty high because it provides important amino acids that are easily incorporated into the body, but most commercial beef comes with a helping of steroids, antibiotics, and hormones that you certainly don't need or want. Choose protein sources that are both high on the scales of bioavailability and also low on the scales of pollutants and contaminants. Examples include grass-fed beef, free range chicken and turkey, eggs, and wild salmon.

Ingredients

Turkey

2 tablespoons (40 g) honey mustard
½ teaspoon ground cumin
½ teaspoon curry powder
¼ teaspoon allspice
1 tablespoon (6 g) orange zest
Salt and fresh ground pepper, to taste
1 boneless, skinless turkey tenderloin
    (2 pounds or 900 g)

Salsa

2 cups (200 g) fresh cranberries
    (or 1 bag [8 ounces] frozen,
    unsweetened, thawed)
1 large navel orange, peeled and halved
1 small jalapeño, stemmed and roughly
    chopped, optional
¼ cup (85 g) raw honey, or to taste

From Chef Jeannette

To Complete the Meal: Scrub four garnet yams (or regular sweet potatoes if you can't find yams) well, pierce once with a fork, and place them in a microwave oven. Microwave on high for about 5 minutes. Remove the yams and place them on a sheet of aluminum foil (to catch any drippings) on the rack next to the turkey. Cook with the turkey for 30 minutes or until soft to the squeeze. Serve with a sprinkle of salt and a tiny touch of butter or ghee.

One Main, Two Meals II

From Dr. Jonny: Let's talk turkey. If you're looking for a healthy, low-calorie, generally excellent all-around protein source, look no further. It's not hard to find free-range turkey, and even the regular kind tends to be less loaded with the chemicals and hormones put into factory-farmed beef. Cranberries are another of these great fruits that don't get enough attention, although that's beginning to change. They're high in antioxidants and anti-inflammatory properties, low in calories, and they bring a terrific taste to almost anything they're added to (especially turkey). And for the second meal you've got barley, a "good carb" because it's a great source of both soluble and insoluble fiber, which makes it a terrific grain for the heart. For those who are concerned about cholesterol, barley is a great way to bring it down naturally. In fact, the U.S. Food and Drug Administration recently gave food companies the okay to make a health claim on foods containing barley! And soup is a proven weight-loss food, adding to this recipe's healthy résumé.

Easy Roasted Turkey Tenderloin with Cranberry Salsa

Preheat the oven to 400°F (200°C, gas mark 6). Spray a roasting pan with high-heat cooking oil.

In a small bowl, mix together the honey mustard, cumin, curry, allspice, and zest and set aside.

Lightly salt and pepper the turkey tenderloin and coat it evenly with the honey-mustard mixture (use your hands or a brush). Roast the turkey uncovered for about 35 minutes or until an instant-read thermometer inserted into the thickest part of the meat reads 160°F (71°C). Remove the turkey and let it rest for at least 5 minutes before slicing. Slice half of the turkey thinly for tonight's meal, and shred or dice the other half into bite-size cubes (for tomorrow's soup).

Once the turkey is in the oven, prepare the salsa and let it rest while the meat is cooking so the flavors can develop. Place the cranberries, orange, jalapeño, if using, and honey in a blender or food processor and blend well, to the consistency of relish. Serve the salsa with the sliced turkey.

Yield: 4 servings plus extra relish
Per Serving: 437 Calories; 15g Fat (31.3% calories from fat); 46g Protein; 30g Carbohydrate; 3g Dietary Fiber; 132mg Cholesterol; 253mg Sodium

Ingredients

1½ tablespoons (25 ml) olive oil

1½ cups (240 g) prepared diced onion (or 1 yellow onion, diced)

1½ cups (165 g) prepared shredded carrots (or grate 2 whole carrots)

6 cups (1.5 L) chicken broth

½ teaspoon salt

½ teaspoon pepper

½ teaspoon dried thyme

2 tablespoons (28 ml) mirin

¾ cup (150 g) quick-cooking pearl barley

1½ (195 g) cups frozen corn

1 pound (455 g) leftover (or precooked cooked) turkey, shredded or cubed

½ cup (75 g) golden raisins

Low-Cal Turkey Barley Soup

Heat the oil in large, heavy-bottom soup pot over medium heat. Add the onion and carrots and sauté for about 5 minutes. Add the chicken broth, increase the heat to high, and bring to a boil. Add the salt, pepper, thyme, mirin, and barley, reduce the heat, and simmer for 10 minutes. Add the corn, turkey, and raisins, and simmer for about 5 minutes or until the veggies and barley are tender.

Yield: 4 servings

Per Serving: 329 Calories; 11g Fat (28.6% calories from fat); 21g Protein; 38g Carbohydrate; 6g Dietary Fiber; 41mg Cholesterol; 996mg Sodium

From Chef Jeannette

Planned Leftovers: This soup makes a big pot. If you aren't serving company, freeze the extras for a third meal. Cool it thoroughly in the fridge, then freeze it in a tempered-glass container, such as Pyrex. Cover the surface of the soup with a layer of microwave-safe plastic wrap and seal it with the lid, squeezing out any excess air. You should leave about an inch (2.5 cm) of space for expansion: It will expand as it freezes.

To Complete the Meal: Serve soup with a salad of crunchy greens, such as romaine hearts, diced green apples, raisins, toasted sliced almonds or chopped walnuts, and a light fruity prepared vinaigrette, such as pomegranate. (Or use our recipe for a quick apple dressing on page 48.)

If You Have 10 More Minutes: To add additional fiber to the soup for more staying power on a cold night, add 1½ cups (186 g) of ¾-inch (1.5 cm) cubes of any peeled and seeded winter squash (e.g., prepared butternut). Add the squash when you add the broth and simmer it for an extra 10 minutes before you add the barley—you may need to add a bit more broth.

Meat

No mystery meat here! Chef Jeannette's iron-rich, grass-fed beef recipes sizzle with Latin and South American flavors that put your favorite Mexican restaurant's calorie-laden menu to shame. With super-healthy additions like chile peppers, olives, cumin, and fire-roasted tomatoes, these recipes will satisfy your taste buds without breaking the calorie bank.

Totally Fast Tamale Bake

Almost-Instant, Iron-Rich Picadillo

One-Pot Fiber Fiesta Taco Soup

Wild about Venison Stew with Savory Mushrooms

Totally Fast Tamale Bake

From Dr. Jonny: Nothing personal, Taco Bell, but this recipe has you beat on every count, starting with taste and ending with nutrition. With this recipe, the term "healthy fast food" is no longer an oxymoron! It's light, tasty, easy to prepare, and with its combination of chili powder, corn, and cumin, distinctly Mexican. Loaded with fiber and protein, it also contains healthy compounds called phenols from the black olives, blood pressure–lowering garlic, and cancer-fighting antioxidants such as lycopene from the tomatoes. Best of all, because you make it yourself, you get to choose the protein source—grass-fed beef (instead of mystery meat), turkey, or even a vegan option! Take that, Taco Bell chihuahua!

Ingredients

1½ cups (240 g) prepared diced onion (or 1 yellow onion, diced)

2 teaspoons prepared minced garlic (or 3 cloves, minced)

1½ cups (225 g) prepared diced tricolor peppers (or 1 green or red bell pepper, seeded and diced)

1 pound (455 g) leanest ground beef, turkey, or vegan "beef crumbles" (12-ounce [340 g] bag)

½ teaspoon salt

1 can (15 ounces or 425 g) black beans, drained and rinsed

2 cans (14.5 ounces or 413 g) fire-roasted diced tomatoes, undrained

½ cup (50 g) sliced black olives, optional

2 cups (260 g) frozen corn

1 tablespoon (7.5 g) chili powder, or to taste

1 teaspoon ground cumin

¼ teaspoon ancho chile pepper (or cayenne)

½ cup (70 g) cornmeal

Preheat the oven to 350°F (180°C, gas mark 4).

Lightly spray a 9 × 13-inch (23 × 33 cm) baking dish with olive oil and set aside.

Heat the oil in a large skillet over medium-high heat. Add the onion, garlic, bell pepper, meat, and salt, and sauté until no pink remains, 6 to 7 minutes. (If using veggie crumbles, add 1 to 2 tablespoons (15 to 28 ml) olive oil and sauté the onion and pepper for 5 minutes, then add the "beef crumbles" and cook for about 2 minutes, stirring constantly to prevent sticking. If the crumbles are frozen, no need to thaw ahead.) Drain the meat and spoon into a large bowl. Add the beans, tomatoes, olives, if using, corn, chili powder, cumin, chile pepper, and cornmeal, and stir gently to mix well. Spoon into the prepared baking dish. Bake uncovered for 40 minutes.

Yield: about 8 servings

Per serving: 140 Calories; 4g Fat (23.6% calories from fat); 10g Protein; 17g Carbohydrate; 4g Dietary Fiber; 20mg Cholesterol; 269mg Sodium

From Chef Jeannette

If You Have 5 More Minutes: Sprinkle ½ cup (58 g) of shredded Monterey Jack cheese on top for a shot of calcium.

Planned Leftovers: This recipe makes two dinners for four people. To freeze the leftovers, cool for 2 hours to overnight in the fridge, remove any condensation, lay a layer of microwave-safe plastic over the surface of the casserole, sealing it tightly against the sides to prevent air contact, seal the cover over all, and store in the freezer. When you're ready for round two, thaw the frozen leftovers overnight in the fridge and bake, uncovered, for 10 to 15 minutes at 350°F (180°C, gas mark 4) or until heated through.

To Complete the Meal: Serve this with a generous helping of steamed broccoli.

Almost-Instant, Iron-Rich Picadillo

From Dr. Jonny: Picadillo is a traditional Latin American dish also found in the Philippines, where it goes by the name of *giniling*. Chef Jeannette calls it Latin American chili. It's usually made with ground meat and tomatoes and other regional ingredients. Picadillo has been called "a party on your tongue" as it contains a mix of both sweet and *picante* (translated: hot!) flavors. Our version is made of lean ground beef (grass-fed, please!), pimiento olives, and iron-rich raisins. And let me say a word about plantains. Plantains could be thought of as a cousin to the sweet, overripe bananas we usually consume in the United States, except that they tend to be much lower in sugar, somewhat higher in fiber, and loaded with vitamin A and potassium. We suggest you plan ahead—take the time to make the plantains. They're supersimple to prepare but need a little cooking time. It's worth it.

Ingredients

2 teaspoons olive oil

1 cup (160 g) prepared diced onion (or 1 small yellow onion, diced)

½ cup (75 g) prepared diced tricolor peppers (in the refrigerated section)

2 teaspoons prepared minced garlic (or 3 large cloves, minced)

1 pound (455 g) leanest ground beef (96 percent)

1 can (14.5 ounces or 413 g) diced tomatoes (great with fire-roasted), undrained

½ cup (50 g) pimiento-stuffed olives, roughly chopped

⅓ cup (50 g) raisins

3 tablespoons (27 g) capers

¼ teaspoon salt

¼ teaspoon ground cinnamon

¼ teaspoon ground cloves

1 bay leaf, optional

Heat the oil in a Dutch oven over medium-high heat. Add the onion, peppers, garlic, and beef and sauté for 5 minutes or until nearly cooked through (very little pink remaining). Drain any excess oil, if necessary. Add the tomatoes, olives, raisins, capers, salt, cinnamon, cloves, and bay leaf, if using, stir gently to combine, and bring to a boil.

Reduce the heat, cover, and cook for about 20 minutes or until all veggies are tender and the beef is cooked through. Stir in a little beef broth or water if the liquid level drops too low. Remove the bay leaf, if using, before serving.

Yield: 4 servings

Per Serving: 382 Calories; 23g Fat (54.8% calories from fat); 23g Protein; 20g Carbohydrate; 3g Dietary Fiber; 78mg Cholesterol; 478mg Sodium

From Chef Jeannette

To Complete the Meal: Serve with green brown rice (see page 200 for recipe).

If You Have 45 Extra Minutes: Bake two fully ripe plantains in their skins (they will look almost black when fully ripened). Place them on a baking sheet and bake for 40 to 45 minutes or until very soft. Carefully slice off each end and slit each peel down the length of the plantain. Open and scoop out the hot fruit and mash it lightly with a little coconut oil or butter, and salt and fresh ground pepper, to taste. Find plantains in large grocery stores or Latin American markets.

Variation Tip: For a slightly leaner meat and different nutrient profile, substitute lean ground turkey for the beef.

Ingredients

2 teaspoons olive oil

1 pound (455 g) lean ground turkey (or veggie "beef crumbles," such as Quorn Meatless Soy-Free Grounds, 12-ounce [340 g] bag frozen, no need to thaw)*

1 teaspoon prepared minced garlic (or 2 cloves, minced), optional

½ teaspoon salt

½ teaspoon ground black pepper

2 cups (260 g) frozen corn

1 can (15 ounces or 425 g) kidney beans, undrained

1 can (15 ounces or 425 g) pinto beans, undrained

1 can (15 ounces or 425 g) black beans, undrained

2 cans (14.5 ounces or 413 g each) fire-roasted diced tomatoes, undrained

1 small can diced green chiles, undrained

1 packet (1 ounce or 28 g) high-quality taco seasoning (we like Simply Organic Southwest Taco Seasoning)

1 packet (1 ounce or 28 g) high-quality ranch dressing (we like Simply Organic Ranch Dressing)

One-Pot Fiber Fiesta Taco Soup

From Dr. Jonny: The featured ingredient in this tasty, tangy soup is canned beans! Now I know I've railed against canned foods before, calling them inferior nutritionally, but there are exceptions to the "no cans" rule, and beans are one of them (along with pineapples and pumpkin). Beans hold their nutritional value very well, and it's easy to find all kinds of varieties of canned beans that are organic and made without added salt or preservatives—a godsend for quick cooking. This trifecta of bean soup is filling, but much lighter in calories than the taco soup that you'd get in a typical Mexican restaurant. But it's no lightweight when it comes to flavor—your whole family will love this one!

Heat the oil in a large soup pot over medium heat. Add the turkey, garlic, if using, salt, and pepper, and mix well. Cook, stirring frequently, until there is no pink left in the turkey, about 8 minutes. Add the corn, three types of beans, tomatoes, chiles, and taco and ranch seasoning packets, and mix well.

Fill one empty can with water and add that in twice (two cans' worth). Increase the heat and bring to a boil. Lower the heat, cover, and simmer for 30 minutes.

Yield: about 12 servings

Per Serving: 460 Calories; 5g Fat (10.4% calories from fat); 31g Protein; 74g Carbohydrate; 24g Dietary Fiber; 30mg Cholesterol; 468mg Sodium

*If you use the "beef crumbles," skip the browning step and add them when you add the corn and canned veggies

From Chef Jeannette

Flawless Freezing: Cool the portion of food you would like to freeze completely in the refrigerator—overnight is best. Remove any condensation and store it in a freezer-safe container with at least an inch (2.5 cm) of space between the top of a liquid and the lid (½-inch [1 cm] for solids). To protect against ice crystals, lay a sheet of microwave-safe plastic wrap right on the surface of the chilled food, sealing it on the sides and blocking all air contact. Squeeze out the air, seal the lid, and store in the freezer. Thaw overnight in the fridge before warming for use the next time. If you take these careful steps to freeze it, it will taste just as fresh as when you cooked it.

To Complete the Meal: Top with a little shredded Jack or Cheddar cheese for increased protein, calcium, and vitamin D. My son likes to crumble baked corn chips on his, like Mexi-croutons. Add a light green salad with diced bell peppers and a Mexican-style vinaigrette to finish (we like Newman's Own Lighten Up Light Lime Vinaigrette).

If You Have 10 More Minutes: Add a diced zucchini or yellow squash, and a seeded and diced red or orange bell pepper. You can also add a bag of fresh baby spinach or thawed frozen spinach. Just drop them in the soup when you add the beans. If I have fresh cilantro on hand, I'll throw in a good handful of that at the end of cook time, as well.

When Choosing Canned Beans: My family is originally from the South, and I grew up eating this classic, easy "canned soup." Because the beans are undrained and unrinsed, it's even more important to choose high-quality, organic versions with absolutely no chemical additives or salt. Our favorite canned beans are from Eden Organics. The linings on their cans are BPA-free, and they cook their beans with a little kombu (sea vegetable) to naturally improve their digestibility.

Wild about Venison Stew with Savory Mushrooms

Ingredients

2 tablespoons corn or olive oil, divided

¾ pound (340 g) boneless venison meat, cut into ½-inch (1 cm) cubes

½ teaspoon salt

½ teaspoon cracked black pepper

2 shallots, roughly chopped

2 teaspoons prepared minced garlic (or 3 cloves, crushed and chopped)

3 ounces (85 g) wild mushrooms, presliced, if possible (morel, shiitake, cremini, etc.)

1½ teaspoons dried thyme (if time, better with 1½ tablespoons [3.6 g] chopped fresh)

4 cups (950 ml) beef broth plus extra, if necessary

2 tablespoons (18 g) cornmeal

1 can (14 ounces) hominy, drained and rinsed

2 cups (260 g) frozen corn kernels

From Chef Jeannette

To Complete the Meal: Prepare the broccoli jalapeño cornbread on page 206 (from Real Men's Jalapeño Cornbread Chili), or, for a faster option, make a watercress salad with green onions, chopped tomatoes, and a prepared tomato vinaigrette.

Variation Tip: If you can't get venison in your area, substitute lamb for a slightly different flavor and nutrient profile and start checking at 15 minutes of cook time for doneness. If you can't find hominy, use 4 cups (520 g) of fresh or frozen corn instead of 2.

If You Have 15 More Minutes: For a fresher taste, use raw corn right off the cob instead of frozen. Shuck four medium ears of fresh corn, plant the ear vertically on its widest end, and slice the kernels off with a sharp knife lengthwise on four sides of the ear, working from the top down. Put the fresh kernels into the soup about 15 minutes before the end of cook time to soften.

From Dr. Jonny: Whenever I talk to audiences about why I don't believe in making food low fat (or worse, no fat), I point out that our Paleolithic ancestors didn't eat low-fat caribou. Game meat is a whole different animal from the processed meats that give meat-eating a bad name. Venison is naturally low in calories, high in protein, and virtually never filled with all the chemical garbage found in factory-farmed meat. Hominy, corn without the germ, is especially popular in the South, and in New Orleans the whole kernels are still referred to as "big hominy" and the ground ones as "little hominy." In most of the South, in fact, *hominy* has became synonymous with "hominy grits" or just plain grits. In any case, this stew hits the spot on a cold night. The sweetness of the corn mellows the natural gaminess of the venison—a perfect balance!

Heat 1 tablespoon oil in a Dutch oven over medium-high heat. Add the venison cubes, season with salt and pepper, and brown lightly on all sides for 3 to 4 minutes, draining off excess fat. Remove from the pan, set aside, reduce the heat to medium, and add the remaining tablespoon of oil, shallots, garlic, mushrooms, and thyme, and sauté for 3 minutes or until the mushrooms release their juices. Add the venison the back to the pan and add the broth, cornmeal, and hominy. Reduce the heat, cover, and simmer on low heat for 25 to 30 minutes, stirring occasionally, or until the meat is fork tender. Add the corn and extra broth or water if soup is too thick, and simmer for 2 to 3 minutes more or until the corn is tender. Adjust the seasonings, if necessary.

Yield: 4 to 6 servings

Per Serving: 228 Calories; 7g Fat (26.9% calories from fat); 22g Protein; 19g Carbohydrate; 3g Dietary Fiber; 48mg Cholesterol; 1205mg Sodium

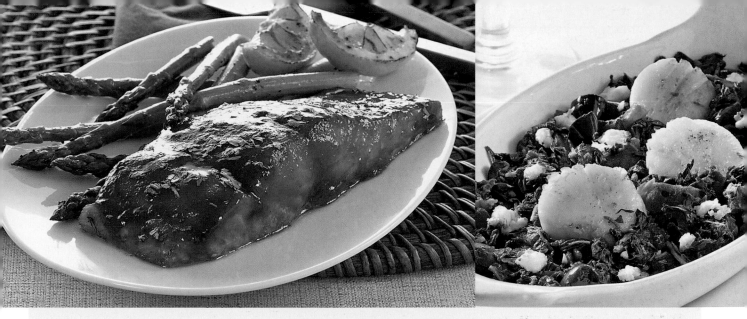

Seafood

Fish is not only an excellent source of protein, it's also one of the quickest foods on the planet to prepare, as evidenced by this fabulous foursome. Flavors from heart-healthy olive oil, the superfood coconut milk, and garlic—one of the oldest medicinal foods on Earth—enhance and enrich these dishes. Add vegetable superstars like spinach and cauliflower and you'll love these delicious, nutritious offerings.

Tasty, Time-Saving Tuna in Comforting
  Coconut Milk

15-Minute German Potato Salmon Salad

Heart-Healthy Harissa Roasted Salmon
  with Lemon Asparagus

Awesome Antioxidant Scallops
  Mediterranean

Ingredients

2 tablespoons (28 ml) olive oil

1½ cups (240 g) prepared diced onion (or 1 sweet onion, diced)

1 cup (130 g) thin-sliced carrot coins, about 2 peeled carrots (or prepared shredded carrots, or prepared diced red pepper)

1 teaspoon curry powder

¼ teaspoon turmeric

¼ teaspoon ground nutmeg

3 cups (300 g) small cauliflower florets, ½ inch (1 cm), (about 2 pounds or 900 g precut fresh, or 1 medium head, chopped)

1 can (15 ounces or 425 g) light coconut milk

¾ teaspoon salt

1 can (7 ounces or 195 g) tuna fish in water, drained and flaked (you can also use salmon—we like Vital Choice)

From Chef Jeannette

To Complete the Meal: Add a healthy serving of steamed sugar snap peas or a small salad of fresh tropical fruits.

Superspeed Tip: To prepare this dish in half the time, omit the carrots and sauté the onions for 3 minutes. Using one 15-ounce (425 g) bag of frozen cauliflower florets (unthawed) in place of the fresh, add all ingredients from curry powder through tuna fish to the Dutch oven. Simmer for 7 to 8 minutes or until the cauliflower is hot and tender. Add 1 cup (130 g) of frozen peas for the last minute of cook time.

Tasty, Time-Saving Tuna in Comforting Coconut Milk

From Dr. Jonny: This is one of those recipes that literally made my mouth start to water as soon as I read the title. I love coconut, which I consider a superfood, and the idea of cauliflower simmering in a coconut sauce got my taste buds going! The recipe features one of the greatest superspices on the planet, turmeric, which is tremendously anti-inflammatory—it's also good for the liver. Cauliflower is one of the few exceptions to the "don't eat anything white" rule. It's a member of the brassica family of vegetable royalty and loaded with plant compounds called indoles, which have significant anticancer activity. The Vital Choice tuna (or salmon) adds a ton of clean protein to the mix. Creamy, warming, and satisfying, this is healthy comfort food at its best!

Heat the oil in a large Dutch oven over medium heat. Add the onion and carrots and sauté for 4 minutes. Add the curry, turmeric, and nutmeg, and sauté for 1 minute, stirring well to coat. Add the cauliflower, coconut milk, and salt, stirring gently to combine well. Increase the heat to bring just to a boil. Reduce the heat and cook uncovered until the cauliflower is tender, about 30 minutes. Add the tuna and gently stir it in for the last 10 minutes of cook time.

Yield: 4 servings

Per Serving: 231 Calories; 13g Fat (47.1% calories from fat); 16g Protein; 16g Carbohydrate; 4g Dietary Fiber; 15mg Cholesterol; 627mg Sodium

15-Minute German Potato Salmon Salad

From Dr. Jonny: I get all my salmon from Alaska, direct from Vital Choice, this terrific company of third-generation Alaskan fishermen who are as an environmentally and nutritionally conscious a group as I've ever seen. They ship me the absolute finest and tastiest fish I've ever eaten. So I'm constantly ordering salmon and looking for new ways to serve it. This is one I honestly would never have thought of (which is why Chef Jeannette is the chef in this partnership!). Here's a satisfying potato salad with an interesting twist and a trace of the Germanic. It's a hearty meal that also works cold, and, unlike "traditional" potato salad, is loaded with protein and omega-3 fats. By the way, some of the prep time for this one happens at the end of the very short cooking time, rather than at the beginning.

Ingredients

1¼ pounds (567 g) small baby Yukon Gold potatoes, unpeeled, halved, or quartered if larger than golf balls

2 tablespoons (30 g) Greek yogurt

2 tablespoons (28 ml) olive oil

1 tablespoon (15 g) Dijon mustard

1½ tablespoons (25 ml) apple cider vinegar

1 tablespoon (11 g) mustard seeds

½ teaspoon salt

½ teaspoon cracked black pepper

1 cup (160 g) sliced scallions

2 cups (40 g) baby arugula or baby spinach

2 cans (6 ounces or 170 g each) smoked wild Alaskan salmon, drained (e.g., Vital Choice Smoked Wild Red Salmon, or use regular skinless, boneless)

In a large saucepan, combine the potatoes and enough water to generously cover the potatoes.

Bring to a boil over high heat, lower the heat, partially cover, and simmer for about 15 minutes or until the potatoes are fork-tender. Drain.

While the potatoes are cooking, in a small bowl, mix together the yogurt, olive oil, mustard, vinegar, mustard seeds, salt, and pepper.

Put the cooked potatoes in a large bowl and stir in the scallions and arugula to wilt, partially crushing the potatoes. Fold in the salmon and dressing and mix gently to coat.

Adjust the seasonings, if necessary, and serve warm.

Yield: 4 servings

Per Serving: 309 Calories; 11g Fat (33.3% calories from fat); 21g Protein; 30g Carbohydrate; 3g Dietary Fiber; 21mg Cholesterol; 1006mg Sodium

Heart-Healthy Harissa Roasted Salmon with Lemon Asparagus

Ingredients

2 teaspoons olive oil, divided
2 teaspoons harissa paste,* or to taste
2 tablespoons (40 g) honey
2 salmon steaks (10 ounces or 280 g each)
1 pound (455 g) female asparagus (the
    thicker ones), trimmed and sliced into
    2-inch (5 cm) pieces
¼ teaspoon salt
¼ teaspoon black pepper
1 lemon, quartered
¼ cup (4 g) chopped fresh cilantro, optional

From Dr. Jonny: I confess: I didn't know what harissa was when we started this book. So I did what I always do and went to the trusty Googles. A few minutes later I had a pretty good idea that whatever else it was, harissa was hot! Technically it's a hot chili sauce that's common in North Africa, made from tomatoes, paprika, and red hot chile peppers (the food, not the band!). Yes, it's got a fiery bite, but as Chef Jeannette points out below, it's really a complex flavor, not at all like straight-up pepper. The lemon and honey calm its fiery edge in this true one-pot meal. Worth noting is that asparagus is one of the highest-protein vegetables as well as one of the lowest-calorie ones. A mere cup of asparagus contains only 40 calories and more than 4 grams of protein, not to mention 1.5 mg of iron and more than 400 mg of heart-healthy potassium (take that, bananas!).

Preheat the oven to 400°F (200°C, gas mark 6). Line a shallow roasting pan with foil and set aside.

In a small bowl, mix together 1 teaspoon of the olive oil, harissa paste, and honey. Brush the fish all over with the mixture and lay the fillets on one side of the prepared pan. In a medium bowl, toss the asparagus with remaining teaspoon of olive oil, salt, and pepper, and arrange on the other side of the pan. Nestle the lemon quarters among the fillets and asparagus. Roast for 10 to 12 minutes or until the fish is just cooked through. To serve, divide each fillet in half and remove the center bones (and skin, if desired), add one quarter of the asparagus and one quarter of the roasted lemon, garnishing with the cilantro, if using.

Yield: 4 servings
Per Serving: 218 Calories; 7g Fat (29.5% calories from fat); 28g Protein; 10g Carbohydrate; trace Dietary Fiber; 73mg Cholesterol; 229mg Sodium

*Harissa paste is a very pungent chili paste—a little goes a long way! It contains several spices, including garlic, and has a distinctive flavor. Look for it in tubes or jars in Middle Eastern markets and gourmet grocers.

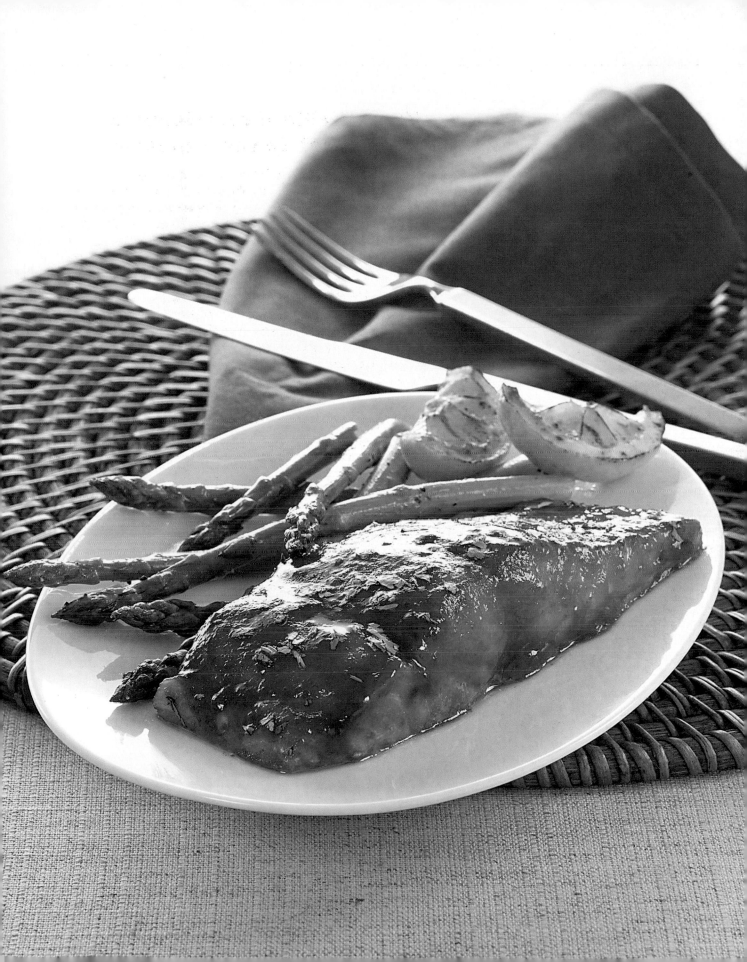

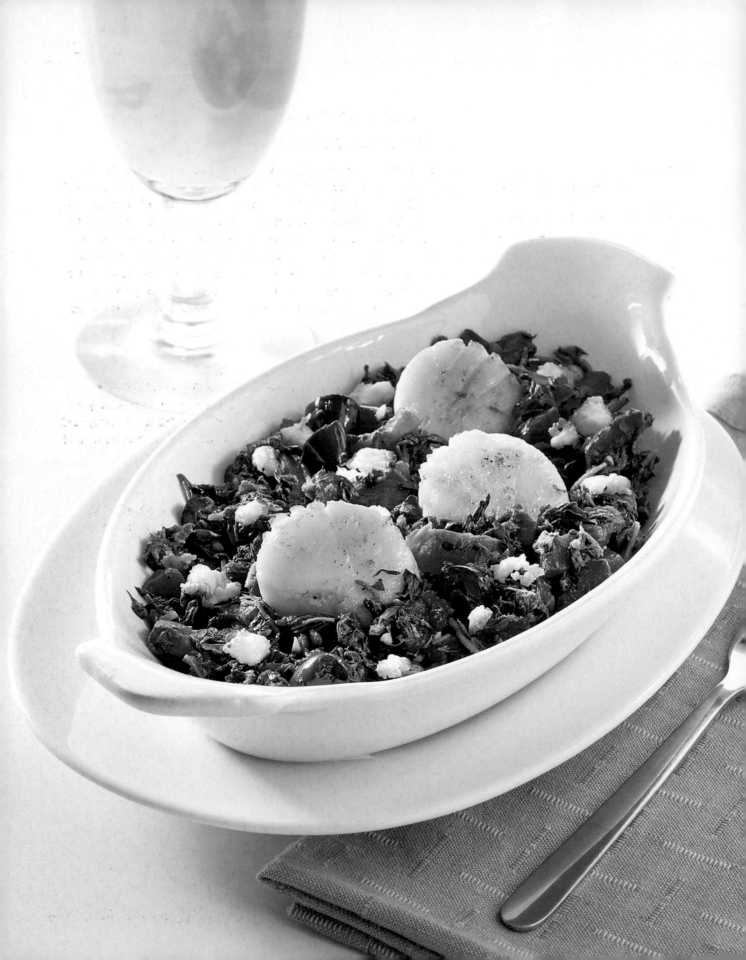

Awesome Antioxidant Scallops Mediterranean

Ingredients

1 can (14.5 ounces or 413 g) diced tomatoes, drained

1 package (10 ounces or 280 g) chopped frozen spinach, thawed and drained (pressing against sieve to remove excess moisture)

2 tablespoons (28 ml) dry white wine

2 roasted red peppers, diced

1/3 cup (33 g) pitted, halved, Kalamata olives

1 1/2 teaspoons prepared minced garlic (or 2 cloves, minced)

2 teaspoons dried basil

1/4 teaspoon salt

1/4 teaspoon fresh ground black pepper

1 1/2 pounds (710 g) sea scallops

4 ounces (115 g) crumbled feta cheese

From Chef Jeannette

If You Have 5 More Minutes: Drizzle a teaspoon or two of olive oil over the casserole just before baking and garnish with 1/4 cup (15 g) of chopped parsley and few squeezes of fresh lemon juice before serving.

From Dr. Jonny: It's hard to argue with the success of the Mediterranean diet for improving health and reducing the risk of really bad stuff happening. Although the Mediterranean diet has a lot of variations, all focus heavily on fruits, vegetables, nuts, oils such as olive oil, and a ton of fish. This kind of diet has been shown to reduce heart disease and, more recently, the risk of strokes and ultimately, dementia. This dish is classic Mediterranean fare—high-quality protein from the sea mixed with high-antioxidant vegetables such as tomatoes and spinach and topped with feta, the classic Mediterranean cheese. Did I mention that it tastes great, too?

Preheat the oven to 450°F (230°C, gas mark 8).

Lightly spray a 7 × 11-inch (18 × 28 cm) baking pan with olive oil.

In a medium bowl, mix together the tomatoes, spinach, wine, peppers, olives, garlic, basil, salt, and pepper until combined. Fold in the scallops and pour into the prepared dish. Sprinkle evenly with the feta. Cook for 15 to 20 minutes or until just browned.

Yield: 4 servings

Per Serving: 306 Calories; 10g Fat (30.4% calories from fat); 37g Protein; 16g Carbohydrate; 4g Dietary Fiber; 84mg Cholesterol; 937mg Sodium

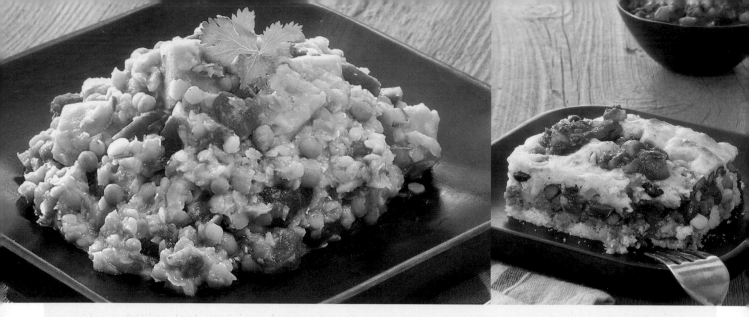

Meatless

Talk about comfort food! Here's pizza, pasta, and pudding—with all the flavor and none of the guilt! These easy and robust dishes get their protein from beans, cheese, tofu, eggs, and yogurt. Good-for-you grains such as whole wheat pasta and rolled oats add fiber and avoid the high-glycemic load of more traditional offerings.

Portobello Power Pizza in a Snap

Robust Red Lentil Curry-in-a-Hurry

One-Pot Red-Beans-and-Greens with a Kick

Fantastic Feta-Chickpea Casserole

Fiber-Friendly Protein Pasta

Easy Everyday Enchiladas

Zippy Zucchini Lasagna

Super Low-Cal Curried Zucchini Soup

Healthy Jalapeño Cornbread Chili

Low-Sugar, High-Protein Indian Pudding

Healthy Start Breakfast Bake

Ingredients

2 tablespoons (28 ml) olive oil

3 cloves garlic

2 portobello mushroom caps, stemmed, halved, and sliced into strips (about ⅓ inch [0.7 cm] thick)

Pinch salt

1 whole-grain, premade, thin pizza crust (10 ounces or 280 g), about 12 inches or 30 cm (we like Rustic Pizza organics)

¾ cup (184 g) premade pizza sauce with Italian herbs (we like Muir Glen—one 15-ounce [425 g] can makes 2 pizzas), or to taste (I prefer extra sauce and less cheese!)

1 cup (100 g) halved or sliced ripe pitted black olives

⅔ cup (75 g) shredded mozzarella cheese (or can use Manchego sheep cheese), or to taste

Sprinkling fresh grated Parmesan, optional

From Chef Jeannette

Variation Tip: This basic formula works well with many combinations. Try shredded cooked chicken with caramelized onions and wilted baby spinach over a light glazing of barbecue sauce (page 44) and grated Cheddar.

Superspeed Tip: Use any combination of ingredients that require no precooking. For instance, try raw baby arugula (or baby spinach) mixed into the tomato sauce, sliced artichoke hearts, and soaked sun-dried tomato strips with a combo of feta and shredded mozzarella.

To Complete the Meal: Serve with a side of Greek or Caesar salad.

Portobello Power Pizza in a Snap

From Dr. Jonny: Remember the famous "pizza study" that the media was buzzing about a couple of years ago? Seems that men who ate ten or more servings of foods with cooked tomatoes, such as pizza, had a lower risk of prostate cancer. That sounded like really good news for pizza lovers, but the fact is that it wasn't the pizza that lowered the risk, it was the cooked tomatoes (which most guys consumed in the form of pizza and spaghetti sauce). Not that there's anything wrong with pizza per se. But really, who needs all the bad stuff that goes with greasy, commercial, traditional pizza—white flour crust, cheap oil, and a ton of calories? Certainly not you or me. But there's a great solution: the Portobello Pizza in a Snap! Instead of greasy meat and poor-quality cheese, you get a delicious, light, whole-grain thin-crust masterpiece you can make in minutes. Seriously. See Chef Jeannette's notes about customizing this base with your own favorite nutrient-packed toppings. Try including my favorite—pineapple.

Preheat the oven to 450°F (230°C, gas mark 8).

Heat the oil in a large sauté pan over medium heat. Add the garlic and sauté for 1 minute. Add the mushrooms and salt, and stir gently to coat (give mushrooms space, so they can brown properly). Sauté the mushrooms, turning often to brown evenly, until soft and wilted, about 7 minutes. They will drink all the oil quickly at first, then release their delicious juices.

Lightly oil a baking sheet (or use a pizza stone) and place the crust in the center. Spread the sauce evenly around the crust, leaving a border at the edge, and place the mushrooms into the sauce, spacing them apart evenly. Sprinkle on the olives and top with the cheeses. Reduce the oven temperature to 425°F (220°C, gas mark 7) and cook the pizza for 10 to 12 minutes until the cheese is melted and the edges are lightly browned.

Yield: 4 servings

Per Serving: 200 Calories; 16g Fat (66.1% calories from fat); 7g Protein; 11g Carbohydrate; 2g Dietary Fiber; 17mg Cholesterol; 623mg Sodium

Ingredients

3 cups (710 ml) low-sodium vegetable or chicken broth

1 tablespoon (15 g) Thai green curry paste (e.g., Thai Kitchen)

1 can (14.5 ounces or 413 g) diced tomatoes

1½ cups (288 g) dried red lentils, rinsed and drained

1 large sweet potato, peeled and diced into ½-inch (1 cm) cubes

½ teaspoon salt, or to taste

1 cup (130 g) frozen peas

1 cup (235 ml) low-fat coconut milk

⅓ cup (13 g) chopped fresh cilantro or slivered fresh basil, optional

From Chef Jeannette

To Complete the Meal: Serve with steamed broccoli and tomato wedges with a squeeze of lime juice and a sprinkle of salt.

Robust Red Lentil Curry-in-a-Hurry

From Dr. Jonny: About every month or so a magazine or website asks me to compose a list of top "superfoods"; I usually mix and match from the foods in my book *The 150 Healthiest Foods on Earth*, but I almost always include beans. Technically, the term *legumes* includes beans, lentils, and peas, but from a health perspective, beans and lentils are almost the same. Lentils are a dieter's dream, and eating lentils on a regular basis is associated with significantly lower rates of cancer and heart disease. I especially like red lentils and I love curry and its nice dose of the anti-inflammatory superspice turmeric. This is a mellow (for curry!) and satisfying dish—once you try it, you'll wind up eating it often!

Heat the broth in a large soup pot over high heat. Whisk in the curry paste to dissolve, add the tomatoes, lentils, and potato, and bring to a boil. Reduce the heat to a simmer, cover, and cook for 15 minutes or until the vegetables and lentils are tender—watch the liquid level. Stir in the salt, peas, and coconut milk until smooth and cook for 2 minutes or until heated through. Adjust the seasonings to taste and stir in the cilantro just before serving, if using.

Yield: 4 to 6 servings
Per Serving: 285 Calories; 5g Fat (14.4% calories from fat); 19g Protein; 46g Carbohydrate; 18g Dietary Fiber; trace Cholesterol; 313mg Sodium

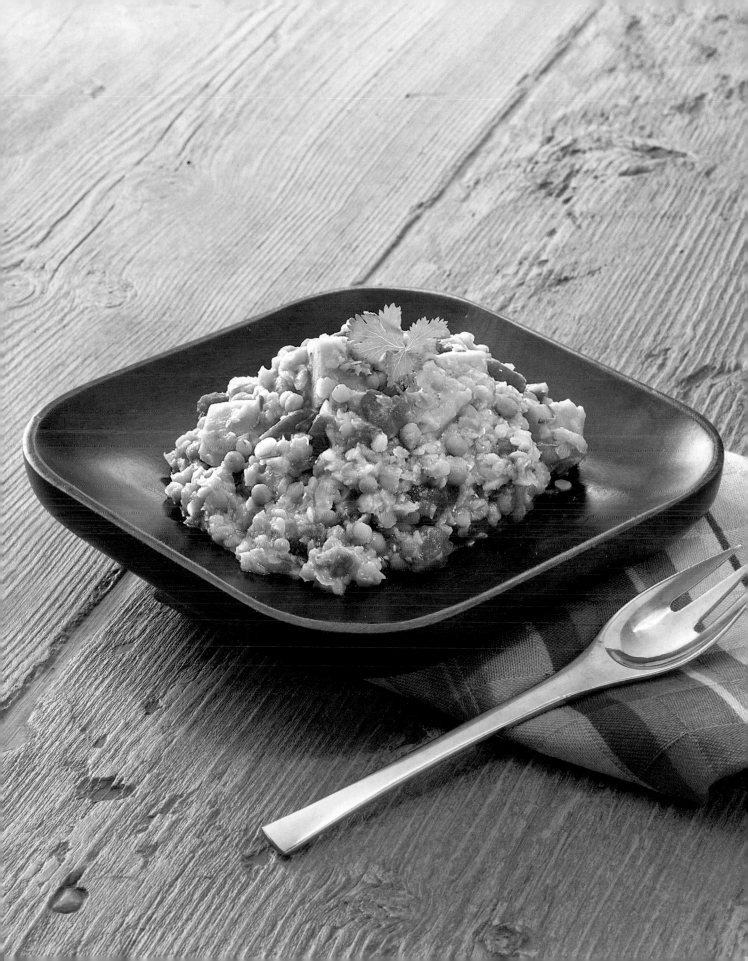

Ingredients

2¼ cups (535 ml) low-sodium chicken or
   vegetable broth
1 teaspoon olive oil
½ teaspoon salt
½ teaspoon chipotle pepper (or red pepper
   flakes), or to taste
1 cup (195 g) quick-cooking (parboiled)
   brown rice
2 packed cups (110 g) stemmed, shredded
   collard greens*
2 tablespoons (32 g) tomato paste
3 drops liquid smoke, optional
2 to 3 sprays Bragg Liquid Aminos, optional,
   to taste
1 can (15 ounces or 425 g) red beans,
   drained and rinsed

From Chef Jeannette

To Complete the Meal: This is a true one-pot meal and can stand alone as a light meal as far as macronutrient balance. If you want a little something extra, try a light salad of grated carrots and jicama dressed in fresh lime juice, olive oil, and fresh cilantro.

One-Pot Red-Beans-and-Greens with a Kick

From Dr. Jonny: Probably the most traditional food pairing in the world is beans and rice, and for good reason. The amino acids in the two foods complement each other perfectly, making a complete protein. Let's not forget the high amount of fiber in the beans. Chef Jeannette has upped the ante even further by adding collard greens, a staple of my "soul food" youth. Well, maybe I'm exaggerating, as I grew up Jewish, but collard greens were among my favorite dishes that my Southern friends served, and I love them to this day. You'll love them too in this tasty, filling entrée.

Bring the broth to a boil over high heat in a large saucepan. Add the oil, salt, pepper, and brown rice, stirring lightly to mix. Reduce the heat and simmer, covered, for 10 minutes. Stir in the shredded collards and cook for 10 more minutes. Add the tomato paste, liquid smoke, and liquid aminos, if using, stirring well to combine. Gently fold in the beans, remove from the heat, and rest it for 5 minutes. Season to taste with additional liquid aminos or chipotle pepper, if necessary. Fluff with a fork and serve.

Yield: 4 servings
Per Serving: 462 Calories; 2g Fat (4.4% calories from fat); 33g Protein; 80g Carbohydrate; 28g Dietary Fiber; trace Cholesterol; 655mg Sodium

*To shred the collards, stack them neatly on top of each other on your cutting board, run your knife down either side of the tough stem sections in a V, and pull the stems out. Or save these to dice and cook later; they actually have a higher mineral concentration than the leaves themselves. Fold the leaves over and roll them up like a cigar. Run the cigar through the grating attachment on your food processor, or to shred by hand, slice the "cigar" in half the long way. Holding the two rolled halves together, thinly slice the leaves along the width, and chop the slices roughly.

Fantastic Feta-Chickpea Casserole

Ingredients

2 tablespoons (28 ml) coconut oil (or olive)

1 large yellow onion, diced (or 2 cups [320 g] diced prepared)

1 can (15 ounces or 425 g) chickpeas, drained and rinsed

3 cloves garlic, minced (or 1½ teaspoons prepared)

1 tablespoon (2.4 g) minced fresh thyme (or ¾ teaspoon dried)

½ cup (75 g) crumbled feta cheese

1 tablespoon (15 ml) lemon juice

3 eggs, lightly beaten

½ teaspoon salt

½ teaspoon cracked black pepper

From Chef Jeannette

To Complete the Meal: Serve with shredded zucchini and tomatoes. Using the grating attachment on your food processor, shred two medium zucchini. Heat 2 teaspoons of olive oil and 1 minced clove (or 1 teaspoon prepared minced) garlic in a large sauté pan over medium and add the shredded zucchini. Cover and cook for about 4 minutes, stirring occasionally. Remove the lid, add 1 cup (180 g) of grape tomatoes, sprinkle with salt and fresh ground pepper to taste, stir well, and re-cover for 2 minutes. Remove the lid, stir, and test for tenderness and seasonings. If the zucchini is very juicy, drain and discard the extra liquids, if desired. Season to taste and continue cooking for another minute or so until tender, if required.

From Dr. Jonny: Chickpeas are one of the great utilitarian foods that deliver an awful lot of nutritional bang for the proverbial buck. Not only are they a great source of vegetarian protein (about 12 grams per cup!) but they are also a magnificent source of fiber (almost 11 grams for the same cup, more than 20 grams for a 15-ounce [425 g] can!) And let's be honest—almost none of us gets enough fiber. Virtually every health organization on the planet recommends between 25 and 38 grams a day, but the average American gets between 4 and 11 grams. Higher-fiber diets are associated with lower rates of heart disease and diabetes, and fiber helps you feel full longer, making it less likely that you'll overeat. A half cup of feta cheese adds an additional 11 grams of protein to the protein you've got in the eggs and beans, not to mention a whopping 370 mg of calcium. And I'm biased—put feta cheese on almost anything and I'll eat it—but when you taste the combo of garbanzo beans and feta, you'll see what I'm talking about.

Preheat the oven to 350°F (180°C, gas mark 4).

Lightly spray a 7 × 11-inch (18 × 28 cm) baking dish with cooking oil.

Heat the oil in a large skillet over medium heat. Add the onion and sauté until softened, about 5 minutes.

While the onion is cooking, mash the chickpeas coarsely in a large bowl with a potato masher or a large fork until they form a chunky paste (or you can do this in about 10 seconds in the food processor).

Add the garlic and thyme to the sautéing onions and sauté for 1 minute. Reduce the heat to medium-low and stir in the prepared chickpeas. Cook, stirring often, for about 5 minutes. Remove from the heat and spoon into a large bowl. Stir in the feta cheese, lemon juice, eggs, salt, and pepper. Spoon into the prepared baking pan and bake for about 20 minutes or until lightly browned on top.

Yield: 4 servings

Per Serving: 368 Calories; 17g Fat (40.8% calories from fat); 18g Protein; 38g Carbohydrate; 5g Dietary Fiber; 176mg Cholesterol; 538mg Sodium

Fiber-Friendly Protein Pasta

Ingredients

1 bottle (32 ounces or 905 g) tomato vegetable juice (e.g., Knudsen's Very Veggie Organic)

2 cups (475 ml) low-sodium vegetable broth (or chicken broth or water)

2 tablespoons (28 ml) mirin (or use 1 tablespoon [20 g] honey)

2 teaspoons dried basil

2 teaspoons dried oregano

1 tablespoon (9 g) garlic granules (or 1 tablespoon [10 g] prepared minced garlic)

¾ teaspoon red pepper flakes

1¾ cups (336 g) dried brown lentils, rinsed and drained

1 tablespoon (15 ml) sherry, optional

8 ounces (225 g) any style whole grain pasta (e.g., Barilla Plus)

From Chef Jeannette

If You Have 5 More Minutes: Add one 10-ounce [280 g] bag of shredded carrots and/or 2 cups (320 g) of prepared diced onions (or slice one large Vidalia) when you stir in the lentils for more veggie power.

From Dr. Jonny: Ah, pasta. The first food to go on a low-carb diet, yet one of the most beloved comfort foods on the planet. (As a kid, I loved plain old white spaghetti with ketchup, butter, and grated cheese.) But that blue-box white pasta I enjoyed as a kid—the basic pasta everyone eats, minus, of course, the ketchup—is really not what we'd call a "good carb." It's high on the glycemic scale, meaning it raises your blood sugar high and fast, which is bad news for people trying to control their weight and people with blood sugar issues in general. It is high in calories in conventional-size portions. And the heavily sugared sauces don't help matters much. But we do love our pasta, so we've come up with a way to enjoy it guilt free. Barilla Plus pasta is high in fiber, higher in protein, and our version adds lentils for fiber, antioxidants, and a lower blood sugar response. Added bonus: the powerful antioxidant *lycopene* (from the vegetable juice). The recipe is vegan and cholesterol-free (for those who are concerned about those things). Want more calcium? Just sprinkle with a little crumbled feta or freshly grated Parmesan cheese.

In a large soup pot, combine the veggie juice, broth, mirin, basil, oregano, garlic, and pepper and mix well to combine. Stir in the lentils and heat over high heat. When the soup is boiling, reduce the heat, cover, and simmer for about 40 minutes or until the lentils are tender. In the last 10 minutes of cook time, stir in the sherry, if using, and prepare the pasta al dente according to the package directions. Serve the sauce over the hot pasta.

Yield: 4 full servings plus 4 of sauce to freeze—will need another 8 ounces (225 g) of pasta to complete the meal

Fiber-Friendly Protein Pasta
Per Serving: 389 Calories; 2g Fat (3.9% calories from fat); 21g Protein; 73g Carbohydrate; 16g Dietary Fiber; 0mg Cholesterol; 438mg Sodium

Fiber-Friendly Protein Pasta (Sauce)
Per Serving: 178 Calories; 1g Fat (3.8% calories from fat); 13g Protein; 31g Carbohydrate; 14g Dietary Fiber; 0mg Cholesterol; 434mg Sodium

Ingredients

2 tablespoons (28 ml) olive oil

1 cup (160 g) prepared diced onion

1 cup (75 g) prepared diced tricolor peppers

1 package (12 ounces or 340 g) frozen vegan "beef" crumbles (e.g., Quorn Meatless and Soy-Free Grounds)

1 packet (1 ounce or 28 g) high-quality taco seasoning (e.g., Simply Organic Southwest Taco Seasoning)

½ cup (235 ml) water

2 bottles (8 ounces or 225 g each) natural enchilada sauce

8 whole grain wraps (8 inches or 20 cm) or soft corn tortillas (e.g., the 12-ounce package of whole-grain Wrap-itz by Tamxico's)

1 can (16 ounces or 455 g) nonfat, vegetarian refried beans

2 cups (225 g) shredded Mexi-mix cheese, divided

From Chef Jeannette

Planned Leftovers: Cover the glass dish with plastic wrap, laying it on the surface of the cheese and sealing the edges to minimize air contact. Seal with a cover (or use aluminum foil) and store in the freezer until ready to use. Thaw overnight and bake, uncovered, for 30 minutes as directed above.

Easy Everyday Enchiladas

From Dr. Jonny: Enchiladas are always a crowd-pleaser. This special "Planned Leftovers" version is perfect for a Super Bowl party or for dinner tonight and a heat-and-eat next month! By using whole-grain wraps, vegetarian refried beans, vegan "beef" crumbles, and tricolor peppers, you wind up with an enchilada that's just as tasty as Taco Bell (maybe more!) but with less than half the fat and, I venture to say, twice the nutrition. This is a taste of the Southwest that will please just about anyone. Once you make it, it keeps really well and can fill in for a meal or a snack anytime. Even for breakfast!

Preheat the oven to 350°F (180°C, gas mark 4).

Spray two 7 × 11-inch (18 × 28 cm) Pyrex (or other tempered glass) baking dishes lightly with olive oil and set aside.

Heat the oil in a large skillet over medium heat. Add the onion and peppers and cook for 4 minutes, stirring frequently. Add the crumbles, taco seasoning, and water to the dish, stirring well to incorporate, and simmer for about 6 minutes.

Toward the end of the cooking time, set up your enchilada station: Pour a little enchilada sauce into the bottom of each dish and spread it evenly to form a thin layer. Lay your wraps, beans, and half the cheese out near your oven. When the grounds mix is ready, evenly divide the ingredients among the middle of eight wraps in this order: layer of beans, layer of crumbles, sprinkling of cheese. Then fold the far edge of the wrap toward you, up and over the filling. Tuck in the two sides and fold the full section toward you to close the wrap. Lay the wrap seam-side down on the sauce in the prepared baking dish, nestling the wraps together, four to a dish. Pour the remainder of the enchilada sauce evenly over the enchiladas in both dishes and top each with half of the remaining cheese. Bake each dish for 30 minutes.

Yield: 4 servings

Per Serving: 586 Calories; 26g Fat (37.0% calories from fat); 24g Protein; 75g Carbohydrate; 16g Dietary Fiber; 37mg Cholesterol; 1626mg Sodium

Ingredients

1 small sweet potato, peeled and cut in half
lengthwise (or use unpeeled Yukon Gold)

1 medium zucchini, stemmed

1 medium Vidalia or yellow onion

1 jar (24 ounces or 680 g) high-quality pasta
sauce (e.g., Rao's Homemade Arrabiata
for a spicier bite or Amy's Family
Marinara for a milder basil flavor)

1 package (12 ounces or 340 g) frozen vegan
"beef" crumbles (e.g., Quorn Meatless
and Soy Free Grounds), thawed (microwave in a covered glass dish with
2 tablespoons (28 ml) water for 1 to 2
minutes until warm)

1½ cups (175 g) shredded mozzarella cheese

From Chef Jeannette

To Complete the Meal: Add a salad with
hearts of romaine, sliced radishes, diced
red onion, sliced mushrooms, and grated
carrots. Dress lightly with olive oil, fresh-
squeezed lemon juice, and sprinkles of
dried oregano, basil, and garlic granules
(or use a high-quality prepared Italian or
balsamic vinaigrette).

If You Have 15 More Minutes: To beef up
your iron or B$_{12}$ levels, sauté 1 pound
(455 g) of lean ground turkey or 96
percent lean ground beef with a little salt
and fresh ground pepper until cooked
through and use it in place of the veggie
crumbles (drain off any oils first).

Also, for higher nutrient content,
use a homemade red sauce in place of
prepared. See our recipe for no-cook
marinara on page 144, and beef it up with
½ teaspoon of red pepper flakes.

Zippy Zucchini Lasagna

From Dr. Jonny: This incredible, rich dish preserves the classic flavor
of lasagna while lightening up the carb load (not to mention the prep
time) by simply skipping the noodles. But you'll hardly notice. The layers of hearty sweet potatoes will make you forget you ever cared about
pasta in the first place (okay, maybe not, but close). Sweet potatoes
are loaded with nutrients, especially vitamin A and beta-carotene, and
while they're not exactly a "low-carb" diet staple, they're a lot better than white potatoes from a nutritional point of view. Mixed with
cheese, onions, and veggies, the overall dish has a low glycemic load
and won't put you in blood sugar hell. It may, however, put you in taste
bud heaven!

Preheat the oven to 350°F (180°C, gas mark 4).

Lightly spray a 7 × 11-inch (18 × 28 cm) baking dish with olive oil.

Using a mandoline, slice the potato halves into thin half-moon slices,
the zucchini into thin slices lengthwise, and the onion into thin rounds.
(Or use the slicing attachment on a food processor—just slice the potato
into thirds and zucchini in half *lengthwise*, to fit, and make half-moon slices.
It's easiest to slice the onion into thin rounds by hand.)

Spread a thin layer of sauce on the bottom of the baking dish and cover
with a layer of half the sweet potatoes. Make a layer with half the zucchini
and cover with a layer of half the onion. Cover with half the crumbles, half
the sauce, and half the cheese. Repeat the layers in that order with remaining ingredients, making sure all crumbles are covered by sauce to prevent
scorching. Bake uncovered for 45 minutes or until the veggies are tender.

Yield: 4 servings

Per Serving: 239 Calories; 12g Fat (43.4% calories from fat); 18g Protein;
18g Carbohydrate; 5g Dietary Fiber; 39mg Cholesterol; 280mg Sodium

Super Low-Cal Curried Zucchini Soup

From Dr. Jonny: Here's one thing to know about soup—it's one of the best diet aids in the world. Studies by Barbara Rolls, Ph.D., at Penn State University show that people who eat a vegetable-based soup before dinner consume significantly fewer calories during the dinner itself. It seems to be a great way to blunt your appetite. But that's not the only reason to eat this great-tasting, superlow-calorie soup. It's loaded with cancer-fighting onions, blood pressure–lowering garlic, heart-healthy olive oil, and nutritious zucchini, which are loaded with vitamin A and potassium.

Ingredients

1 tablespoon (15 ml) olive oil

2 cups (320 g) prepared chopped onion (or 1 large sweet onion, chopped)

3 teaspoons prepared minced garlic (or 4 cloves, minced)

2 teaspoons curry powder

3/4 teaspoon dried dill (or 1 to 2 tablespoons [4 to 8 g] fresh, added at end of cook time)

1/2 teaspoon salt, or to taste

1/2 teaspoon cracked black pepper

3 medium zucchini, thinly sliced or grated (use the slicing or grating attachment on a food processor to do this in a snap)

3 cups (710 ml) chicken or vegetable broth

1 package (8 ounces or 225 g) Tofu Shirataki fettuccine, rinsed and drained*

1 1/2 cups (345 g) plain low-fat yogurt

Heat the oil in a soup pot over medium heat. Add the onion and sauté for 5 minutes. Add the garlic, curry, turmeric, dried dill, salt, pepper, and zucchini, and sauté for 2 minutes, turning and stirring frequently to coat. Add the broth, increase the heat to high, and bring to a boil. Reduce the heat, cover, and simmer for 6 to 8 minutes until tender (will take less time if zucchini is grated). Puree the soup with an immersion wand or in a blender (carefully!) and return to the heat. Add the fresh dill now, if using. Add the noodles and simmer for 1 minute. Stir in the yogurt.

Yield: 4 to 6 servings

Per Serving: 140 Calories; 3g Fat (21.9% calories from fat); 7g Protein; 21g Carbohydrate; 4g Dietary Fiber; 1mg Cholesterol; 608mg Sodium

*Find Tofu Shirataki fettuccine in the refrigerated section of natural food stores and high-end grocers. At 40 calories, 6 carb grams (4 of them fiber), and 4 grams of protein for the *entire package*, these precooked noodles are a kind of fast-food, low-carb, low-cal miracle! They are also very inexpensive. To use them, drain the water they come in and rinse. They have a bit of a fishy odor, so parboil them for 2 to 3 minutes to remove it. But if I'm putting them into a cooked product, I just rinse and use. This is not a delicate noodle; it has a firm bite, al dente, so you really feel like you're eating something. Use them in other light, brothy soups to give them a toothier feel without changing the carb or calorie count much. How many noodles can you say *that* about?

From Chef Jeannette

If You Have 5 More Minutes: Add 2 tablespoons (28 ml) of fresh-squeezed lemon juice and/or a couple of dashes of hot pepper sauce for a flavor boost and a blast of vitamin C and capsaicin.

Superspeed Tip: Skip the sauté step and omit the oil. Just add all the ingredients through pepper and proceed as instructed. You may need a couple of extra minutes of simmer time for the veggies to soften.

Variation Tip: Use yellow squash in place of the zucchini, and 1/4 cup (10 g) of fresh basil (or 1 teaspoon dried) in place of the dill, but the squash will need about 10 minutes more cooking time to soften.

To Complete the Meal: Serve this dish as is for light fare, or with a piece of light protein, such as grilled chicken or a couple of boiled eggs.

Ingredients

1½ tablespoons (21 g) butter or nonhydrogenated omega-3 vegetable oil spread (e.g., Earth Balance)

2½ cups (312 g) whole-grain cornbread/muffin mix (e.g., Bob's Red Mill Stone Ground Cornbread Mix)

4 eggs

8 ounces (225 g) cottage cheese, about 1 cup

½ cup (120 ml) any milk (cow's, unsweetened plain, soy, almond, etc.)

1 to 2 tablespoons (9 to 18 g) canned chopped jalapeño, drained (or can use fresh, seeded), or to taste

1 package (14 ounces or 400 g) refrigerated vegan "beef" (e.g., Gimme Lean Meatless Beef–or use 1 pound [455 g] cooked lean ground beef or turkey)

1 jar (16 ounces or 455 g) salsa

1 can (15 ounces or 425 g) kidney beans, drained and rinsed

1 can (15 ounces or 425 g) black beans, drained and rinsed

1 cup (130 g) frozen corn, optional

½ cup (50 g) chopped green or Spanish olives, pitted, optional

1½ cups (173 g) shredded Monterey Jack cheese

From Chef Jeannette

If You Have 5 More Minutes: For more veggies, thaw and add a box of frozen chopped broccoli to the cornbread mix.

To Complete the Meal: Serve with a plate of steamed fresh greens, such as spinach or collards.

Healthy Jalapeño Cornbread Chili

From Dr. Jonny: This is what I call "Mexi-comfort" food at its best! It's high in protein and fiber, which you don't often see, and it's flavorful, warming, and filling. You can make it three different ways, all of them good, all of them with specific advantages. For you vegetarians (or even omnivores who want an occasional change from animal protein), the featured veggie option is superb. The beef version is fine as long as you use grass-fed beef. (We love the stuff from U.S. Wellness Meats, which is linked on my website, www.jonnybowden.com, under Online Store/Healthy Foods. See Nutritional Note on page 59.) Ground turkey is a little lighter, but equally high in protein. In any of its versions, this dish will make the grade with the guys on Superb Bowl Sunday! (Just don't tell them it's healthy!)

Preheat the oven to 400°F (200°C, gas mark 6). Place the butter in a 9 × 13-inch (23 × 33 cm) baking pan and place in the oven until the butter is melted, about 5 minutes, then remove, swirl the butter to coat the bottom, and set aside.

While the butter is melting, in a large bowl, combine the cornbread mix, eggs, cottage cheese, milk, and jalapeño and mix until just combined. Spread a thin layer of the corn bread batter over the bottom of the prepared pan. Working with wet fingers, break up and drop the faux "beef" evenly over the batter, and pour the salsa over all. Pour the two beans and corn evenly over the salsa. Sprinkle the olives over the beans and corn, if using. Sprinkle the cheese over all, and top with the remaining batter. Use a wet spoon or wet fingers to spread the batter over the top. It will be sticky and may not cover the entire surface. Bake for 30 to 35 minutes or until the cornbread is cooked through.

Yield: 9 to 12 servings

Per Serving: 339 Calories; 13g Fat (33.3% calories from fat); 21g Protein; 36g Carbohydrate; 7g Dietary Fiber; 120mg Cholesterol; 876mg Sodium

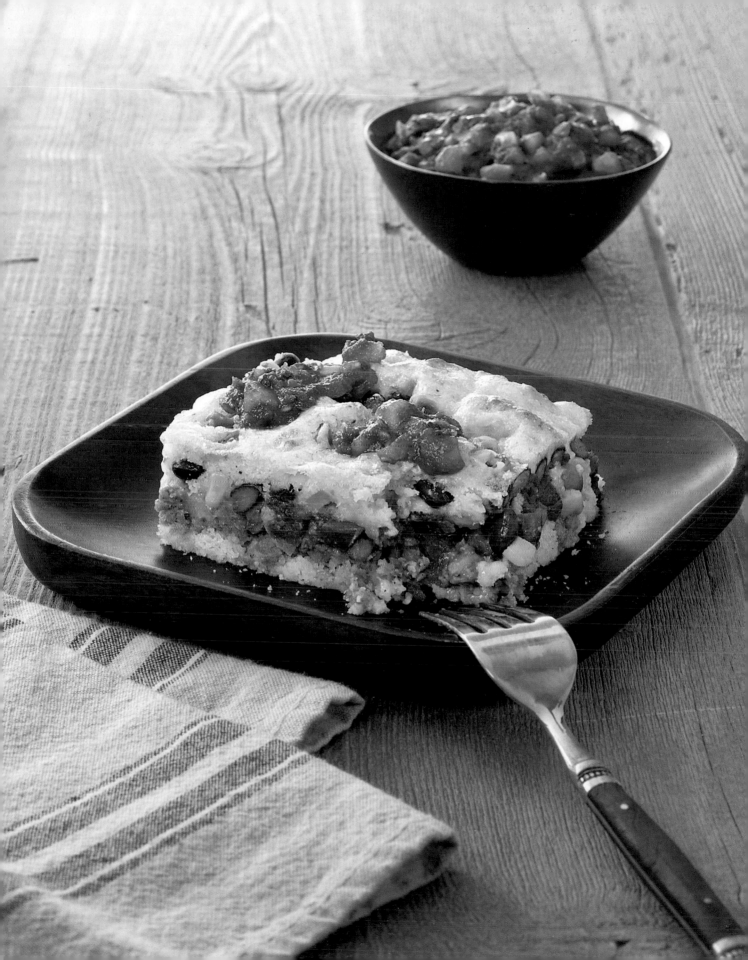

Low-Sugar, High-Protein Indian Pudding

Ingredients

2 cups (275 ml) milk (unsweetened vanilla, soy, or almond milk, or cow's)

½ cup (70 g) cornmeal

⅓ cup (113 g) blackstrap molasses

¼ cup (85 g) 100 percent maple syrup

1 teaspoon ground ginger

½ teaspoon ground cinnamon

¼ teaspoon ground nutmeg

1 cup (460 g) firm silken tofu

⅓ cup (37 g) toasted sliced almonds

⅓ cup (50 g) dried currants

From Chef Jeannette

This is a less sweet, more protein-rich version of the traditional Native American dish, which makes it a good candidate for breakfast or a hearty snack, as well as a lightly sweet dessert. Try it with other nuts or chopped dried fruits.

To Complete the Meal: Serve with vegan or low-fat chicken sausage or vegan, tempeh, or nitrate-free turkey bacon to increase the protein even more and balance the sweetness of the pudding with a salty meat.

From Dr. Jonny: Anything that has "pudding" in the title of the recipe gets my attention. It's been a favorite food of mine since childhood, when my mother used to make it from a mix. So Indian Pudding? I'm paying attention. This recipe not only tastes like pudding but is surprisingly high in vegetarian protein from the soymilk and tofu, which also gives it a creamier texture than traditional Indian pudding. Blackstrap molasses is one of the few really healthy sweeteners, loaded with potassium, calcium, magnesium, and iron. This delicious pudding is warm, dense, and soothing, with a touch of sweet, warming spices. My mother would have loved it, even if though it doesn't come out of a box!

Preheat the oven to 350°F (180°C, gas mark 4).

Spray an 8 × 8-inch (20 × 20 cm) baking pan with almond or olive oil and set aside.

In a medium saucepan, whisk together the milk, cornmeal, molasses, syrup, ginger, cinnamon, and nutmeg. Bring just to a boil over medium-high heat, stirring continuously in the last minute or so as it starts to thicken and steam. (If using cow's milk, don't let it come to a boil—remove from the heat just before.)

While the cornmeal mixture is heating, blend the tofu with an immersion wand or in a food processor until smooth and creamy. Once the pan is off the heat, whisk in the blended tofu until well incorporated, and stir in the almonds and currants. Pour the mixture into the prepared pan and bake for about 40 minutes. You can eat it piping hot and wet, or allow it to cool—it will continue to set as it cools.

Yield: 6 servings

Per Serving: 273 Calories; 9g Fat (27.6% calories from fat); 10g Protein; 41g Carbohydrate; 3g Dietary Fiber; 6mg Cholesterol; 42mg Sodium

Ingredients

4 eggs

½ cup (115 g) low-fat cottage cheese, small curd (or feta)

1 teaspoon dried basil

½ teaspoon dried oregano

½ teaspoon salt

3 to 4 hot dashes hot pepper sauce, to taste, plus more to serve

2 cups (240 g) grated zucchini (about 2 small)

⅓ cup (37 g) sun-dried tomato strips, in oil, well drained

1 cup (80 g) whole rolled oats

¼ cup (25 g) grated Parmesan cheese

Healthy Start Breakfast Bake

From Dr. Jonny: For me as a nutritionist and as a functioning, busy person, there are two big challenges with breakfast. One is getting enough high-quality protein (which keeps you full, boosts your metabolism, and contributes to weight loss), and two is making sure the meal doesn't spike my blood sugar so that I'm starving at 11 a.m. This breakfast bake addresses both issues. Everything is low glycemic (meaning your blood sugar will be squarely in the "zone" of sustained energy, no cravings), the vegetables are filled with antioxidants, the oats provide fiber (and help fill you up even more), and the protein is from two of the best sources on earth—whole eggs and cottage (or feta) cheese. Extra nutritional points for the calcium in the cheese! Even more extra points for how good this tastes!

Preheat the oven to 350°F (180°C, gas mark 4).

Spray an 8 × 8-inch (20 × 20 cm) baking pan with olive oil. Set aside.

In the mixer, beat the eggs, cottage cheese, basil, oregano, salt, and pepper together until well blended, 30 to 60 seconds.

Stir in the zucchini, tomatoes, and oats. Pour into the prepared baking dish. Sprinkle with Parmesan and bake for 30 to 35 minutes until lightly browned.

Serve with extra hot sauce to taste, if desired.

Yield: 4 servings

Per Serving: 234 Calories; 9g Fat (33.3% calories from fat); 18g Protein; 22g Carbohydrate; 4g Dietary Fiber; 218mg Cholesterol; 778mg Sodium

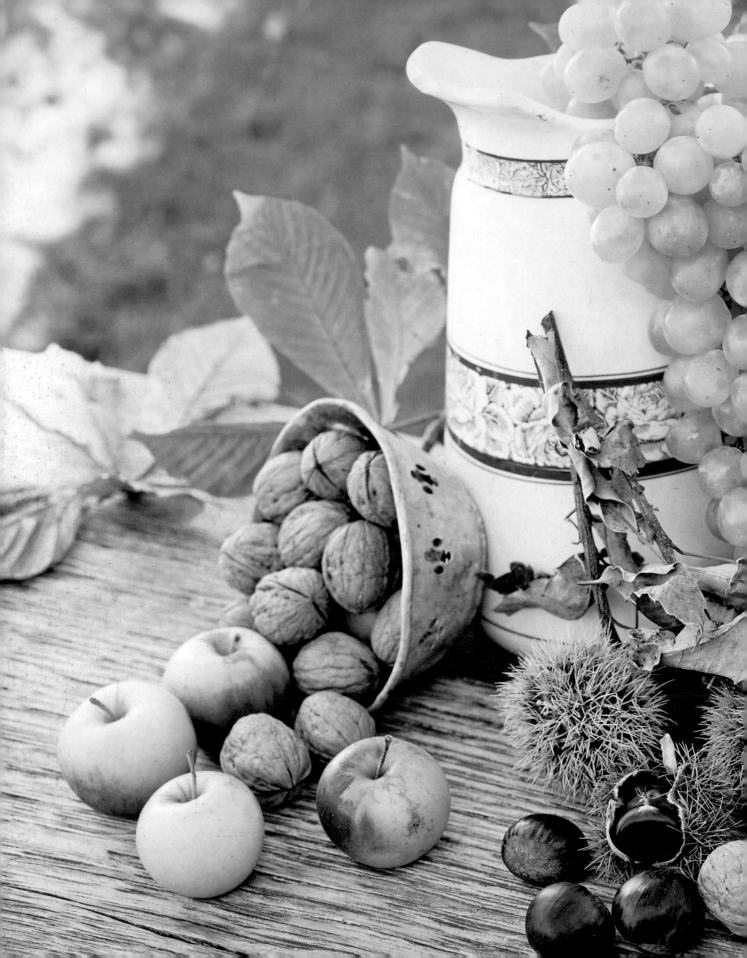

3 | The 25 Healthiest Quick Snacks

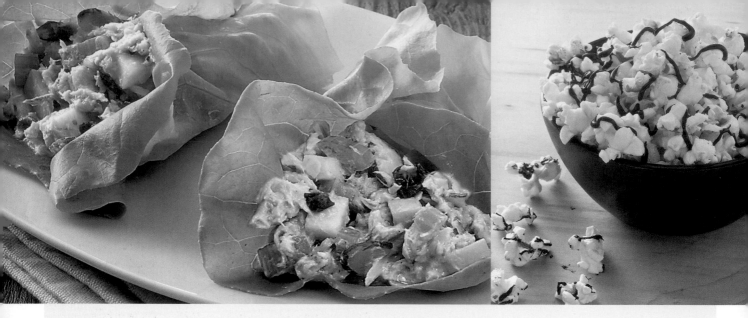

Savory

Looking for something to tide you over between meals? Unlike most commercial, packaged snacks, our savory snack recipes are carefully nutritionally balanced to minimize blood sugar impact and maximize nutrient density for the calories. Any of these can stand alone, and many can serve as mini-meals in a pinch. With a wide spectrum of options to choose from, you will be sure to find something to tickle your fancy...and your taste buds!

Cashew Miso Spread in a Whirl

Awesome Autumn Bean Dip

Creamy Low-Fat Waldorf Slaw in Seconds

Presto Popcorn

Crunchy, Curried, Good-for-You-
     Garbanzos

Ga-Ga for Fresh Gazpacho

Zesty and Heart-Healthy Mixed Nuts

Vitamin D-Cal Booster:
     Anchovy Cheese Spread

Low-Cal Tuna-Cranberry Lettuce Wraps

Polyunsaturated Party:
     Lox Canapés with Avocado Miso

Low-Carb Pesto Pizza

Quick Cottage Cheese Salad

Cashew Miso Spread in a Whirl

From Dr. Jonny: Fermented foods such as miso are among the healthiest in the world. Why? Because natural fermentation produces live bacteria known as probiotics, which are like diesel fuel for your digestive system—they make everything run better, help keep pathogens at bay, crowd out "bad" bacteria such as yeast, and generally support and boost your immune system. And everyone knows by now the benefits of nuts. In one major Harvard University study, people who ate nuts five times a week had significantly lower rates of heart disease. They also were better able to control their weight! Taste-wise, the mellow saltiness of fresh miso paste is a perfect complement to the light sweetness of the cashew butter. Great stuff! Hint: Try spreading it on a celery stick.

Combine all ingredients in a food processor or in a small bowl (and use immersion blender) and process until smooth.

Yield: about ¾ cup
Per Serving: 134 Calories; 11g Fat (68.1% calories from fat); 4g Protein; 7g Carbohydrate; 1g Dietary Fiber; 0mg Cholesterol; 149mg Sodium

Ingredients
½ cup roasted cashew butter
1½ tablespoons (24 g) mellow white miso
½ teaspoon onion powder
¼ cup (60 ml) warm water

From Chef Jeannette

To Complete the Snack: Enjoy this lightning-quick spread with crudités or cooked veggies, spread on whole-grain crackers, or thin it out with a touch more water and mix it into cooked shredded chicken for a quick chicken salad.

⭐ # Awesome Autumn Bean Dip

Ingredients

1 can (15 ounces or 425 g) Great Northern
 beans, drained and rinsed
1 can (15 ounces or 425 g) pumpkin puree
3 tablespoons (45 g) tahini
3 tablespoons (45 ml) fresh-squeezed
 lemon juice
1½ teaspoons ground cumin
½ teaspoon ground coriander
1 teaspoon salt
½ teaspoon ancho chile pepper
 (or cayenne), or to taste
2 cups (260 g) baby carrots
2 cups (150 g) sugar snap peas
2 cups (220 g) sliced crisp apples
2 cups (220 g) sliced crisp pears

From Chef Jeannette

If you don't want so much, simply cut all
the ingredients in half. I made it generous
so you could use the whole can of beans
and the whole can of pumpkin. You can
also batch and freeze some for a quick
healthy snack anytime!

From Dr. Jonny: From time to time I get asked by magazines to put together a list of superfoods that no one thinks are superfoods. You know the type of article: "Foods You Should Be Eating but Aren't," "Surprising Superfoods," or something along those lines. Well, whenever I have to write one of those articles I always include pumpkin. We never seem to think of pumpkin except around holiday time, but really, we should. It's a high-fiber, low-calorie food that's loaded with nutrients such as vitamin A, and it's one of the few exceptions to the rule about canned fruits and vegetables never being any good (the other exceptions are pineapples and beans, if you really want to know). So mix that fabulous pumpkin with some Great Northern beans and you've got a high-fiber dip that tastes terrific. Its gorgeous orange color makes it all the more appealing. This makes a superquick, satisfying snack for the family or a great healthy appetizer for company!

Process the beans in a food processor until nearly smooth, scraping down the sides, as necessary. Add the pumpkin, tahini, lemon juice, cumin, coriander, salt, and chile pepper and process until smooth, scraping down the sides periodically. Serve with crudités on the side.

Yield: 8 to 10 servings
Per Serving: 228 Calories; 3g Fat (12.4% calories from fat); 11g Protein; 41g Carbohydrate; 12g Dietary Fiber; 0mg Cholesterol; 236mg Sodium

Creamy Low-Fat Waldorf Slaw in Seconds

Ingredients

½ cup (115 g) plain low-fat yogurt

1 to 2 tablespoons (14 to 28 g) vegan mayonnaise (e.g., Nayonaise or Veganaise) to taste, optional

1 tablespoon (20 g) raw honey, or to taste

1 bag (12 ounces or 340 g) slaw veggies (shredded cabbage and carrots)

2 large green apples, cored and chopped, unpeeled

½ cup (75 g) raisins

½ cup (60 g) chopped toasted walnuts

From Dr. Jonny: With all the raging controversies in the nutrition world it's always nice to find one thing that absolutely everyone—from Ornish to Atkins—agrees on, and that's this: the value of fruits, vegetables, and nuts. A study that followed more than 80,000 people for 30 years found that those who consistently ate nuts (5 ounces or 140 g a week) had a 35 percent lower risk of cardiovascular disease; other studies have found similar benefits. And it's accepted by just about everyone that diets high in fruits and vegetables are associated with lower rates of heart disease and stroke. So now that you're sold—as if you weren't already—here's a great way to get the trifecta of nutrition (fruits, veggies, and nuts) in one single, easy-to-make dish. It's a speedy, healthy twist on the popular classic Waldorf salad, dressed lightly with another superstar health food: yogurt. No need to ever feel guilty indulging in this one!

In a small bowl, whisk together the yogurt, mayo, if using, and honey. In a salad bowl, toss together the slaw veggies, apples, raisins, and walnuts. Dress to taste and toss lightly to combine.

Yield: 4 servings
Per Serving: 238 Calories; 9g Fat (32.3% calories from fat); 7g Protein; 36g Carbohydrate; 5g Dietary Fiber; 4mg Cholesterol; 77mg Sodium

Ingredients

Base Popcorn

2 tablespoons (28 ml) high-heat oil

1/2 cup (100 g) dried organic popping corn

Cocoa-Nut Corn

2 tablespoons (28 ml) coconut oil for popping corn

2 tablespoons (22 g) high-quality dark chocolate chips

2 tablespoons (28 ml) light coconut milk

Salty Spicy Corn

2 tablespoons (28 ml) avocado oil for popping corn

5 to 6 spritzes of Bragg Liquid Aminos, or to taste (Bragg 6-ounce [175 ml] spray bottle)

4 to 5 shots hot pepper sauce, or to taste

Variation Tip: Add 1/2 teaspoon ground cinnamon to the chocolate mix to reduce the blood sugar impact of the chips. Also try adding 1/4 cup (21 g) unsweetened dried or shaved coconut and/or 1/2 cup (55 g) toasted sliced almonds.

Presto Popcorn

From Dr. Jonny: There's a lot not to like about movie popcorn; for example, everything! The average portion is at least 1,000 calories (no, that's not a misprint), the fake butter is a chemical nightmare, and there are trans fats lurking everywhere. Compare that to popcorn made with organic (non-GMO) corn and a decent oil. (Feel free to melt a little real organic butter and drizzle it before eating; I promise not to tell.) High in fiber, low in calories, this terrific basic popcorn can be flavored in multiple ways: Use one of the unique combinations suggested below or use your own imagination and enjoy!

Base Popcorn

Place the oil and corn in a stovetop popcorn maker over medium heat, turning a couple of times to distribute. Once the first kernels start to pop, usually at 4 to 5 minutes, turn the crank continuously for 60 to 90 seconds or until the kernels are all popped (there are about 5 seconds of silence after a pop). If the crank gets stuck, just turn it the opposite way until the jam is freed up. Empty the popcorn into a large bowl and top with your choice of toppings below.

Yield: about 14 cups dry (4 servings of 3½ cups); moist mixtures will "collapse" the kernels somewhat and yield less volume

Per Serving: 60 Calories; 7g Fat (100.0% calories from fat); 0g Protein; trace Carbohydrate; trace Dietary Fiber; 0mg Cholesterol; trace Sodium. Exchanges: 1½ Fat.

Cocoa-Nut Corn

Melt the chocolate chips in a double boiler or in a microwave (about 1 minute at 80 percent power), stir well, and whisk in the coconut milk until smooth. Pour over the popcorn and toss well with clean hands to coat.

Salty Spicy Corn

Empty the popped corn into a bowl and spritz the aminos directly onto the popcorn. Add the hot sauce and toss the popcorn thoroughly with a big spoon to coat evenly.

(continued on page 218)

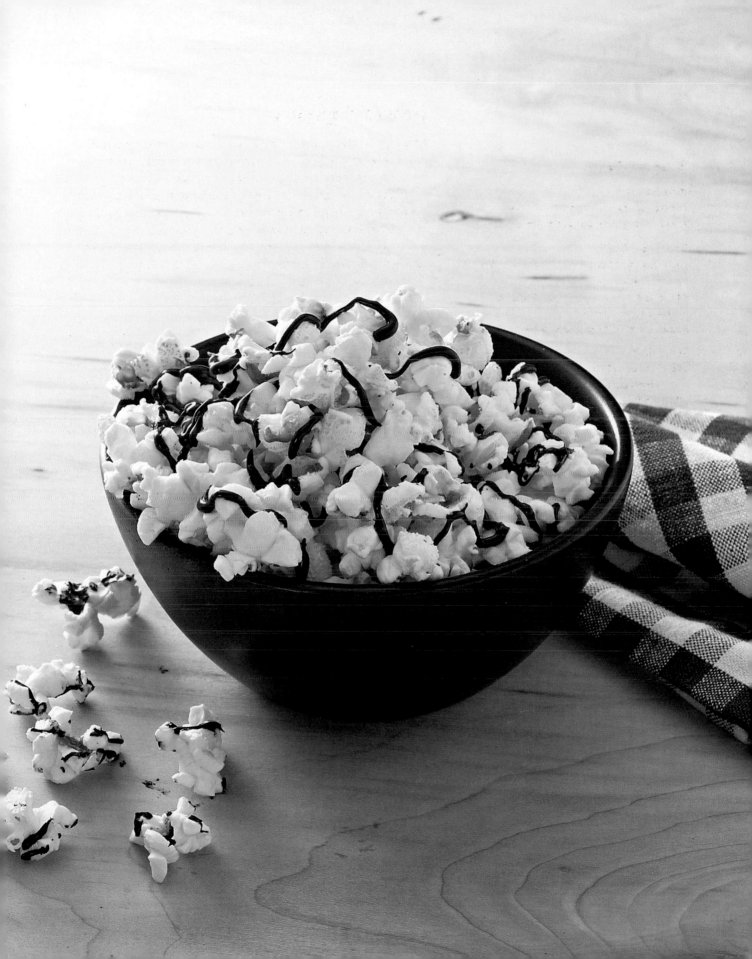

Curried Corn

2 tablespoons (28 ml) coconut oil,
    for popping corn

1 tablespoon ghee

1 teaspoon curry powder

½ teaspoon cumin seeds

¼ teaspoon salt

Pinch cayenne pepper, or to taste

1 tablespoon (20 g) honey

⅓ cup (48 g) roasted peanuts, optional

⅓ cup (50 g) raisins, optional

Superspeed Tip: For a faster, lower-calorie option, omit the oil and use an air popper or microwave bags of plain, unsalted organic corn. Then follow the directions for a flavor concept.

Curried Corn

While the corn is cooking, melt the ghee over medium heat in a small pan. Add the curry powder, cumin seeds, salt, and cayenne. Stir well to coat and sauté for about 2 minutes until very aromatic and cumin seeds are lightly toasted but not scorched. Remove from the heat and stir in the honey until melted and well incorporated. Empty the popped corn into a bowl, pour the curry mixture over the popcorn, and toss thoroughly with a spoon until evenly coated. Add the peanuts and raisins, if using, and toss lightly to combine (the nuts and raisins will drop to the bottom of the bowl).

Three Superspeed Variations

1. Toss the hot popped corn with 1 tablespoon (15 ml) of warm olive oil, ¼ to ⅓ cup (25 to 33 g) fresh-grated Parmesan cheese, and cracked pepper, to taste.

2. Drizzle 3 tablespoons (48 g) warm, low-sugar barbecue sauce over popped corn and toss thoroughly with hands to coat. (See recipe for quick barbecue sauce on page 44.)

3. Drizzle the popped corn with 2 tablespoons (28 ml) warm rosemary or garlic olive oil, sprinkle with a few pinches of salt, and toss thoroughly to combine. (See recipe for homemade rosemary garlic oil on page 122.)

Crunchy, Curried, Good-for-You-Garbanzos

Ingredients

1 teaspoon ground cumin
½ teaspoon curry powder
½ teaspoon chili powder
½ teaspoon garlic granules
¼ teaspoon cayenne pepper
¼ teaspoon powdered ginger
¼ teaspoon ground cinnamon
½ teaspoon salt
1 can (15 ounces or 425 g) chickpeas, drained and rinsed
1 tablespoon (15 ml) coconut oil, warmed to liquid (we like Barlean's)

From Dr. Jonny: So if you've read *The 150 Healthiest Foods on Earth* or any of my other food or recipe books, you're probably already aware that I hold chickpeas, also known as garbanzo beans, in very high regard! One of the earliest cultivated vegetables, chickpeas are high in protein (12 grams per cup) as well as in fiber (11 grams per cup). You don't see many foods that have nearly equal amounts of protein and fiber, not to mention a healthy amount of potassium, some calcium, iron, and other assorted minerals and vitamins. Beans consistently place near the top of the lists when foods are rated for antioxidant power. And here's another thing about chickpeas specifically: You know that sort of mealy texture they have when you eat them normally? It's not there when you roast them. Instead they become delightfully crunchy, almost like nuts. Add in those pungent curry spices that taste as good as they smell and you have a tasty, unique snack.

Preheat the oven to 450°F (230°C, gas mark 8).

Place all the spices through salt in a medium bowl and mix to combine.

Roll the chickpeas in a paper towel to remove excess moisture. Add the chickpeas and oil to the spice bowl and toss gently to coat evenly. Spread the chickpeas out in a single layer on a shallow roasting pan or baking sheet with edges. Roast for 35 to 40 minutes, turning at 10 and 25 minutes, until just browned and slightly shrunken but not scorched.

Allow them to rest for at least 10 minutes in the pan before eating or storing (in the pantry for up to 48 hours or in the fridge for up to 4 days—they will lose some of their crunch).

Yield: 4 to 6 servings
Per Serving: 281 Calories; 7g Fat (20.9% calories from fat); 14g Protein; 44g Carbohydrate; 13g Dietary Fiber; 0mg Cholesterol; 198mg Sodium

Ingredients

1 cup (170 g) ripe honeydew melon chunks (or cantaloupe)

2 medium lemon cucumbers, peeled, quartered, and seeded (or 1 small ultrafresh cucumber, peeled, seeded, and coarsely chopped)

4 medium ripe yellow or orange tomatoes, quartered (or another sweet, low-acid heirloom variety)

2 tablespoons (28 ml) olive oil, plus more if desired

¼ teaspoon salt, or to taste

Generous squeeze of fresh lime or lemon juice, optional

Fresh ground black pepper, optional

1 large heirloom tomato, chopped (zebra, if you can find them)

¼ cup (10 g) lemon basil, snipped into ribbons or confetti (or regular basil)

From Chef Jeannette

This is a high-summer soup designed to feature the just-picked flavors of fresh farmer's market produce. Eating raw seasonal produce with light preparation maximizes the life energy in the plants. As Dr. Liz Lipski, author and certified clinical nutritionist, says, "The life in food gives us life." This smooth gazpacho is like a summer salad puree.

Ga-Ga for Fresh Gazpacho

From Dr. Jonny: Gazpacho is a perfect example of the concept of synergy, especially as it relates to nutrition. For example, tomatoes, the base of the whole shebang, are rich in an antioxidant called *lycopene*, which is absorbed more easily in the presence of fat (like the olive oil in this recipe). This delicious gazpacho has a hint of sweetness from the melon, which nicely mellows the natural acid of the tomatoes. And cucumber, though it's mostly water, adds a refreshing cool taste. Not only that, it has more potassium than a banana (444 mg versus 422 mg) and is also a good source of silica, a trace mineral that contributes to the strength of our connective tissue. It's high fiber and high water content make this a very low-calorie—and nutritious—dish!

Process the honeydew, cucumber, and tomatoes in a blender or food processor to desired consistency. Add the olive oil and salt, and process briefly to mix, adjusting amounts to taste, if necessary. Pour into a bowl and stir in the citrus juice, to taste, if using. Gently stir in the pepper, if using, tomato chunks, and basil, adjusting the seasoning to taste. Garnish with extra basil, if desired. Serve at room temperature or well chilled.

Yield: 4 to 6 servings

Per Serving: 81 Calories; 5g Fat (47.7% calories from fat); 2g Protein; 10g Carbohydrate; 3g Dietary Fiber; 0mg Cholesterol; 101mg Sodium

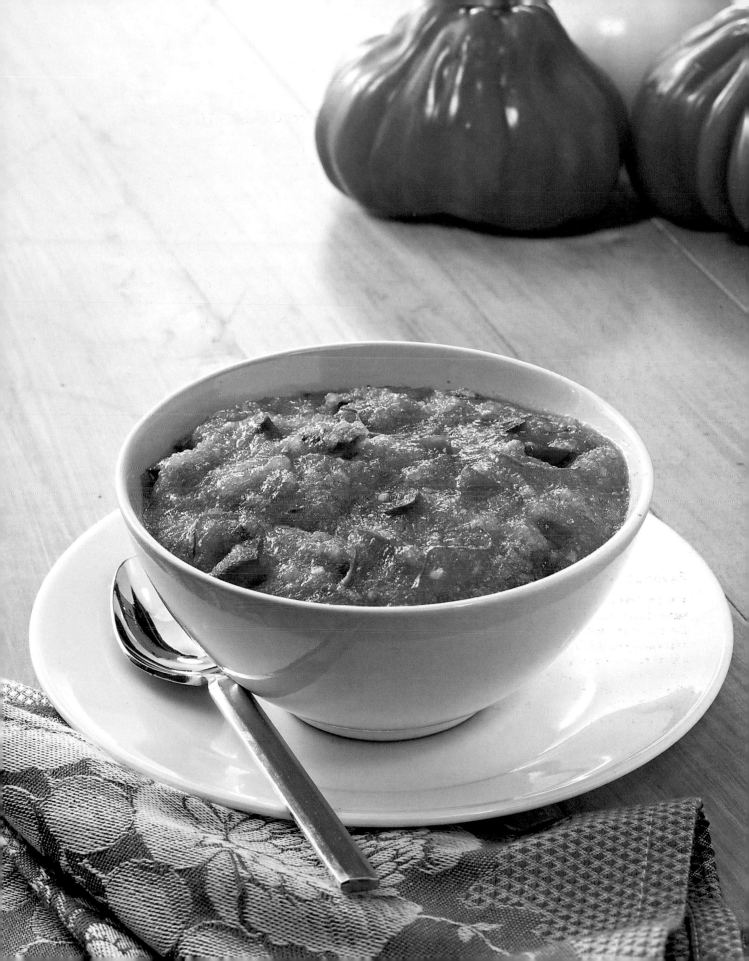

Zesty and Heart-Healthy Mixed Nuts

Ingredients

1 teaspoon Dijon mustard

1 tablespoon (20 g) 100 percent maple syrup

1½ cups (218 g) unsalted mixed nuts (raw or roasted)

2 tablespoons (14 g) high-quality natural ranch salad dressing mix (e.g., Simply Organic)

From Dr. Jonny: Just as I was writing the introduction to this tasty recipe, two new studies on nuts were published. One, in the *Archives of Internal Medicine*, examined the data from 25 different studies on nut consumption. The results? "Diets enriched with nuts significantly improved total and LDL cholesterol and lowered triglycerides in those with initially high levels," according to one of the studies. Translated: Nuts of all kinds are really good for you. This tantalizing combo of sweet and savory flavors has a light mustard bite. Your only challenge will be to not eat the whole cup and a half at once!

In a large bowl, whisk together the mustard and syrup, add the nuts, and mix well to coat. Add the dressing mix and stir gently to combine.

Spray a large skillet lightly with olive oil and heat at just under medium heat. Add the nuts, spread into a single layer, and cook, turning occasionally, for 5 to 6 minutes or until glazed and hot. Cool, break them up, and store in an airtight container in the refrigerator.

Yield: 6 servings

Per Serving: 269 Calories; 23g Fat (76.8% calories from fat); 5g Protein; 10g Carbohydrate; 3g Dietary Fiber; 1mg Cholesterol; 73mg Sodium

Vitamin D-Cal Booster: Anchovy Cheese Spread

Ingredients

6 anchovy fillets, well drained

2 cloves garlic, crushed

Zest of 1 lemon plus 1 tablespoon (15 ml) juice

1/3 cup (77 g) plain low-fat yogurt

1 package (8 ounces or 225 g) Neufchâtel cheese

1 cup (150 g) feta cheese

1/4 teaspoon cracked black pepper, or to taste

4 dashes hot sauce, or to taste

2/3 cup (110 g) sliced scallions

6 cups (780 g) assorted crudités (carrot sticks, celery sticks, zucchini sticks, grape tomatoes, blanched broccoli florets, etc.)

From Dr. Jonny: Think of anchovies and the first thing that usually comes to mind is pizza. Or maybe antipasto. But the truth is, these sometimes strong-tasting little fish are remarkably low in calories and unlikely to contain mercury or other contaminants found in fish higher on the food chain. In this unusual and tasty spread, Chef Jeannette has combined the fish with Neufchâtel cheese—high in calcium and lower in calories than cream cheese without sacrificing any flavor or mouthfeel—to make a spread that is rich in flavor but not overly fishy. The spread is as healthy as you can get, combining yogurt (with its generous helping of protein and probiotics), feta cheese (high in calcium), and raw garlic, long known for its multiple health benefits, which include lowering blood pressure and reducing the risk of some cancers. Best of all, it tastes great. Note: Try spreading on whole-grain crackers or even on celery!

Place the anchovy fillets, garlic, lemon juice, zest, and yogurt in a food processor and process until smooth. Add the cheeses, pepper, and hot sauce and process until smooth, scraping down the sides as necessary. Add the scallions and pulse or stir until just combined. Serve at room temperature with crudités.

Yield: about 3 cups dip plus veggies

Per Serving: 68 Calories; 4g Fat (53.7% calories from fat); 3g Protein; 5g Carbohydrate; 1g Dietary Fiber; 16mg Cholesterol; 183mg Sodium

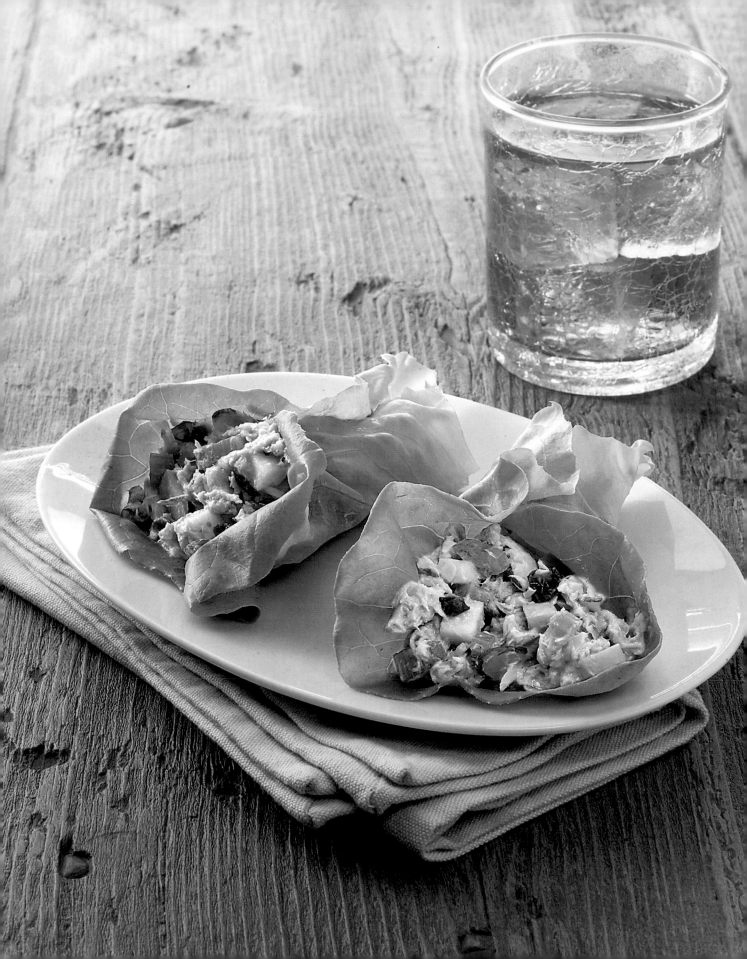

Low-Cal Tuna-Cranberry Lettuce Wraps

Ingredients

1 to 2 tablespoons (33 g) prepared, juice-sweetened cranberry sauce (e.g., Knudsen's), to taste

2 tablespoons (30 g) plain low-fat yogurt (regular or Greek—use only 1 tablespoon if not adding celery and apple)

1 can (7 ounces or 195 g) tuna fish in water, drained and flaked (e.g., Vital Choice)

⅓ cup (40 g) diced celery, optional

⅓ cup (42 g) diced green apple, optional

2 tablespoons (18 g) sliced toasted almonds

Large, fresh lettuce leaves

From Dr. Jonny: Canned tuna is one of the great nutritional bargains of all time. (There are caveats, but I'll get to those in a moment.) Tuna is high in protein, relatively low in calories, easily available, and mixes well with lots of foods. It also has a nice dose of niacin and vitamin B_{12}, and the all-important mineral selenium. The only concern is mercury, but interestingly enough, this is a bigger problem with the more expensive kinds (such as albacore)—the chunk light is a better choice! Buying tuna packed in water rather than oil reduces the total calories of the dish. This recipe is definitely an unusual combo, but the sweet tart bite of the cranberry perfectly complements, and brightens, the taste of the tuna. Hint: Try ordering a six-pack of canned tuna from the same place I got mine, Vital Choice (available through a link on my website, www .jonnybowden.com, under "Shopping: Healthy Food"). You'll never feel the same way about "store bought" again. Enjoy!

In a medium bowl, mix together the cranberry sauce and yogurt. Add the tuna, celery, if using, apple, if using, and almonds, and mix gently to combine well. Spoon a few tablespoons of tuna into each lettuce leaf, roll it up, and serve.

Yield: 2 generous portions
Per Serving: 211 Calories; 6g Fat (23.9% calories from fat); 28g Protein; 12g Carbohydrate; 2g Dietary Fiber; 30mg Cholesterol; 363mg Sodium

Polyunsaturated Party: Lox Canapés with Avocado Miso

Ingredients

1 large, ripe Hass avocado, peeled, pitted, and roughly chopped

1 tablespoon (16 g) sweet white miso

1 large cucumber, peeled and sliced thickly OR 8 slices whole-grain cocktail bread (e.g., Rubschlager Rye)

4 ounces (115 g) thinly sliced lox (e.g., Vital Choice)

From Dr. Jonny: I grew up in a middle-class Jewish household in New York City, so I was hardly a stranger to lox. But up till my teens I still thought it was some kind of red stuff that was covered with weird little miniature olives that old folks like my grandparents used to love. Especially with cream cheese on a bagel from Zabar's. Now I know that lox is salmon fillet that has been cured and sometimes cold-smoked, a process that doesn't actually cook the fish and results in a characteristic smooth texture. (And the "miniature olives" were capers, in case you hadn't guessed.) Anyway, lox is a great way to get your salmon fix, and with it all the healthy things salmon is known for—omega-3 fats, for example, and antioxidants such as astaxanthin. Add to the mix avocado (for more wonderfully healthy fat, this time of the monounsaturated variety) and the probiotics from fermented miso and you've got a fresh-tasting snack brimming with health!

Using a fork or immersion blender, mash together the avocado and miso in a small bowl until smooth and bright green. Spread a thick layer of avocado miso onto the cucumber or bread slices and top with a layer of lox. Serve at room temperature.

Yield: 2 to 4 servings

Per Serving: 133 Calories; 9g Fat (59.6% calories from fat); 7g Protein; 7g Carbohydrate; 2g Dietary Fiber; 7mg Cholesterol; 727mg Sodium

Low-Carb Pesto Pizza

Ingredients

1 whole or sprouted-grain wrap

1½ tablespoons (23 g) prepared pesto (great with arugula pesto leftovers from Calcium-Rich Caprese Salad on page 154, or use sun-dried tomato paste)

4 slices heirloom tomato

¼ cup (33 g) thawed frozen corn

2 tablespoons (10 g) fresh-grated Parmesan cheese

1 teaspoon olive oil

Fresh basil, optional for garnish

From Dr. Jonny: Ask me my five greatest guilty pleasures in the food kingdom, and pizza is going to be on the list. I don't have it often, and when I do, I try to get the healthiest kind, but it's not always easy. The problem with generic pizza is that it's mostly dough—starchy, processed carbs of the worst kind. The cheese and oil have more fat than most people are comfortable with, and the quality of these ingredients used in your normal pizza parlor isn't the greatest. Here's the solution: Lighten up on the cheese (and the other fats) and lighten up on the carbs by using the ultimate thin crust—a whole-grain wrap. Then customize toppings to your heart's content! Pineapple, peppers, mushrooms, spinach, onions, chicken...it's all good and makes a perfect snack or mini-meal anytime!

Preheat the oven to 400°F (200°C, gas mark 6). Lay the wrap out on a baking sheet. Spread the wrap evenly with the pesto. Lay the tomato slices in a single layer on the top. Scatter the corn evenly over the pizza and top with the Parmesan. Drizzle the olive oil over the Parmesan. Snip the basil over the Parmesan, if using.

Cook for 8 to 10 minutes until hot and crispy.

Yield: 1 serving

Per Serving: 472 Calories; 24g Fat (43.8% calories from fat); 19g Protein; 51g Carbohydrate; 11g Dietary Fiber; 15mg Cholesterol; 540mg Sodium

Quick Cottage Cheese Salad

Ingredients

8 ounces (225 g) low-fat, small-curd cottage cheese

2 to 3 teaspoons prepared horseradish, to taste

1 teaspoon Dijon mustard

2 teaspoons lemon juice

1/4 teaspoon each salt and fresh-ground pepper

1 cup (180 g) halved cherry tomatoes

1 stalk celery, thinly sliced

1 tablespoon (5 g) crushed walnuts, optional

From Dr. Jonny: Cottage cheese was named for the cottages in which it was traditionally made. It comes from the cheese curd, but because it is only drained, not dried, it retains a good deal of its whey content (remember Miss Muffett and her curds and whey?). Whey is one of the most bioavailable sources of protein, and cottage cheese is, not surprisingly, high in protein (more than 12½ grams for 4 ounces [115 g] of cheese) and very low in carbs (roughly 1 gram of carbs per ounce of cheese). Even the full-fat kind, which has only 2 more grams of fat than the 2 percent kind, is low in calories (111 calories for 4 ounces [115 g]) and a good source of calcium, phosphorus, and potassium. Best of all, high-quality, traditionally made cottage cheese is fermented and thus teeming with beneficial bacteria (called probiotics) similar to that found in yogurt. Cottage cheese is also easier to digest than typical dairy products, such as milk. Tip: Include the optional walnuts for extra minerals and plant-based omega-3 fats!

Gently mix all ingredients together and enjoy.

Yield: 1 serving

Per Serving: 287 Calories; 8g Fat (24.5% calories from fat); 34g Protein; 21g Carbohydrate; 3g Dietary Fiber; 19mg Cholesterol; 1576mg Sodium

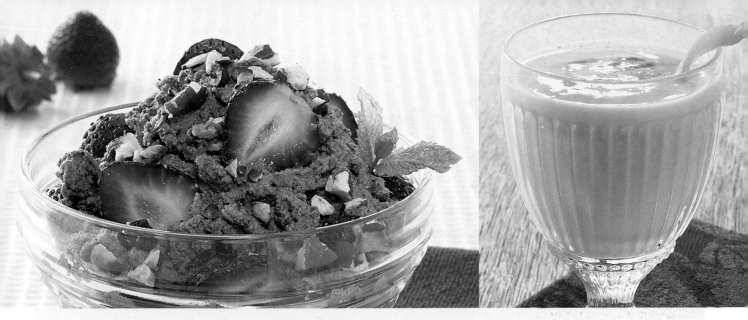

Sweet

These delicious snacks are sure to satisfy your sweet tooth, but they won't spike your blood sugar or crash your energy like those afternoon donuts so popular at the office. The Heart-Lovin' Lemon Zinger Truffles will hit the spot when you want something sweet-tart, but they also provide some serious staying power with a high dose of both soluble and insoluble fiber. Is it chocolate you crave? Nothing beats our Sinless Strawberry Dark Chocolate Ricotta Dream for a rich-tasting, high-protein snack (or perfect dessert) that really satisfies.

Antioxidant Cocoa Oal Dreams

No-Fuss, Fast, and Healthy Chocolate
    Cherry Frosty

Fiber Bonanza:
    Oat Bran Kheer on the Quick

Sinless Strawberry Dark Chocolate Ricotta
    Dream

Low-Fat Pumpkin Pie Dip

Instant Pudding Series:
    Slimming Sweet Potato-Chocolate
    Whip

    Peanut Butter Protein Power

Light Honey Melon Salad with Chèvre and
    Pistachios

Coconut Mango Low-Sugar Lassi

Apple-a-Day Wine-Marinated Fruit Mix

Super Simple Vitamin C Citrus with Mint

Nutty Fruit Bars I:
    Healthy Bite Cherry Chewies

Nutty Fruit Bars II:
    Heart-Lovin' Lemon Zinger Truffles

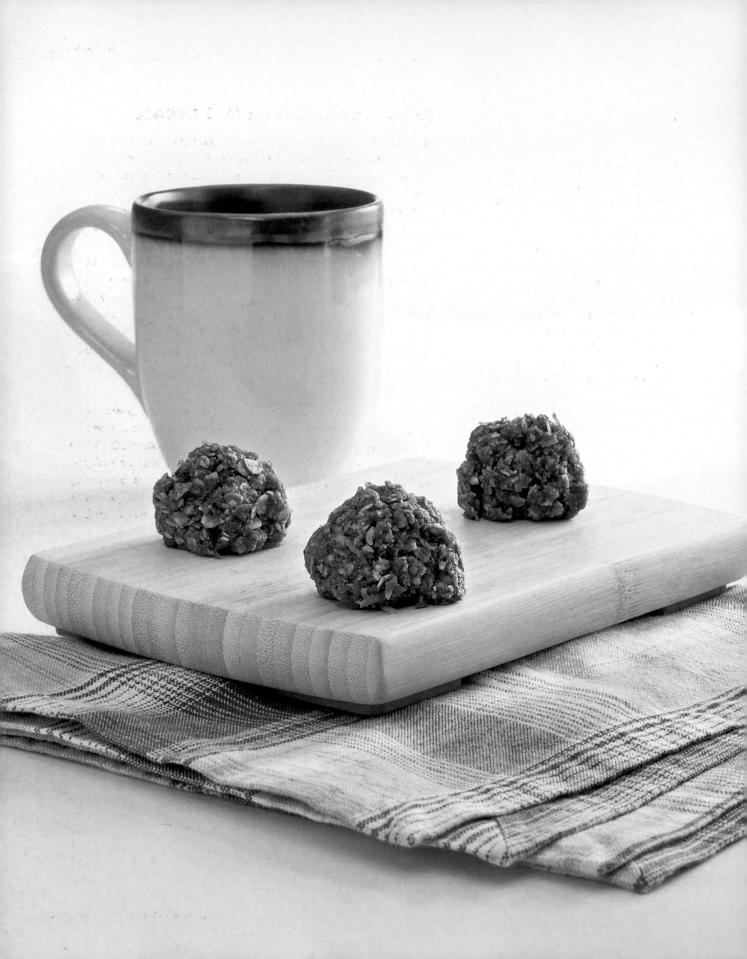

Ingredients

¼ cup (60 ml) milk (use cow's, or unsweetened vanilla almond, soy, or rice milk)

¼ cup (60 ml) coconut oil

⅓ cup (64 g) xylitol

¼ cup (65 g) natural peanut butter

2 tablespoons (10 g) unsweetened cocoa powder

½ teaspoon vanilla extract

1½ cups (120 g) quick-cooking oats

½ cup (40 g) dried unsweetened coconut

½ cup (47 g) almond meal (prepared—we like Bob's Red Mill—or process raw or blanched almonds very finely in a food processor)

Antioxidant Cocoa Oat Dreams

From Dr. Jonny: When Chef Jeannette and I wrote our first cookbook, *The Healthiest Meals on Earth*, one of the biggest surprises was the popularity of the Real-Food Brownies, whose main ingredient is garbanzo beans. I have a feeling this dish is going to be this year's Real-Food Brownies. I guarantee you'll have a hard time finding a chocolate dessert that tastes this good while being this good for you. When making it, avoid using the popular brands of peanut butter, which sometimes contain trans fats and more often, too much sugar. Instead use the kind that comes right out of the grinder, or one of the "natural" brands, without added sugar. Chocolaty, peanuty, sweet, and chewy—it's a dessert eater's dream and will hit the spot anytime you're hankering for a sweet treat. Note: If you want to eat these cookie-style, no problemo. Plan ahead so they can set up in the fridge (takes about an hour)—or (my fave) enjoy them warm, with a spoon, right out of the bowl. Delish.

Place the milk, coconut oil, xylitol, peanut butter, and cocoa powder in a small saucepan over medium heat. Stir frequently to mix until melted and well incorporated. Remove from the heat and stir in the vanilla. While the cocoa sauce is melting, place the oats, coconut, and almond meal in a large bowl and mix lightly with a fork. Pour the cocoa mixture over the dry mix and mix well with a fork until well incorporated. Form into loose balls (about a large tablespoon each) onto waxed paper. Refrigerate for 30 minutes to 1 hour to firm them up.

Yield: 25 dreams
Per Serving: 84 Calories; 6g Fat (58.7% calories from fat); 2g Protein; 7g Carbohydrate; 1g Dietary Fiber; trace Cholesterol; 14mg Sodium

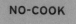

No-Fuss, Fast, and Healthy Chocolate Cherry Frosty

Ingredients

2 cups (450 ml) unsweetened chocolate almond milk (e.g., Blue Diamond Natural)

3 scoops unsweetened vanilla whey protein powder

2½ tablespoons (12 g) raw cacao powder (or 2 tablespoons [10 g] unsweetened cocoa powder), to taste

1 frozen banana (or to taste, for sweetness and creaminess)

1½ cups (233 g) frozen pitted sweet cherries

2 drops vanilla extract

From Dr. Jonny: Who among us doesn't remember the fabulous taste and texture of a milk shake? They were a favorite "drugstore" order back in the days when you could still get a chocolate egg cream at the local "soda shoppe." (Yes, I'm dating myself, but so what?) Chef Jeannette has come up with a winner here: raw cacao, rich with blood-pressure-lowering flavanols, immune-system boosting whey protein powder, and a good old potassium-rich banana. This is so darn yummy, cool, frosty, and rich, it'll beat the pants off a standard boring milk shake on a hot afternoon.

Place all ingredients into a powerful blender and process until smooth.

Yield: 4 frosties

Per Serving: 150 Calories; 2g Fat (10.4% calories from fat); 13g Protein; 23g Carbohydrate; 2g Dietary Fiber; 23mg Cholesterol; 35mg Sodium

Fiber Bonanza:
Oat Bran Kheer on the Quick

Ingredients

1 can (13.5 ounces or 385 g) light coconut milk

1 cup (235 ml) milk (cow's, unsweetened vanilla soy, or almond milk)

2 tablespoons (30 g) erythritol or xylitol

¼ cup (35 g) raisins

½ teaspoon ground cardamom

1 cup (100 g) oat bran

¼ cup (28 g) sliced toasted almonds

¼ cup shelled roasted pistachios

From Dr. Jonny: Here's another Indian delicacy I had never heard of until Chef Jeannette turned me on to it. Kheer is a warmly spiced Indian pudding usually made with rice, but this pumped-up version uses oat bran as a base instead. It's much faster to prepare, much lower in glycemic impact (meaning it doesn't raise your blood sugar very high nor very quickly), and it's simply loaded with fiber. Oat bran has a terrific reputation for lowering cholesterol, but it does even more than that for the heart. Oat bran contains antioxidant compounds called *avenanthramides* that actually help prevent the LDL cholesterol from being damaged by free radicals; it's only when cholesterol is damaged (or oxidized) that it becomes a problem in the body, so the ability of oat bran to help prevent this damage is one of its most important benefits for the heart! The fat from coconut and nuts gets a thumbs-up for health, and you even get a dollop of protein from the milk. You can use either xylitol or erythritol as a sweetener—both are sugar alcohols with minimal impact on blood sugar, and both taste exactly the same as white sugar with none of the negatives. And by the way, this dish makes a great breakfast, not to mention a fabulous "anytime" snack. Tasty, satisfying, and good for you too!

Combine the coconut milk, milk, sweetener, raisins, and cardamom in a large saucepan over medium-high heat and bring to a boil, whisking frequently. When the mixture reaches a boil, turn the heat down to low and whisk in the oat bran for 10 seconds. Remove from the heat and stir in both nuts. The cereal will continue to thicken as it cools. Serve hot.

Yield: 4 to 6 servings (about 3 cups)
Per Serving: 225 Calories; 14g Fat (45.2% calories from fat); 8g Protein; 29g Carbohydrate; 5g Dietary Fiber; 5mg Cholesterol; 39mg Sodium

Sinless Strawberry Dark Chocolate Ricotta Dream

Ingredients

¼ cup (44 g) high-quality dark chocolate chips (try grain sweetened for best health impact or Callebaut for high-end cocoa bliss)

1 cup (250 g) fresh, low-fat ricotta cheese

2 cups (340 g) fresh sliced strawberries

¼ cup (30 g) crushed toasted walnuts, optional

From Chef Jeannette

Variation Tip: Use any seasonal fruit in place of the strawberries. This dessert is also wonderful (and antioxidant loaded!) with fresh raspberries. While lacking the benefits of cacao–for those of you who don't like dark chocolate (there must be someone out there)–try high-quality white chocolate chips for an alternative protein-packed snack. Try the white version with 1 teaspoon lemon zest, ½ teaspoon vanilla extract, and fresh blueberries.

From Dr. Jonny: Want to perform your own little mind-body experiment to see how what we think affects our physiology? Good. Think of dark chocolate swirled with strawberries, walnuts, and creamy ricotta cheese. Now notice what's happening: We call that mouthwatering, and your mouth watered just by thinking about the ingredients in one of my absolute favorite desserts by Chef Jeannette. And this just happens to be a dessert you don't have to feel guilty about eating. Dark chocolate is rich in blood-pressure-lowering flavanols while ricotta cheese is high in protein, calcium, and vitamin D. The strawberries have a cancer-fighting chemical called *ellagic acid* not to mention a host of antioxidants and phytochemicals. And the walnuts are a good source of plant-based omega-3 fats, fiber, and minerals. The taste—well, let me just say three words: *rich*, *creamy*, *satisfying*. This baby will nip a chocolate craving in the bud with far more nourishment that any conventional dessert.

In a medium glass bowl, melt the chocolate chips at 75 percent power in a microwave in 30-second intervals until soft, and stir gently. You can also melt them in a double boiler over medium heat (or use a metal mixing bowl set into a medium saucepan with 1 inch [2.5 cm] of water). Add the ricotta and stir until well incorporated. Top with the strawberries and sprinkle the walnuts over all.

Yield: 4 servings

Per Serving: 208 Calories; 13g Fat (51.9% calories from fat); 10g Protein; 17g Carbohydrate; 3g Dietary Fiber; 19mg Cholesterol; 80mg Sodium

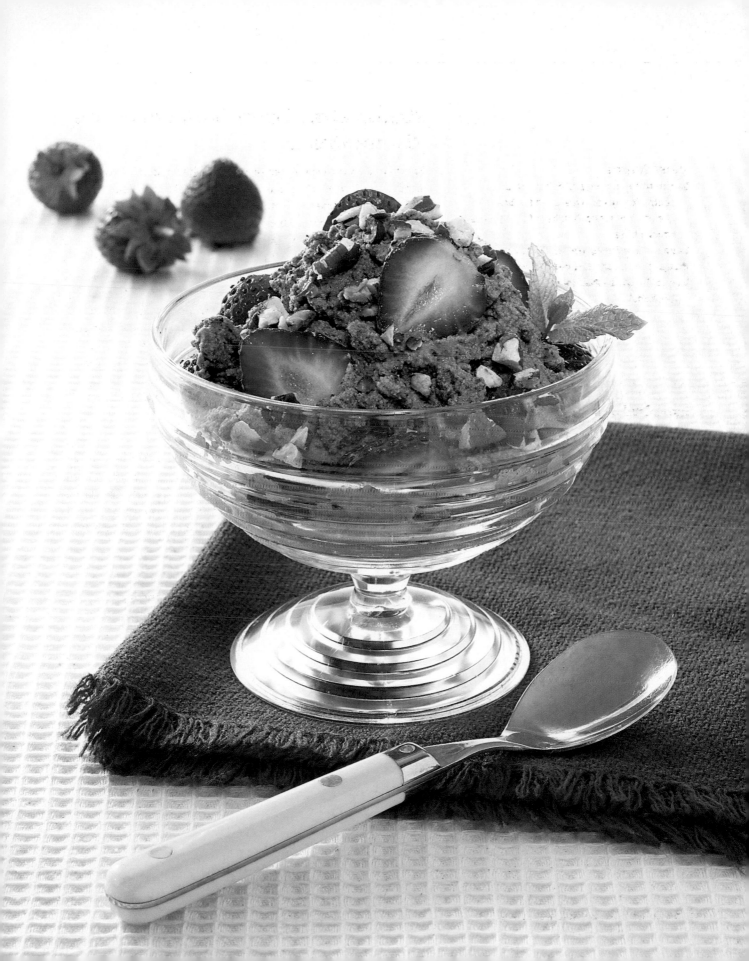

Dark Chocolate—Good for Your Heart in Many Ways

Dark chocolate is loaded with compounds known as flavonoids. These nutritive compounds, found in plant foods, are nature's way of protecting the plants from environmental toxins. Flavonoids offer similar protection to our bodies, often functioning as antioxidants and anti-inflammatory agents. The particular subclass of flavonoids found in cocoa are called flavanols, and their claim to fame is the ability to prevent fatty substances in the bloodstream from clogging up your arteries. That's a good thing. By reducing the ability to form clots, you also reduce the risk of stroke and heart attack!

Flavanols also raise the level of a terrific compound in the body called nitric oxide, which is critical for both healthy circulation and healthy blood pressure. In fact, one study showed that dark chocolate was able to lower blood pressure, and it's probably because of the positive effect of cocoa flavanols on nitric oxide.

As an added benefit, dark chocolate is a good source of magnesium, another heart-healthy mineral!

Ingredients

1 package (12.3 ounces or 350 g) soft silken tofu

1 large ripe banana, mashed

1 can (15 ounces or 425 g) pumpkin puree

1/3 cup (113 g) maple syrup, or to taste

2 teaspoons pumpkin pie spice

1 teaspoon ground cinnamon

1/2 teaspoon vanilla extract, optional

From Chef Jeannette

To Complete the Snack: This dip is fabulous with sliced fall fruit such as pears and apples. It also makes a delicious, low-glycemic cold pudding with berries. For a special treat, serve it up with high-quality, low-sugar, whole-grain ginger snaps—yum!

Low-Fat Pumpkin Pie Dip

From Dr. Jonny: I'm such a huge fan of pumpkin I'm always including it on lists I'm asked to do by the magazines, lists that include "superfoods you didn't know about" or "great foods for weight loss." Why? Because this underappreciated vegetable is loaded with vitamin A, low in sugar and calories, and high in fiber. Not to mention it's associated with some of the best eating holidays! Problem is it usually comes in the form of a high-calorie pie, which, if bought commercially, nearly always is loaded with trans fats and sugar. So here's the perfect way to eat this fabulous veggie—high in protein (from the silken tofu, which, together with the mashed banana, gives this dip the most luscious creamy texture), pretty low in sugar (for a dish this delicious), and yet just as typically "pumpkin pie" tasting as the most fattening holiday dessert. Best of all, it's built for speed—you can whip this up in just about the time it takes to open a can! I love this dip!

Blend the tofu in a food processor for about 15 seconds or until smooth. Add the banana, pumpkin, syrup, spice, and vanilla, if using, and process until smooth, scraping down the sides as necessary.

Yield: about 3 cups
Per Serving: 82 Calories; 2g Fat (17.9% calories from fat); 3g Protein; 14g Carbohydrate; 2g Dietary Fiber; 0mg Cholesterol; 5mg Sodium

Instant Pudding Series:
Slimming Sweet Potato–Chocolate Whip

From Dr. Jonny: I had a few favorite dishes as a kid, and one of them was pudding. Chocolate pudding. Which my mother sometimes burned, leaving a thick little film on the top, which I absolutely loved to peel off and eat separately. So when I see a dish with "pudding" in the title and "chocolate" in the description, I'm in. This isn't exactly chocolate pudding, but it's a brilliant twist on the traditional version, using sweet potato puree as the base, sweetening it with maple syrup, and flavoring it with real, high-quality cocoa. The incredible ease of making this dish and the speed with which it comes together make it a winner. It's low glycemic (meaning it doesn't knock your blood sugar for a loop), high in fiber, and loaded with nutrients such as beta-carotene and eye-healthy lutein and zeaxanthin from the sweet potato. Best of all the taste is heavenly. Note: Grade B maple syrup sounds like it's not as good as grade A, but it's actually better and has more minerals!

Ingredients

1 can (15 ounces or 425 g) high-quality sweet potato puree (e.g., Farmer's Market Organic)*

¼ cup (20 g) high-quality cocoa (e.g., Ghirardelli), sifted

1 tablespoon (20 g) maple syrup (or melted frozen apple or orange juice concentrate)

½ teaspoon vanilla extract

½ teaspoon orange extract (or vanilla)

¾ teaspoon orange zest, optional

Place all the ingredients into the bowl of a mixer and whip at medium speed until perfectly smooth.

Yield: about 1⅔ cups (roughly 4 servings)
Per Serving: 107 Calories; 1g Fat (7.1% calories from fat); 2g Protein; 25g Carbohydrate; 4g Dietary Fiber; 0mg Cholesterol; 11mg Sodium

*The quality of the ingredients definitely counts with this recipe. Choosing an organic puree will help to ensure a more flavorful, nutrient-rich base.

Ingredients

1 package (12.3 ounces or 350 g) silken tofu

1 ripe banana, peeled*

¼ cup (60 ml) unsweetened vanilla almond
milk (or soy or cow's)

⅓ cup (87 g) peanut butter (or nut or seed
butter of your choice)

1 teaspoon ground cinnamon

Peanut Butter Protein Power

From Dr. Jonny: Who doesn't like peanut butter and banana? Raise your hands, please. No hands? Not surprised. You've probably thrown together a peanut butter and banana sandwich at some point in your life either for yourself, your kids, or someone in your family, and why not? The combination of protein and carbs is a winner—good fat, lots of potassium, and a ton of taste. Well, Chef Jeannette has taken that fabulous taste and transported it into a pudding. Loaded with protein and high-quality fats, this lightly sweet, dense, and creamy concoction hits the spot every single time. A satisfying snack if there ever was one!

Process the tofu and banana together in a food processor until smooth. Add the milk, nut butter, and cinnamon and process until well incorporated and smooth.

Yield: about 2 cups (4 servings)

Per Serving: 234 Calories; 16g Fat (56.8% calories from fat); 13g Protein; 14g Carbohydrate; 3g Dietary Fiber; 2mg Cholesterol; 116mg Sodium

*Use a larger banana for a sweeter flavor, smaller for less. To boost the sweetness even more, add raw honey 1 teaspoon at a time until you hit your mark

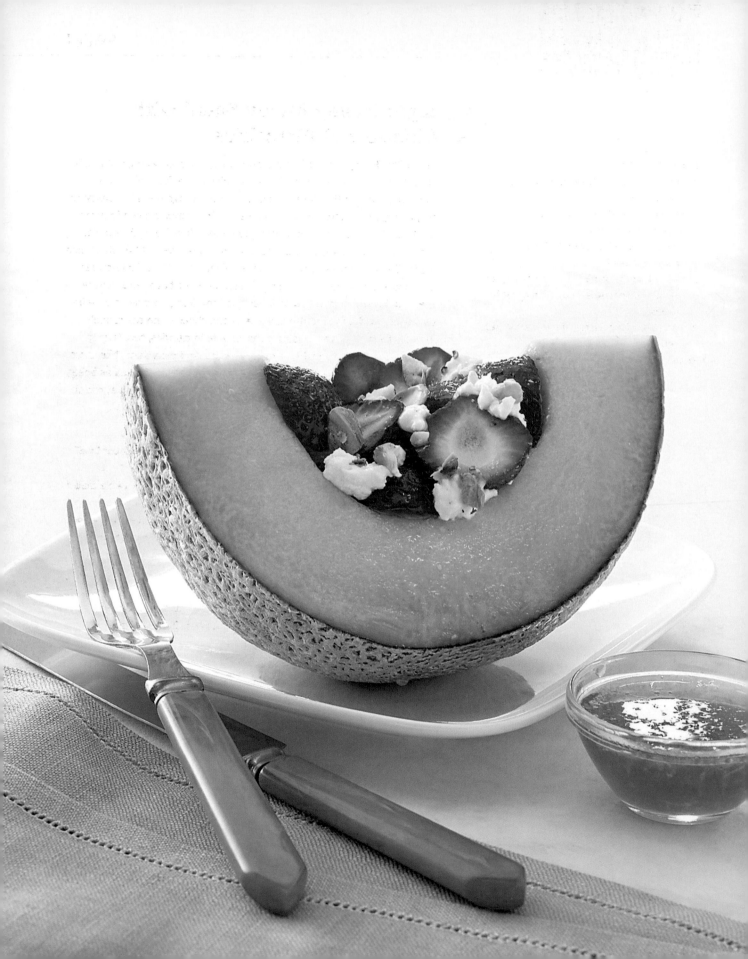

Light Honey Melon Salad with Chèvre and Pistachios

Ingredients

3 tablespoons (45 ml) fresh-squeezed lemon juice

2 tablespoons (40 g) raw honey

1 teaspoon lemon zest

¼ cup (31 g) roasted, salted, shelled pistachio meats

1 ripe cantaloupe or ½ large ripe honeydew melon, unpeeled, seeded, and cut into 4 slices

2 cups (290 g) ripe strawberries, stemmed and halved

¼ cup (38 g) chèvre

From Dr. Jonny: In my humble opinion, great chefs and great musicians have a lot in common. Great musicians take the same twelve tones that exist in the Western scales and rearrange them in constantly surprising, novel, interesting ways that ordinary mortals would never think of. Chefs do the same with ingredients. I love honeydew melon (and cantaloupe, too), but never in a million years would I think of pairing it with goat cheese and pistachios. (That's why Chef Jeannette is the chef and I'm the nutritionist!) What a burst of flavor and texture! Fresh, light, and sweet, this dish has got something for everyone—the sweetness of the melon, the tartness of the cheese, and the crunchiness of the nuts. It's surprisingly reasonable in calories, too, largely because the salad is mostly water by weight. And pistachios, like most nuts, are high in minerals (potassium and phosphorus) as well as being a good source of heart-healthy monounsaturated fat. Note: Get melon at the peak of the summer season so it's bursting with flavor!

In a small bowl, whisk together the lemon juice, honey, and zest until well incorporated.

In a sandwich-size plastic bag, lightly crush the pistachios with a mallet or rolling pin.

Lay out the melon slices and fill with even portions of the strawberry halves. Dot evenly with chèvre and drizzle the dressing over all, to taste. Top with the crushed pistachios.

Yield: 4 servings

Per Serving: 152 Calories; 4g Fat (24.3% calories from fat); 4g Protein; 27g Carbohydrate; 3g Dietary Fiber; 4mg Cholesterol; 49mg Sodium

Coconut Mango Low-Sugar Lassi

From Dr. Jonny: Ever hear of traditional Indian lassi? No? I'm not surprised. I confess I'd never heard of it either, but from what folks tell me it's delicious. Problem is, it's also loaded with white sugar. Chef Jeannette came up with a version that has no added sugar but is still sweet and silky. If you like mangoes—and who doesn't?—you'll love this dish. Mangoes are the most adored fruit in India. Mangoes are used in India as "blood builders," probably because they are high in iron and are considered especially beneficial to women during pregnancy and menstruation. And their high potassium and magnesium content can help with muscle cramps, stress, and even heart problems. They're also high in beta-carotene, the important precursor for vitamin A, and as an added benefit: A single mango has 3.7 grams of fiber! P.S. Don't forget to use yogurt that contains live cultures to get the benefits of probiotics in this tasty drink!

Ingredients

⅓ cup (40 g) dried mangoes, chopped*

3 ripe mangoes, peeled

1 cup (235 ml) light coconut milk
    (or use cow's, unsweetened vanilla soy,
    or almond)

½ cup (115 g) plain low-fat yogurt

2 cups ice cubes

Pinch ground cardamom

In a small bowl cover the dried mangoes with water, soak for 10 minutes, and drain.

While the dried mango is soaking, slice the two "cheeks" (broad sides of pit) and two thinner sides (narrow sides of pit) from each peeled fresh mango. Halve each fruit slice. Add the soaked mango and fresh mango chunks to a powerful blender and process until smooth. Add the coconut milk, yogurt, and ice and process to desired smoothness.

Divide among four glasses and place a pinch of cardamom at the top of each glass.

Yield: 4 servings

Per Serving: 175 Calories; 3g Fat (16.2% calories from fat); 3g Protein; 37g Carbohydrate; 4g Dietary Fiber; 1mg Cholesterol; 42mg Sodium

*Dried mango is tough and leathery. It's easier to use kitchen shears than a knife to snip it into pieces. If you desire more sweetness than that from the dried fruit, add raw honey, 1 teaspoon at a time, until sweet enough.

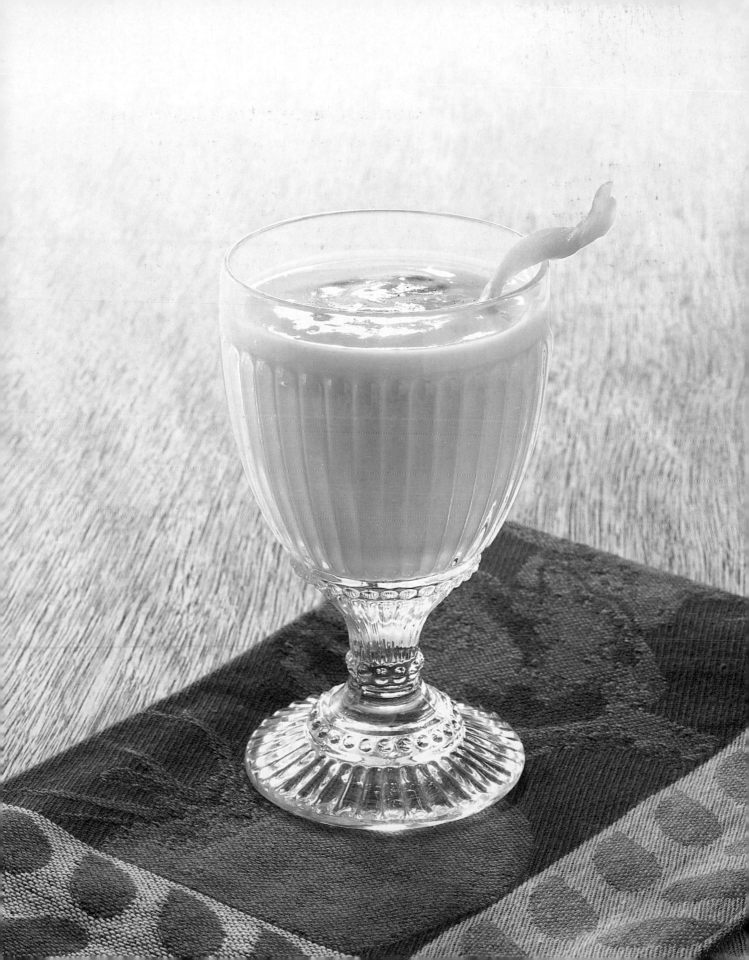

Apple-a-Day Wine-Marinated Fruit Mix

Ingredients

¾ cup (175 ml) fruity red wine

1 teaspoon ground cinnamon

3 tablespoons (36 g) Sucanat

2 large red, crisp apples (try Honeycrisp, Braeburn, or Gala), unpeeled, cored, and quartered

1 cup (100 g) walnuts

From Dr. Jonny: Wine and apples—how can that not be good? We already know red wine is brimming with *resveratrol* (see Nutritional Note opposite), a phenomenal plant polyphenol that's been shown to turn on "longevity" genes in every species studied so far. And apples, well, they're about as perfect a fruit as you can get: high in fiber from pectin, a great source of the anti-inflammatory, anticancer nutrient quercetin, high in bone-protecting boron, and rich in vitamin C. Should I go on? I thought not! Chef Jeannette has given us a lovely way to make a rich, flavorful evening snack, or even a dessert, that's absolutely loaded with nutrients!

In a medium glass container, whisk together the wine, cinnamon, and Sucanat.

Coarsely chop the apples and walnuts in a food processor, scraping down the sides as necessary. Add wine mixture to the container, mix well to incorporate the wine and apples, cover, and marinate for an hour (or up to 3) before serving.

Yield: 4 servings

Per Serving: 225 Calories; 14g Fat (60.6% calories from fat); 6g Protein; 15g Carbohydrate; 3g Dietary Fiber; 0mg Cholesterol; 29mg Sodium

Raise a Glass to Resveratrol

A ton of attention has been focused recently on a little plant chemical called resveratrol, especially among those who are interested in living longer!

To understand exactly how resveratrol exerts its "antiaging magic," we have to go back to a bunch of important studies involving calorically deprived rats. Apparently caloric restriction turns on a set of genes known as the sirtuin genes, which are considered to be major influencers of how long we live. "The sirtuin genes are the holy grail of medicine and nutrition," says my good friend Mark Houston, M.D. "These genes turn on or turn off different metabolic pathways that are designed to promote longevity and health."

But calorie restriction isn't terribly popular, especially among people who like to eat.

That's why there was so much excitement when David Sinclair, M.D., a professor and researcher at Harvard Medical School, discovered that there was another way to turn on these longevity genes, one that wouldn't require you to starve yourself. He and his associates published a now-famous paper reporting that plant compounds known as *polyphenols* could do the job quite well. And the polyphenol that seemed to work best was *resveratrol*.

Resveratrol is found in red wine, the skin of young unripe red grapes, grape seeds, purple grape juice, and to a lesser extent, in peanuts and mulberries. And it may turn out to be the closest thing we have at present to an antiaging elixir. Science and business are taking resveratrol very seriously.

In 2004, a company formed to commercialize Sinclair's research and develop drugs that work with the body's own defenses against aging. That company, Siritis, was purchased by drug manufacturer GlaxoSmithKline in June 2008 for the nifty sum of $720 million.

That may turn out to be a bargain. If resveratrol lives up to its promise, it may not only extend life, but also improve its quality. Resveratrol has been shown in studies to inhibit the growth of several cancer cell lines and tumors. It's also a powerful antioxidant and anti-inflammatory agent. It ramps up detoxification enzymes in the liver (making it easier for your body to get rid of carcinogens) and protects the heart through a number of different mechanisms. It also protects neurons (brain cells). Recent research has even shown that it may reduce insulin resistance, a key factor in metabolic syndrome and type 2 diabetes.

No one I know claims that taking resveratrol will counter the life-shortening effects of a terrible diet, smoking, and lack of exercise. But if you're doing everything else right, a high-quality resveratrol supplement may just give you a real edge in the longevity sweepstakes.

Meanwhile, do as the French do and drink some red wine or include it in your cooking, as Chef Jeannette does in this recipe. If you're not a wine drinker, or even if you are, start making dark grapes part of your diet.

Super Simple Vitamin C Citrus with Mint

Ingredients

2 large pink grapefruit

1 to 2 tablespoons (20 to 40 g) raw honey, or to taste

¼ cup (24 g) chopped fresh mint leaves

From Chef Jeannette

This light, refreshing dish can be chilled in the fridge before serving for extra cooling benefits, or lightly broiled for a richer feel in cooler weather. To broil, before dressing the grapefruit, place the plain halves, cut side up, onto a broiling sheet under high heat for about 5 minutes or until the fruit starts to plump and caramelize. Remove from the heat, dress, and serve. Sprinkle with a bit of cayenne to pop the flavor even more. If you want to forgo the sweetener altogether, nutrition expert Ann Louise Gittleman, Ph.D., C.N.S., recommends spreading 1 teaspoon of olive oil on each cut half and letting it rest (in the fridge) for a few hours to neutralize the natural acid, increasing its sweetness.

From Dr. Jonny: Anyone remember the Mayo Clinic Diet, where you ate grapefruit at every meal supposedly to help lose weight? Well, that diet was never from the Mayo Clinic and was mostly regarded as bogus, but a 2004 study in the Division of Endocrinology at Scripps Clinic in La Jolla, California, showed that eating grapefruit does in fact help with weight loss and insulin resistance. There was a significant difference in weight loss for those who consumed either fresh grapefruit or grapefruit juice over a placebo. Study participants lost an average of 3.6 pounds in 12 weeks, and their insulin resistance improved. The authors concluded that "although the mechanism of this weight loss is unknown, it would appear reasonable to include grapefruit in a weight reduction diet." These scientists know what happened—they're just not sure why. I say "who cares?" Low-calorie, low-glycemic grapefruit with its high vitamin C, antioxidant, and fiber content is a great food. And dressing it simply, as Chef Jeannette has done here, is a light way to mellow this very tart fruit. Enjoy!

Slice the grapefruits in half through the middle (around the "equator"). Run a knife just inside the skin around the segments and then along the side of each individual segment membrane to free the fruit. Squeeze about a tablespoon of juice from each of the four halves into a small bowl. Whisk the honey and mint into the juice. Pour the dressing evenly over each of the four halves and serve.

Yield: 4 servings

Per Serving: 76 Calories; trace Fat (1.3% calories from fat); 1g Protein; 20g Carbohydrate; 2g Dietary Fiber; 0mg Cholesterol; 2mg Sodium

Nutty Fruit Bars I: Healthy Bite Cherry Chewies

Ingredients

½ cup (70 g) loosely packed, pitted dates (8 to 9, or 6 to 7 if using larger Medjool dates)

½ packed cup (60 g) dried, unsweetened sweet cherries or juice-sweetened tart cherries

⅔ cup (97 g) raw almonds

⅓ cup (45 g) pine nuts

1 to 2 tablespoons (15 to 28 ml) water

From Dr. Jonny: This bar is the easiest thing in the world to make. I know because I've made it myself and really, it was a pure pleasure. It's an even greater pleasure to eat. Cherries, almonds, and pine nuts? What in the world could you possibly not like? And here's a secret: These bars were inspired by cherry Larabars, a commercial favorite of both Chef Jeannette and myself. Truth be told, making these cherry delights at home is actually far less expensive, and this version has the added advantage of being lower in sugar. If you're breezing through this book and wondering what recipe to start with, you couldn't do much better than this one! It's simplicity itself, comes together in minutes, and will knock your socks off with its rich, chewy texture and sweet-tart flavor. Worth noting: Although you can use unsweetened sweet cherries, you can also use juice-sweetened tart ones. Both varieties are a good source of anti-inflammatory anthocyanins, but tart cherries have a lot more. Animal studies conducted by University of Michigan researchers suggest that tart cherries can reduce factors linked to heart disease and diabetes.

Place the dates, cherries, almonds, and pine nuts in a food processor and process for 1 to 2 minutes, scraping down the sides a couple of times. The mixture will first come apart and then become finer, finally holding together in a clump of "dough" that will roll around in the processor. If the dough doesn't hold together by 1 minute, add water 1 tablespoon at a time until it does. When the ingredients are well incorporated into a dough, roll the mixture into quarter-size balls or tubelike mini-bars, or flatten it evenly into a 5 × 7-inch (13 × 18 cm) Pyrex dish (3-cup size) and slice (slicing is smoother if the dough is chilled for at least 1 hour). Store in the refrigerator.

Yield: approximately 20 balls or 8 to 10 pan bars

Per Serving: 57 Calories; 3g Fat (50.9% calories from fat); 2g Protein; 6g Carbohydrate; 1g Dietary Fiber; 0mg Cholesterol; 1mg Sodium

Nutty Fruit Bars II: Heart-Lovin' Lemon Zinger Truffles

Ingredients

½ cup (70 g) loosely packed pitted dates (8 or 9, or 6 to 7 if using Medjool—very sweet and creamy, but also large!)

½ cup (85 g) dried apples

½ cup (75 g) raw cashews

¼ cup (20 g) whole rolled oats

2 tablespoons (12 g) oat bran

½ teaspoon ground ginger

2 tablespoons (28 ml) fresh-squeezed lemon juice

1 teaspoon lemon zest

From Dr. Jonny: So here's the deal: Every so often when Chef Jeannette sends me these recipes, she'll tag one with a note that says, "Drop everything and make this! It's amazing!" This recipe came with such a note, so of course, I had to drop everything and make it (my basic rule is to obey every whim of anyone who makes food as well as Chef Jeannette does). Well, she was right. These truffles are amazing, and they come together in minutes. You'll never find an "energy bar" in the supermarket, even the gourmet ones, that tastes as good as these do, and certainly not one that has as much nutrition. High in heart-healthy fiber from the apples and oats, these bars are tangy and fresh tasting with just the right amount of sweetness. You will truly be amazed at how delicious they are!

Place the dates, apples, cashews, oats, oat bran, ginger, lemon juice, and lemon zest in a food processor and pulse a few times to break up the larger pieces. Then process for 1 to 2 minutes, scraping down the sides a couple of times. The mixture will first come apart and then become finer, finally holding together in a clump of "dough" that will roll around in the processor. When the ingredients are well incorporated into a dough, roll the mixture into quarter-size "truffles" or tubelike mini-bars, or flatten it evenly into a 5 × 7-inch (13 × 18 cm) Pyrex dish (3-cup size) and slice (slicing is smoother if the dough is chilled for at least 1 hour).

Yield: approximately 15 large or 20 small truffles or 8 pan bars
Per Serving: 46 Calories; 2g Fat (34.6% calories from fat); 1g Protein; 7g Carbohydrate; 1g Dietary Fiber; 0mg Cholesterol; 5mg Sodium

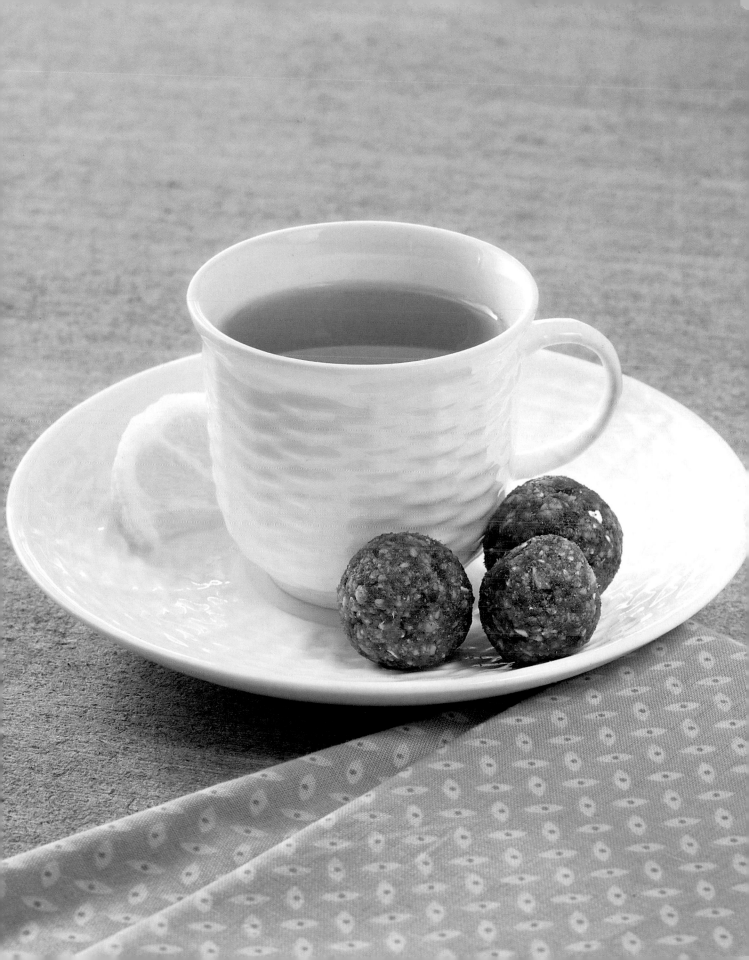

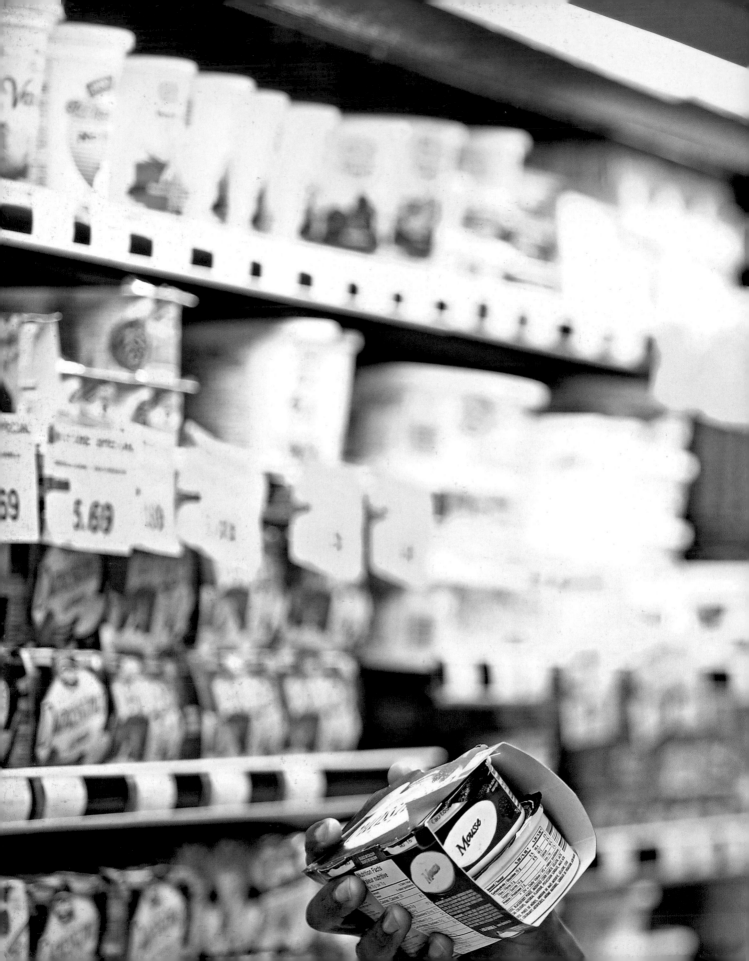

4 | What Nutritional Labels *Really* Mean

Nutritional labels, often confusing for even the most sophisticated consumers, contain a lot of information. Some of it is useful. A good deal of it is not.

Let me explain.

Let's start with the stuff that's helpful to know. How much protein is in a serving size, for example? How many grams of carbohydrates? How much sugar? And of course, how many calories? Assuming you know what these numbers mean, this can be good information to have.

For example, I recently got hold of a nice little package of blackberries, imported from another country where the rules governing nutritional labeling are a little different than they are in the United States. Here's what was on the label:

Nutritional Facts	
Portion	6 oz
Calories	83
Protein	1.7 g
Fat	1.2 g
Carbohydrates	17 g
Calcium	46 mg
Potassium	245 mg
Vitamin A	288 IU
Vitamin C	30 mg

Now as labels go, that's pretty useful, though I would have liked to see fiber listed (the berries are very high in fiber, which you wouldn't know from this label). The choice of calcium, potassium, vitamin A, and vitamin C is fairly arbitrary—what happened to magnesium? Iron? Vitamin B$_{12}$?—but different countries have different regulations about what must be listed on the label. (The U.S. government mandates that food manufacturers list calcium, iron, vitamin A, and vitamin C. Go figure.) All things considered, the imported berry label's not bad.

In the United States, a typical label looks like this:

SAMPLE NUTRITION FACTS LABEL

Nutrition Facts
Serving Size 1 Bar (85g)
Servings Per Container 4

Amount Per Serving

Calories 170 | Calories from Fat 50

	% Daily Value *
Total Fat 0g	9%
Saturated Fat 4g	19%
Trans Fat 0g	
Polyunsaturated Fat 0.5g	
Monounsaturated Fat 1g	
Cholesterol 13mg	4%
Sodium 83mg	3%
Total Carbohydrate 33g	11%
Dietary Fiber 4g	16%
Sugar 25g	
Protein 3g	

Vitamin A 110% • Vitamin C 2%
Calcium 10% • Iron 3%

*Percent Daily Values are based on a 2,000 calorie diet. Your daily values may be higher or lower depending on your calorie needs.

	Calories	2,000	2,500
Total Fat	Less than	65g	80g
Sat Fat	Less than	20g	25g
Cholesterol	Less than	300mg	300mg
Sodium	Less than	2,400mg	2,400mg
Total Carbohydrate		300g	375g
Dietary Fiber		25g	30g

Calories per gram:
Fat 9 • Carbohydrate 4 • Protein 4

The first thing I have a problem with is the "calories from fat" part in the upper right-hand corner. This implies that calories from fat are somehow a bad thing, worse for you than calories from any other source. For example, the calories from fat listed on a tablespoon of fish oil would be 100 percent of the total calories because fish oil is pure fat. So what? Similarly, the calling out of saturated fat for special attention perpetuates the myth that saturated fat is always bad, which it's not.

So if you evaluate our recipes through the lens of "fat is bad," you're likely to be surprised—some of our recipes are indeed higher in fat than you might expect, especially if you buy into the antifat concept. We hope you don't. (Buy into that concept, I mean, because it's boneheadedly wrong.) Fear not because the *quality* of the fat in our recipes is high and the health value is positive, as we note throughout the book. The now-famous disclaimer in all movies and TV productions, "no animals were harmed during the making of this movie," can be aptly paraphrased here: *No harm will come to you from the fat in these recipes.*

On the plus side, the labeling laws mandate that manufacturers list the number of grams of trans fats. Trans fats are almost *always* bad (unlike saturated fat), and you should strive to keep your dietary intake of them as close to zero as possible. If something has trans fats in it, I want to know about it. Even 1 gram is too much.

The laws also mandate labeling sodium, which is something you should pay attention to. Although not everyone is salt sensitive, (meaning their blood sugar goes up in response to sodium,) enough of us are that it's worth knowing about. Current dietary recommendations are to consume no more than 2,300 to 2,400 mg of sodium per day (about the amount in a teaspoon of salt), but the problem is that most of our sodium doesn't come from the saltshaker. It comes from processed foods. If a portion of soup contains 800 mg of sodium, I want to know about it.

The useless and confusing part of the nutrition facts label is that column on the right where it lists % Daily Value. There are many things to dislike about this practice—for instance, everything. The daily value is something almost no one understands, but basically it's the amount of a given nutrient that the U.S. Food and Drug Administration (FDA) thinks you need each day. The *percent* daily value is the *percentage* of that total amount that the food in question provides. The problem is that many nutritionists, myself included, disagree with the government's recommended amounts for many nutrients.

For example, let's take the vitamin C in the generic serving of macaroni and cheese listed on the label above. The FDA's recommended daily intake for vitamin C is 75 to 90 mg, an amount no nutritionist I've ever met thinks is optimal or even adequate. Now let's do some math: The label says a serving of macaroni and cheese contains 2 percent of the daily value for vitamin C. Two percent of 90 mg is…1.8 mg of vitamin C. You can tell from the label that 2 percent is awfully low, and you'd be right in thinking this food has virtually no vitamin C.

Where it gets tricky is this: Let's suppose that macaroni and cheese had 45 mg of vitamin C. Then the label would say it contains 50 percent of your recommended daily intake. You'd be thinking, "Wow, I'm getting a lot of vitamin C in this dish" but in fact you'd be getting a ridiculously low amount (45 mg) that only has a high "percent daily value" because the daily value itself is so low.

It gets even trickier when you're talking about percentages as they relate to carbohydrates, fat, and protein. Again, the FDA makes a ridiculous assumption, which is that the average American diet is either 2,000 calories a day or 2,500. Most Americans eat way more than 2,000 calories a day, which makes the FDA's one-size-fits-all model irrelevant to them.

The agency makes other assumptions about the ideal amount of protein, fat, and carbs that you should consume each day for that amount of calories—assumptions that are, well, highly questionable. (Many researchers believe that 50 grams a day of protein is pathetically low, especially for weight loss purposes, yet that's the amount of the recommended daily value. And many health professionals get apoplectic at the daily value for carbohydrates—an astoundingly high 300 grams a day!) So if the label tells you you're getting 30 percent of the daily value of protein, you might think that's a lot, but it's 30 percent of a very low amount. And a food with a whopping 150 grams of carbs (such as an average restaurant portion of pasta) is "only" half the recommended daily amount for carbohydrates. Give me a break!

My advice: Ignore the *percent daily value* on the nutrition facts label. It's confusing, misleading, and adds almost nothing to your knowledge.

Pay attention, however, to the numbers for calories, protein, carbs, fat, and fiber. And of course to sugar, which is way more important than fat as a health hazard.

Why the RDA Model Doesn't Help You

For those who'd like to know, here are the U.S. Food and Drug Administration's current daily values, or recommended amounts of nutrients (such as vitamins) and macronutrients (protein, fat, carbohydrates) that men and women should consume each day.

They're not all bad, but many are out of date (selenium, vitamin D) and some (300 grams of carbs, 50 grams of protein) are simply out of proportion (carbs are way too high, protein is too low). In my opinion, these values are compromises based on statistical models that have little relevance to the average person. The percent daily value on your nutrition facts label is based entirely on these numbers, and if the numbers are wrong, the percent daily value is next to useless.

THE U.S. FDA'S CURRENT DAILY VALUES	
Nutrient	**Daily Value**
Total fat	65 grams (g)
Saturated fat	20 g
Cholesterol	300 milligrams (mg)
Sodium	2,400 mg
Potassium	3,500 mg
Total carbohydrate	300 g
Dietary fiber	25 g
Protein	50 g
Vitamin A	5,000 international units (IU)
Vitamin C	60 mg
Calcium	1,000 mg
Iron	18 mg
Vitamin D	400 IU

Nutrient	Daily Value
Vitamin E	30 IU
Vitamin K	80 micrograms (mcg)
Thiamin	1.5 mg
Riboflavin	1.7 mg
Niacin	20 mg
Vitamin B$_6$	2 mg
Folate	400 mcg
Vitamin B$_{12}$	6 mcg
Biotin	300 mcg
Pantothenic acid	10 mg
Phosphorus	1,000 mg
Iodine	150 mcg
Magnesium	400 mg
Zinc	15 mg
Selenium	70 mcg
Copper	2 mg
Manganese	2 mg
Chromium	120 mcg
Molybdenum	75 mcg
Chloride	3,400 mg

ACKNOWLEDGMENTS

From Jonny and Jeannette:

Special thanks from both of us to our hardworking agent, Coleen O'Shea; to our favorite editor, Cara Connors; to our organization queen, Tiffany Hill; and to the amazing design and photography team at Fair Winds, especially Michele Lancialtomare and Rachel Sherwood.

In addition, for their indispensable feedback on the recipes, Jeannette would like to extend a warm thank you to her testers, tasters, and clients, including Frank and Karen Knapp, Jodi Bass, Sharon Lavallee, Leslie Lindeman, Judie Porter (thanks, Mom!), Russell and Karen Pet, her Real Food Moms partner, Tracee Yablon Brenner, and her beloveds, Jay, Jesse, and Julian. Kudos and thanks also to John K. Callaghan of Bellevue Wine and Spirits for his perfect wine pairing suggestions, and thanks to my mom and our dear friend Pam Goff for sharing their ideas for quick, tasty meals with me.

ABOUT THE AUTHORS

Jonny Bowden, Ph.D., C.N.S., is a board-certified nutritionist with a master's degree in psychology and a nationally known expert on nutrition, weight loss, and health. A member of the Editorial Advisory Board of *Men's Health* magazine and a health columnist for America Online, he's also written or contributed to articles for dozens of national publications (print and online) including *The New York Times, The Wall Street Journal, Forbes, Time, Oxygen, Marie Claire, W, Remedy, Diabetes Focus, US Weekly, Cosmopolitan, Family Circle, Self, Fitness, Allure, Essence, Men's Health, Weight Watchers, Pilates Style, Prevention, Woman's World, InStyle, Fitness, Natural Health,* and *Shape.* He is the author of *The Most Effective Ways to Live Longer, The 150 Most Effective Ways to Boost Your Energy,* and *The 100 Healthiest Foods to Eat During Pregnancy* (with Allison Tannis, R.D.).

A popular, dynamic, and much sought-after speaker, he's appeared on CNN, Fox News, MSNBC, ABC, NBC, and CBS, and speaks frequently around the country.

In addition to the above, he is the author of the award-winning *Living Low Carb: Controlled Carbohydrate Eating for Long-Term Weight Loss, The Most Effective Natural Cures on Earth, The Healthiest Meals on Earth* (with Jeannette Bessinger), and his acclaimed signature bestseller, *The 150 Healthiest Foods on Earth.*

You can find his DVDs, *The Truth about Weight Loss* and *The 7 Pillars of Longevity,* his popular motivational CDs, free newsletter, free audio programs, and many of the supplements and foods recommended in this book on his website, www.jonnybowden.com.

He lives in Southern California with his beloved animal companions Emily (a pit bull) and Lucy (an Argentine Dogo).

Jeannette Bessinger, C.H.H.C., owner of Balance for Life, LLC, www .balanceforlifellc.com, is a board-certified holistic health coach, award-winning lifestyle and nutrition educator, and personal whole foods chef.

She is coauthor of *The Healthiest Meals on Earth* (with Dr. Jonny) and *Simple Food for Busy Families,* and author of *Great Expectations: Best Food for Your Baby and Toddler.*

Designer and lead facilitator of a long-running and successful hospital-based lifestyle change program, she is a regular consultant and speaker to public and private organizations and coalitions working to improve the health of schools and cities in the United States.

As cofounder of Real Food Moms® (www.realfoodmoms.com), she provides busy moms with quick answers for how to feed their families well.

She lives in Portsmouth, Rhode Island, with her patient husband, two teenagers, three dogs, and pesky cat.

INDEX

Note: Page numbers in italics indicate photographs.

15-Minute German Potato Salmon Salad, 191

15-Minute Low-Cal Shrimp and Citrus Ceviche, 86, *87*

15-Minute Middle Eastern Lamb Chops, 67

A

adzuki beans, 134

allicin, 63

almond meal, 231

almond milk, 239

almonds, 68, 111

  Easy, Appetizing Asian Croquettes, 155

  Fast Fruit n' Fiber Quinoa Salad, 152

  Fiber Bonanza: Oat Bran Kheer on the Quick, 233

  Low-Cal Tuna-Cranberry Lettuce Wraps, 225

  Low-Sugar, High-Protein Indian Pudding, 208

  Nutty Fruit Bars I: Healthy Bite Cherry Chewies, 247

Almost-Instant, Iron-Rich Picadillo, 185

ancho chile peppers, 101, 184, 214

anchovies, 223

anthocyanins, 165

Antioxidant Cocoa Oat Dreams, *230*

Antioxidant Paradise: Teriyaki Salmon with Pineapple, *76*, 77

Anytime Fast Fruity Skillet Cake, 162, *163*

Apple-a-Day Wine-Marinated Fruit Mix, 244

apple cider, 42

Apple Power Breakfast on the Go, 164

apples

  Apple-a-Day Wine-Marinated Fruit Mix, 244

  Apple Power Breakfast on the Go, 164

  Awesome Autumn Bean Dip, 214

  Creamy Low-Fat Waldorf Slaw in Seconds, 215

  Fast Fruit n' Fiber Quinoa Salad, 152

  A Healthier Sandwich: Turkey-Apple De-Light, 53

  Healthy-in-a-Hurry Chicken Apple Sausage and Red Cabbage, 176

  Low-Cal Tuna-Cranberry Lettuce Wraps, 225

  Nutty Fruit Bars II: Heart-Lovin' Lemon Zinger Truffles, 248

  Slimming, Sweet, and Savory Turkey-Apple Sausage, 54

  Smoked Turkey-Apple Cobb Salad in Seconds, 48

apricots, 27, 44–45, 51

artichokes

  In-a-Flash Frittatas I: Heart-Healthy Mediterranean, 125

  Potassium Powerhouse: Quickest Artichoke Pasta, 115

  Simple and Energizing Salad Niçoise, 107

arugula, 77, 115, 154, 191

asparagus, 192

astaxanthin, 112

avocados

  15-Minute Low-Cal Shrimp and Citrus Ceviche, 86

  Avocado Soup with Cheesy Tortillas in No Time, 143

  Crab-Acados, 96

  Game Time Five-Layer Salad, Lightened, 66

  A Healthier Sandwich: Open-Faced Veggie-Max, 149

  Nutrient-Filled Chilled Shrimp Salad, 89

  Polyunsaturated Party: Lox Canapés with Avocado Miso, 226

  Smoked Turkey-Apple Cobb Salad in Seconds, 48

Avocado Soup with Cheesy Tortillas in No Time, *142*, 143

Awesome Antioxidant Scallops Mediterranean, *191*, 192

Awesome Autumn Bean Dip, 214

B

baby spring greens, 113. *See also* spring mix

baking items, 22

balsamic vinegar, 61

bananas

  Low-Fat Pumpkin Pie Dip, 237

  No-Fuss, Fast, and Healthy Chocolate Cherry Frosty, 232

  Peanut Butter Protein Power, 239

barbecue sauce, 44–45

barley

  Fast, Flavorful Fiber: Rosemary Apple-Poached Chicken and Barley, 42

  Low-Cal Turkey Barley Soup, 182

  Quick-Fix Stuffed Peppers with Chèvre, 147

basil, 95, 111

  Awesome Antioxidant Scallops Mediterranean, 192

  Calcium-Rich Caprese Salad in Seconds, 154

  Fiber-Friendly Protein Pasta, 202

  Ga-Ga for Fresh Gazpacho, 220

  Low-Carb Pesto Pizza, 227

bass, 73

beans, 50, 115, 133

  Awesome Autumn Bean Dip, 214

  Black Bean Slenderizer Soup, 151

  Easy, Protein-Rich Tangy Tomato Soup, 150

  Easy Everyday Enchiladas, 203

  Easy One-Pot Chicken Miso Soup, 40

  Effortless Antioxidant Tomato Salad, 122

  Fast and Fiberful Black Bean Salad, 129

  Fiber Fest: Shiitake Adzuki Kasha, 134

  Game Time Five-Layer Salad, Lightened, 66

  A Healthier Sandwich: Open-Faced Veggie-Max, 149

  The Healthiest Minestrone Stew, 140

  Healthy Jalapeño Cornbread Chili, 206

  Lightning-Fast Legume-Pesto Spaghetti, 148

  Low-Cal Sloppy Jo-matoes in Minutes, 131

  Low-Cal Stuffed Collards, 135

  Low-Glycemic Caesar Salad Pizza in a Snap, 136–137

  Not Your Average Penne, 116

  Nourishing Potatoes Series II: Beany Greenie Potato, 144

  One-Pot Fiber Fiesta Taco Soup, 186–187

  One-Pot Red-Beans-and-Greens with a Kick, 200

  Quick and Comforting Black Bean Chili, 132

  Quick and Hearty Vegetable-Bean Quinoa, 124

  Quick Quinoa Burgers, 153

  Simple, Satisfying Southwest Chicken-Pinto Bean Stew, 29

  Simple and Energizing Salad Niçoise, 107

  Totally Fast Tamale Bake, 184

bean sprouts

  Easy Asian Endive Wraps, 47

  Healthy Peanut-Hoisin Beef and Bean Sprouts in Seconds, 60

  Tasty, Time-Saving Thai Shrimp and Rice Noodle Salad, 88

beef

  Almost-Instant, Iron-Rich Picadillo, 185

  Body-Building Broiled Steak with Mushrooms, 58

  Cheater Fajiters, 64

  Game Time Five-Layer Salad, Lightened, 66

  Gorgonzola Beef with Spinach, Super-Fast, 56

  grass-fed, 22, 59

  Healthy Peanut-Hoisin Beef and Bean Sprouts in Seconds, 60

  Iron-Rich Blackstrap Balsamic Steak, 61

  Quick-Sizzle Beef Satay Shish Kebab, 62

  Totally Fast Tamale Bake, 184

beer, 101

bell peppers, 33, 82. *See also specific colors*

  Almost-Instant, Iron-Rich Picadillo, 185

  Cheater Fajiters, 64

  Citrus Jicama Salad, 172

  Easy Everyday Enchiladas, 203

Hundreds of hours of my personal nutritional research reveals...

7 SUPER FOODS
That Could Change Your Life!

Dr. Jonny Bowden says...

"Do you want to know the best foods to eat to live a longer, healthier, happier, and more energized life?

If so then follow the instructions below and I'll send you the 7 Super Foods audio course...for free!"

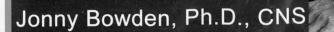

Jonny Bowden, Ph.D., CNS

This **FREE AUDIO COURSE** reveals the best foods to help you...

- **control weight**
- **look & feel younger**
- **prevent disease**
- **extend your life**
- **increase energy levels**

FREE!

Get started by signing up online now!

Simply go to

http://feelyourpower.com

NOW and enter your name and email address.

It's that easy! And you can rest assured that we will keep your email address private. We will NEVER sell or rent your information.

Change your body. Change your life...with Dr. Jonny Bowden!

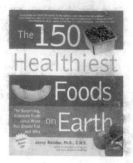

The 150 Healthiest Foods on Earth
The Surprising, Unbiased Truth about What You Should Eat and Why

"The 150 Healthiest Foods on Earth is simply delightful! The information is accurate; the presentation is a visual feast. All in all, reading this book is a very satisfying experience."

—Christiane Northrup, M.D., author of *Mother-Daughter Wisdom, The Wisdom of Menopause, and Women's Bodies, Women's Wisdom*

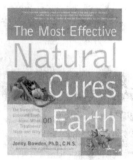

The Most Effective Natural Cures on Earth
The Surprising, Unbiased Truth about What Treatments Work and Why

"I reference this beautifully written and illustrated review of the best cures on the planet so often that it lives on my desk rather than the bookshelf."

—Mehmet C. Oz, M.D., coauthor of *You: The Owner's Manual*

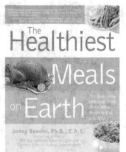

The Healthiest Meals on Earth
The Surprising, Unbiased Truth about What Meals to Eat and Why

"What a simply irresistible book with mouthwatering recipes from all around the world! I plan to use this book as a resource guide and as a gift for all the people I truly care about."

—Ann Louise Gittleman, Ph.D., C.N.S., author of *The Fat Flush Plan and Before the Change*

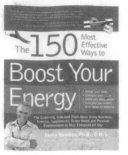

The Most Effective Ways to Boost Your Energy
The Surprising, Unbiased Truth about Using Nutrition, Exercise, Supplements, Stress Relief, and Personal Empowerment to Stay Energized All Day

"Get everyone you love to read my friend Dr. Jonny's brilliance!"

—Mark Victor Hansen, coauthor of *Chicken Soup for the Soul*

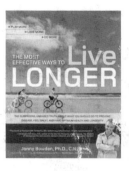

The Most Effective Ways to Live Longer
The Surprising, Unbiased Truth about What You Should Do to Prevent Disease, Feel Great, and Have Optimum Health and Longevity

"A must-read for anyone who wants to live longer! Jonny Bowden takes the lessons we've learned from the world's longest-lived people and offers a research-backed formula for the rest of us to get the most good years out of our lives."

—Dan Buettner, author of *The Blue Zones: Lessons on Living Longer from the People Who've Lived the Longest*

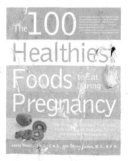

The 100 Healthiest Foods to Eat During Pregnancy
The Surprising, Unbiased Truth about Foods You Should Be Eating During Pregnancy but Probably Aren't

"Another great book from Jonny Bowden! In his signature expert style, Jonny, along with Allison Tannis, recommends the healthiest foods and spices for pregnant women…all pregnant women should read this book."

—Dean Raffleock, D.C., C.C.N., author of *A Natural Guide to Pregnancy and Postpartum Health*